Praise for
The Wise Woman's Guide to Your Healthiest Pregnancy and Birth

"The advice in *The Wise Woman's Guide to Your Healthiest Pregnancy and Birth* is invaluable, hard to find elsewhere, and simply a precious gift to moms and our future generations."

—**Elissa Epel, PhD**, coauthor of
The New York Times bestseller *The Telomere Effect*

"I experienced firsthand Patricia's unparalleled talent, as both an athlete recovering from injury, and as a new mother navigating how to safely regain my strength. This book weaves together the most critical information for any woman embarking on the journey of motherhood, regardless of stage or age. I have no doubt it will become essential reading for generations."

—**Jenna Lee Babin**, journalist and founder of *SmartHer News*

"Having too often witnessed the dis-ease of pregnancy, my hope is that *The Wise Woman's Guide* becomes integrated into all aspects of a woman's clinical care, from preconception to postpartum. This book speaks from a place of wisdom, and its holistic approach has been the spark for innumerable healing journeys in athletes, patients, and especially mothers. The foundational approach to breathing, movement, and nourishment in this book provide the basis for the journey of a lifetime.

—**Brian Hainline, MD**, NCAA chief medical officer,
professor, New York University Department of Neurology,
co-editor, *Neurological Complications of Pregnancy*

"*The Wise Woman's Guide to Your Healthiest Pregnancy and Birth* made me want to have another baby, even though I already have three boys! All too often, pregnancy is a time filled with fear and trepidation when it should be a period of magic, wonder, healthfulness, empowerment, and confidence. The insights, medically founded advice, holistic perspective, and sheer wisdom inside this book are delivered with strength and grace, providing words women must hear as they embark upon pregnancy."

—**Laura Gentile**, senior vice president of
marketing, ESPN, and founder, espnW

"*The Wise Woman's Guide to Your Healthiest Pregnancy and Birth* arms you with powerful information, knowledge, and insights to prepare you for conception, pregnancy, and post-pregnancy on all levels—physically, mentally and emotionally—ultimately allowing you to trust yourself and frankly control all you can. I recommend this book wholeheartedly. It is invaluable and essential, and will leave you empowered and enlightened."

—**Denise Spatafora**, author of
*Better Birth: The Ultimate Guide to Childbirth
from Home Births to Hospitals*

The Wise Woman's Guide to Your Healthiest Pregnancy and Birth

From Preconception to Postpartum

Patricia Ladis, PT, CBBA,
with Anita Sadaty, MD

Health Communications, Inc.
Boca Raton, Florida

www.hcibooks.com

Library of Congress Control Number: 2020948193

© 2021 Patricia Ladis

ISBN-13: 978-07573-2370-6 (Paperback)
ISBN-10: 07573-2370-7 (Paperback)
ISBN-13: 978-07573-2371-3 (ePub)
ISBN-10: 07573-2371-5 (ePub)

HCI, its logos, and marks are trademarks of Health Communications, Inc.

Publisher: Health Communications, Inc.
        1700 NW 2nd Ave.
        Boca Raton, FL 33432-1653

This book is intended as a reference volume only, not as a medical manual. This book is designed to help you make informed decisions but is not a substitute for any approach or treatment that your doctor may prescribe. Should any medical issue arise, we urge you to seek medical help.

Exercise and body mechanics photographs by Chris Trini
Third trimester photographs by Mike Bryan
Diastasis photographs courtesy of Diane Lee
Cover photo © Lois Greenfield
Cover design by Larissa Hise Henoch
Interior design and formatting by Lawna Patterson Oldfield

CONTENTS

To my children, Stel, Dimitri, and Aya,
for their wisdom, teaching me more
than a lifetime's worth.

—P. L.

To my parents,
Dr. Mohamad and Alba Sadaty

—A. S.

ACKNOWLEDGMENTS

I would like to thank my mom, Matina Vahaviolos Ladis, for all her Spartan gynecological, nutritional, and overall health wisdom, and my dad, James Ladis, for his wisdom about agriculture, nature, religion, the arts, and community service.

My amazing and loving husband and soul mate, Nick Pappas, I thank you for your never-ending love, support, and selflessness. The world is lucky to have your leadership in educating the whole child.

Thank you to my sisters, Natasia Brienza and Erica Ladis, for all their support through every twist and turn of life. Thanks to my mother-in-law Mandy Pappas, my sisters-in-law Sophie Pappas and Patty Lafkas, Antigone Stathakis, and my extended family and friends: thank you for always being there for me, for expanding my female tribe—it has been an honor to support you back!

Thank you, Dr. Brian and Pascale Hainline, for supporting me throughout my career and for encouraging me to do this book. My partners at The First 1000 Days of Wellness, Dr. Sergio Pecorelli and Alina Hernandez, have been pioneers and together, we are creating healthy generations to come.

The publishing team has been exceptional, beginning with our agent, Carol Mann. Thanks to Pamela Liflander for helping us get our words on these pages in a creatively magical way. The HCI staff: thank you, Christine Belleris, Allison

Janse, Larissa Henoch, and Lawna Oldfield. Maria Michelle provided beautiful illustrations. Models Vida Dominguez and Jenn Hunter-Marshall were a joy to work with, and we couldn't see their beautiful work without expert photographer Chris Trini. A special thank-you to Nadia Murgasova Bryan for her modeling expertise and Mike Bryan for his impromptu photographic skills to shoot amid the COVID-19 crisis from an iPhone Pro!

I would also like to thank everyone who helped in my research. Agapi Stassinopoulos provided a beautiful meditation, and Arti Panjwani, DO, and Kul Bhushan Anand, MD, for the practice of Ayurveda. Andie (Nancy) Santopietro shared her feng shui wisdom and has been such a support for the past ten years of my life. Patti Wood was so helpful with EMF research. Chantal Traub, Janet Dailey, Yamuna Zake, and Megan Backus shared their experiences and expertise in working with prenatal and postpartum women. And thanks to Gerri Brewster, of NAET, and Katina Mountanos for putting our ancestral high potency antioxidant organic extra virgin Greek Olive Oil on the market for all to enjoy. And to my partner in this project, Dr. Anita Sadaty, for all your wisdom and for taking this leap with me.

I started collecting the wisdom I've poured into this book with my first dance teachers. Vicky Simegiatos and Matina Simegiatos-Sporek piqued my interest in anatomy, movement, and fluidity. Despina Simegiatos and I explored movement in an exciting and rewarding way. One of my mentors, Diane Lee, continues to share her innate wisdom; thank you for pioneering diastasis research and treatment and for being a powerhouse for women's health. LJ Lee: thank you for teaching me how to make thoraxes dance and use my gifts to help more bodies. Peter Litchfield, PhD, and Sandra Reamer taught me about behavioral breathing analysis and capnography so that I could connect with my patients on even deeper levels to amplify their well-being.

I would also like to thank my colleagues Jennifer Green, Stephen Rodriguez, Stephen Cohen, Christine Aziz, Dr. Ted Dugas, Dr. Randi Jaffe, Adrienne McAuley, therapists and staff that I have worked with, Cait Van Damm, Justine Ward, Diana Zotos, Lisa Sottung, Kristine Gneiss, and Liz Simons, for your insights and collaboration on the gold standard of patient care. In the office, Alicia Lewis has always shown her dedication to our patients, my vision, and the practice's administrative needs. Thank you to the Global Wellness Summit and Global Wellness Institute Tribes, particularly the GWI First 1000 Days Initiative Team. Thank you to the ACTIVE MOM research study team; I can't wait to publish our wonderful study about beginning exercise early in postpartum for improved outcomes. Thanks also to all the physicians, chiropractors, physician's assistants, acupuncturists, health coaches, massage therapists, and functional medicine practitioners in my network who have influenced my practice, opened my eyes, and been such amazing practitioners to collaborate with for holistic patient care. Thank you to Lois Greenfield and her amazing dance photography. You made my jump that graces this book's cover look beautiful.

Lastly, thank you to my patients whom I have learned so much from and connected with. You are all truly wise.

—P. L.

I would like to thank my parents, who have been my most ardent supporters and two of the most selfless humans on the planet. The world is a better place with you in it. My father, Dr. Mohamad Sadaty, inspired me to think outside the box and embrace the road less traveled. You have always been my role model and inspiration.

I would like to thank my husband, Daniel Brotman, who has supported and encouraged me to follow my dreams and helped me get through so many difficult and hard choices in my professional life. He is my rock and love. And thanks to my children, Rachel, Sera, and Jackson: you are my greatest gift and achievement in life.

—A. S.

INTRODUCTION

You are a wise woman. You're not wise because you woke up one day and suddenly you knew everything about everything. You're wise because you're curious enough to be holding this book. We're guessing that you want what's best for you and your family. You're willing to make small changes to the way you live as well as take the appropriate steps for optimizing your mind and body, not only during pregnancy, but well beyond birthing.

In the not-too-distant past, wise women like you who were preparing for pregnancy learned from others just like them, right in their community. They would run into their neighbors, friends, and family in their town squares and talk openly about what worked for them during this very special time. But today, the idea of support and community is virtually lost, especially for new mothers. We live more isolated, digital lives, and no longer have the casual meetings that lead to passing down information from woman to woman, generation to generation. Because of this, wise women today who are pregnant, or want to be pregnant, are at a deficit because they have so many questions yet are left to figure everything out on their own.

This is why a wise woman like you instinctively knows that she needs help, and happily, we're here to do just that: support you in every possible way during your pregnancy. The reason is simple—scientifically speaking, support is crucial for every mother-to-be, and its positive effects go far beyond your mental well-being. For example, our colleague Dr. Elissa Epel points out that while nutrition will always be important, one of the most important strategies that helps a woman feel good and safe during her pregnancy is feeling supported by others in her life. Her research and others have shown that high stress during pregnancy is related to shorter telomeres in the baby. And fortunately the opposite is true—feeling positive is related to longer telomeres in the baby.[1]

Outside of giving you a loan, this book can provide a comprehensive support system. Support can mean so many things, and all of them are critical. We're going to share with you a complete program based on the latest, most accurate information to help you make good choices every day of your pregnancy, as well as the wisdom from long ago that we've now come to learn are best practices. Having the right information *at the right time* helps wise women like you understand what is happening to your body during pregnancy. We want you to feel strong and balanced, avoid injury, and recover quickly from any type of delivery. And we want to take the necessary steps to ensure that your baby is healthy throughout its entire life.

The truth is that most American women do not adequately prepare their bodies for pregnancy; they just cross their fingers and hope they will bounce back afterward. This, however, is not the case everywhere. Many places in the developed world put our aspirations into practice. In other countries, pregnant women regularly receive physical therapy treatments as part of routine healthcare and, later, are again supported by physical therapists and home services in order to optimally heal after having their baby. This gap may be one of the reasons that according to 2018 statistics from the Centers for Disease Control (CDC), about *one in ten* US women of childbearing age have difficulty getting pregnant or carrying a pregnancy to term, and *the majority never regain their pre-pregnancy body*. But as a wise woman, you're not going to be just another statistic: you're going to know what to avoid, what to focus on, and the lifestyle adjustments that you need to make before, during, and after pregnancy.

Whether you are picking this book up as you begin to plan your family or if you already are pregnant, you will learn how to strengthen your body, trust your inner wisdom, and take the appropriate steps for preventing injury and chronic disease. This book's unique focus on the physiology of pregnancy—the body's changing structure, musculature, and flexibility—will prepare you for a pain-free pregnancy by providing the exercises and real medical knowledge you need to relax, enjoy, and embrace this beautiful time with confidence and happiness.

We know our program works because we've used it on thousands of our patients and during our own pregnancies. So welcome, wise woman, we're so glad you are here! Now it's time for you to learn a little bit more about us, about your own matrescence—the process of becoming a mother—and our program.

Patricia's Story

As founder of WiseBody PT, the co-founder of First 1000 Days of Wellness, KIMA Center for Physio-therapy & Wellness (2006–2020), and a former professional dancer, Patricia is a physical therapist who specializes in perinatal and postpartum health. Her unique skills include manual therapy, biomechanical analysis, neuromuscular reeducation, joint mobilization, gait (walking and running) training, nerve mobilization, Pilates/Gyrotonic exercises, and core stabilization. These modalities optimize the musculoskeletal system so that women can transition through each stage of pregnancy easily and bounce back after delivery. Patricia is also a Certified Behavioral Breathing Analyst. She analyzes and trains women to optimize their breathing especially when they are pregnant, during childbirth, and postpartum in order to improve their energy level, restore calm, and keep them feeling good during and after pregnancy.

Yet even before all her medical training, Patricia began to understand body mechanics when she joined a professional dance company at the age of fifteen. What most people don't realize is that dancers and injuries go hand in hand: every dancer experiences lots of pain. Luckily, Patricia never had a major injury, partially because she figured out the most effective ways to hold and move her body on and off stage. When she did need to see a physical therapist, Patricia realized that even the ones devoted to dancers rarely looked for the cause of the pain. As a wise woman, she found herself becoming more curious about trying to find real answers to the health issues that she and her dancer friends were facing. After a career in dancing she went to college to become a physical therapist (PT).

Over the years, Patricia's core clients were top athletes and actors as well as dancers, and Patricia became known as the PT who always got women back on the stage post-pregnancy. Today, she not only teaches her patients how the pregnant body changes, she also shares the pearls of wisdom that she learned from her own continuing education with Elizabeth Noble, Diane Lee, and other great researchers as well as what she gleaned from her own Greek heritage. It turns out that the tips her mother and grandmother taught about how to take care of yourself before, during, and after pregnancy are completely aligned with science.

A wise woman and mother of three, Patricia has experienced all types of birth: vaginal, cesarean, and vaginal birth after cesarean (VBAC). She knows how her body felt after each and how she needed to tailor her program after each birth.

Anita's Story

A wise woman in her own right, Dr. Sadaty has learned that better outcomes are possible if women come into labor fully prepared physically, intellectually, and emotionally. Anita is a board-certified obstetrician-gynecologist (ob-gyn) and founder of Redefining Health Medical, a women-focused medical practice that combines conventional medical training with an integrative functional medicine approach. In 2014, she completed her training and certification at the Institution for Functional Medicine and is recognized as an IFM Certified Medical

Practitioner. This advanced training has allowed her to meet the needs of women who embrace a whole-body medical approach to health and healing.

Anita's interest in becoming an ob-gyn began the second she helped with her first delivery in medical school. Beyond the joyous births, she was equally fascinated in the transition points women experience, from puberty to pregnancy to matrescence to menopause.

Her upbringing certainly influenced her decision not only to become a doctor, but one who focused on maintaining the healing traditions of integrative care. Her father was a pediatrician who immigrated to the US from Iran, which at the time was a developing country where infectious disease and childhood illness were very prevalent. Her father had a very reassuring presence about him and had extreme compassion for his patients. When he arrived in America, he was able to apply his training in the rural traditions of medicinal healing to an inner-city environment. As he got older and wiser, as he approached his retirement from his pediatric practice, he discovered the power of natural medicine and an integrating healing technique. He was the one who opened his daughter's eyes to this aspect of healing: that there was more than just the conventional medical model they both learned in medical school.

Anita changed her medical practice to be less reactionary and to focus more on what women need to do before they become pregnant. She found that by focusing on preconception, she could help women make the right choices that most influence not only the outcome of their pregnancy but their overall lasting health and the future health of their children.

What Is Functional Medicine?

Within our own areas of expertise, we both practice a holistic approach to healthcare that is aligned with the tenets of *functional medicine*. As a wise woman, it's no wonder that you are attracted to our outlook. A wise woman wants to go through life in an optimal way. She wants to do everything that she can to really feel good because she's got stuff to do. She doesn't want to be dealing with symptoms that are weighing her down. She wants to honor her own self-discovery, be informed about what's happening, know her options, and be in tune with her changing body.

Functional medicine provides an entirely different way to think about a woman's body during pregnancy. It is a philosophy of medical care that explores the root cause of symptoms and disease rather than prescribing a "pill for every ill." It looks to address all kinds of health issues with the best of preventative wellness therapies that are firmly rooted in lifestyle interventions. These can include easy-to-follow techniques for relieving the stressors that contribute to pain or poor health. What's more, functional medicine strives to provide patients with the most up-to-date clinical research so that they have a better understanding of why these protocols can meet their specific needs.

Functional medicine explains why many of the uncomfortable symptoms that arise during pregnancy may be related to what you're eating, your environment, your mindset, your exercise level, and the various stressful factors you likely have to deal with on a daily basis. Our approach will help you identify what is not supported in your body that is leading to these symptoms and how to adopt better habits so that the symptoms quickly resolve.

And because adopting a healthy lifestyle is an important part of the functional medicine approach, it should be no surprise that developing an appropriate exercise routine for your pregnancy is critical. In fact, having an exercise routine is currently the most research-proven, single largest determining factor in the outcome of having a productive and safe labor and delivery. And while more women are exercising than ever before, very few understand the specific ways they should be supporting and strengthening their organs and muscles before, during, and after pregnancy. Even if you have an exercise routine, the optimal program for pregnant women cannot be found at the gym doing cardio or lifting weights. In order to achieve the best results, you will need to follow a specific routine that can be modified as your body changes.

This book is meant to provide the fundamental knowledge to prevent disease and pain before, during, and after pregnancy. The hope is that together, we can restore and create a new version of the ancient wisdom that was passed down through generations for this transitional time of life.

How This Book Works

This book begins during the critical six months prior to conception because how you and your partner choose to live, eat, and exercise *before* you become pregnant has an enormous impact on the health of your baby. Until recently, the commonly accepted medical wisdom was that pregnancy is the only period of time in which a mother's behavior affects the fetus. We now know through the study of *epigenetics*—how our genes affect our health—that the health of both the mother *and* father *before* pregnancy can influence their offspring's genetic expression. The healthier partners are before conceiving, the healthier their baby will be.

This period of time is known as *preconception*, and we're excited to be one of the first resources that holistically support it. You'll learn about the many reasons why you want to lower inflammation throughout your body before you conceive: the less inflamed you are, the stronger and healthier you will be, leading to enhanced overall health for your baby. And starting the right exercise program at this time will give you the ability to carry your baby with ease, leading to a positive pregnancy and birthing experience. And if you are having fertility issues, addressing your mind and body during preconception may lead to better outcomes.

However, if you are already pregnant, don't feel like you have missed your opportunity. If you're picking up this book when you are pregnant, you can always optimize your choices while you're pregnant and afterward, and possibly learn a thing or two before your next pregnancy.

The material is divided into seven chapters: preconception, first trimester, second trimester, third trimester, delivery, the first forty days after delivery, and beyond. We know that the first forty days following childbirth need to be treated in a very specific way so that you can rest and recuperate, and set the tone for your metabolic, hormonal, and physical health for the rest of your life. Afterward, you can start our appropriate exercise program so you can create a better-than-before-baby body.

Ideally, we want you to read through the entire book during preconception and return to it during each stage of pregnancy and postpartum. Each chapter begins with a clear and easy-to-follow summary that acts like a mini table of contents, so a wise woman like you can find the information you need quickly, before diving into the details, or easily refer back to when you want to reread a section. The resources section includes helpful web addresses to many of our favorite brands and additional educational insights mentioned throughout the book.

The chapters feature the following five sections:

- **Your Body.** A wise woman needs to prepare her mind and body for pregnancy. These sections provide thoroughly researched medical information that is tailored for each unique stage and focuses on your changing body and optimizing overall health. It will include lifestyle suggestions that are most favorable to adopt in order to prevent issues and help to optimize your body so it's primed to have a healthy pregnancy and create a healthy baby. Your health and well-being during every stage is directly connected to the growth and health of your baby and influences their disease risk for years to come.
- **Restorative Breathing.** Here's a fact: 100 percent of pregnant women have a breathing dysfunction because they cannot access their diaphragm in order to breathe properly. These sections will train you to breathe efficiently during pregnancy so that you can compensate in a positive way. Without these lessons, you may inadvertently

overcompensate and develop pain and muscle tension, fatigue, nausea, and even brain fog and anxiety. These techniques will also allow you to manipulate your breath during labor and delivery.

◆ **Movement.** Every wise woman, regardless of her current fitness level, must strengthen the deep muscles that support her abdominals, spine, and pelvis in order to ensure a pregnancy and delivery free from unnecessary pain and injury. The movement sections will teach you how to work these specific muscles in advance to be ready for your changing body. It features complete instructions for dynamic exercises and dance movements accompanied by clear photographs that will instruct you on proper form. Each exercise will fully explain how muscles should be activated to develop *eccentric strength*. The exercises can all be done at home, require minimal equipment, and are appropriate for anyone, including women who haven't exercised in the past.

We will also once and for all shatter the recurring myths and misconceptions surrounding when to exercise during pregnancy. For example, in 2018, the *New York Times* ran an article that highlighted a "multimillion-dollar trial launched by the federal government" that showed that women who started a diet and exercise program during the second trimester helped them avoid excess weight gain during their pregnancies. Yet these same women were not able to lower their rate of gestational diabetes, hypertension, and outcomes.[2] We know the reason: they started exercising too late! According to the most progressive science, the best time to start exercising in order to prevent chronic diseases is during preconception.

◆ **Nourishment.** A wise woman doesn't want to count calories. Instead, she wants a comprehensive nutrition program that establishes ideal eating patterns and food choices that best support conception, pregnancy, breastfeeding, and getting your pre-baby body back. In these sections, you will learn to focus on healthy, high quality foods that are the right combination of fats, carbohydrates, and proteins for the stage of pregnancy you are currently in. You'll also learn how to apply these lessons to a variety of dietary restrictions. When you can't get all of the micronutrients you need from your food, we'll provide information on the best clean supplements. What's more, we will teach you how to make wise food choices based on your hereditary background and what is local and seasonally available in the region you currently live in.

- ◆ **Wisdom.** We want to teach you how to optimally experience this special time. Each chapter will include what we call "pearls of wisdom" gleaned from historical as well as multicultural perspectives that are backed by the latest science. These range from different techniques for improving sleep and continuing sexual activity to setting up a personal team and planning for the future.

Let's Get Started

We're so thrilled that you are ready to have a baby. Our mission is to empower you to trust your body, listen to it, and take natural steps that are right for you to improve your health and your baby's. Everything we've included in this book is meant to lower your stress level and give you the confidence to be a wise woman: informed, supported, empowered, and ready to face the future. This program is rooted in science and practiced on thousands of women, so we are confident that it will enhance your pregnancy in every possible way. Our patients routinely tell us how comforted they feel to get well-rounded answers to their burning questions as they understand the *why* behind our recommendations that comes from both family/ancestral stories and scientific studies. It takes seventeen years for the latest research to make it into the mainstream medical system, yet we know that you don't have time to wait! The lifestyle medicine featured in this book has been proven to amplify health and have a positive impact on the next *two* generations—meaning your children and their children. Let's begin this journey together.

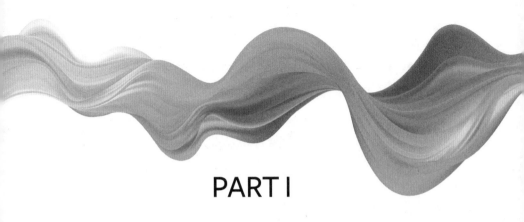

PART I

Preconception:
A Six-Month Head Start

One of the most important messages of this book has nothing to do with the forty weeks of pregnancy. In fact, the six months prior to conception, known as *preconception,* may be more important to your baby's health and wellness than how you live during pregnancy. The truth is, the health and lifestyle choices of *both men and women* during preconception can impact your child's health for a lifetime.

In this section, you will learn how to optimally prepare the body and mind and create the best environment for conception. This includes understanding your current physical health as well as what you interact with in your home and office. We must uncover and then enhance, or as we like to say, *amplify,* exactly what we are putting inside our bodies, what we are applying on our bodies (skin care, body creams, toothpastes), what we are cooking with, what we are storing foods in, what we are thinking, how much we are exercising, and if we are making time every day for rest, relaxation, and doing the things that bring us joy.

The goal of this exploration is to lower inflammation. If you are not feeling your best, chances are that inflammation may be the underlying cause. Inflammation in either partner can prevent you from becoming pregnant, can affect the health of your baby, and can influence how you will feel once you become pregnant.

YOUR BODY:

RESTORATIVE BREATHING:

MOVEMENT:

NOURISHMENT:

CONCEPTION:

WISDOM:

YOUR BODY

Experts in the medical community used to believe that pregnancy was the only period of time in which a mother's behavior affects her baby. Even today, most new moms think that when a woman leads a normal life and eats good quality food during pregnancy, she has done enough. So here's your first surprise: this is not always the case.

The truth is, according to researchers, the first phase of human development, beginning with preconception, sets the stage for 70 percent of an individual's future health.[1] As Dr. Sergio Pecorelli, an internationally renowned obstetrics, gynecology, and preventative medicine expert says, an unhealthy start to life reduces our children's *biological reserves*: the ability to cope with later experiences or exposures resiliently. No matter what you do during pregnancy or how your children choose to live into adulthood, their health outcomes have been predetermined by the choices you and your partner make before you even conceive. That's a serious responsibility!

Here's the science: the lifestyle choices you make every day directly affect your *epigenetics*: the biological mechanism that influences how genes are expressed. Epigenetics is a relatively new field of study. When scientists first discovered the genome—the building blocks of life that make us unique—they believed it was primarily made up of our DNA, the genes we inherited from both of our biological parents. Today we know that only 2 percent of the genome is comprised of genes. The rest is RNA, which is not part of the genetic code, yet plays a major role in how genes are expressed or mutated. As Dr. Pecorelli says, the genes that we inherit are written with ink, while their epigenetics are written with a pencil.

Epigenetic influences change naturally as we age and are in turn influenced by our current health. Yet the primary influencer of epigenetics is our environment, which includes everything that surrounds you and affects your daily life. It's the air you breathe and the water you drink, the quality of your food, whether or not you exercise, smoke, drink, or take drugs. It also includes your emotional life and the amount of stress you have to deal with at home and at work. In fact, if you fight with your partner often, the environmental effect is just as detrimental to your health as being surrounded by air pollution.[2]

Optimizing your environment can therefore positively influence your epigenetics. For instance, if you live a sedentary life, your RNA may turn on inherited genes that lead to obesity or cardiovascular disease. But if you decide to start exercising, the epigenetic expression of your RNA changes, and your risk for developing these same illnesses can be reversed. This is how we know that the lifestyle choices we make today can help or harm us now, and for our lifetime.

During conception, our genes are encoded in the germ cells: the egg or *ova* for women and sperm for men. Women are born with all of their eggs housed in their ovaries. Typically, one is released every month between puberty and menopause. While these eggs each hold a copy of the mother's genetic code, they are not fully matured until ovulation. Therefore, there is plenty of time to impact your egg's genetic expression before conception.

But did you know that the father's health has a *greater* impact on predicting the health of the baby than the mother's? It's true: when it comes to epigenetics, the real burden is on the father. If the father's sperm are suboptimal, the baby is at high risk for illness later in life. Chronic disorders like obesity and diabetes, as well as many brain diseases, including Alzheimer's disease, have a very powerful link to the quality of your man's sperm. It is also thought that sperm are more sensitive to the environment than eggs.

So how do you make the most of what you've got in terms of passing on the best possible health outcomes to your child? The answer is simple: before you even try to get pregnant, take a good look at how you and your partner are living and start cleaning it up. We want those germ cells to be as healthy as possible before conception so that their outcome—your baby—will then be as healthy as possible. Amplifying your well-being through exercise, following a healthy diet, and avoiding toxins and stress are the effective strategies to prevent dysfunctional epigenetic changes. By taking responsibility for your health and your environment during preconception, you and your partner are removing the risks and increasing the odds that your child will have a long and healthy life.

Preconception Lasts Six Months

The preconception period—defined as the six months before you plan on conceiving—allows the time necessary for behavioral interventions to positively affect your germ cells. While women release an egg every twenty-eight days, men produce sperm in a ninety-day cycle. Six months of preconception allows for two full cycles to create clean and healthy sperm. Six months is also a reasonable time for women to deal with their own environment and create new habits that can last throughout pregnancy.

The Functional Medicine Approach to Preconception

The healthy habits we discuss in this chapter share a single purpose: to help you and your partner reduce inflammation. Inflammation is the natural response of the immune system to a perceived threat, such as an infection, injury, stress, exposure to toxins, or even poor diet. When faced with a threat, the immune system starts a process that both destroys the threat and creates a healing barrier between it and the rest of the body. This barrier is the inflammation, which is bringing more nourishment and immune activity to the site of injury or infection. Sometimes you can see and feel inflammation, like when you notice tenderness, redness, and swelling surrounding a cut. But most often inflammation occurs internally, and you aren't aware of it.

Inflammation isn't a problem unless the inflammatory response won't turn off. When it persists, it damages the body and causes illness. Chronic inflammation is linked to many of the most dangerous illnesses, like heart disease, diabetes, and cancer. It can affect your thinking and your mood. It's also linked to infertility. According to the Duke University Fertility Center, lowering inflammation is the best way for you to increase the likelihood that you will get pregnant, develop a healthy placenta during pregnancy, and stay pregnant. For men, diseases related to chronic inflammation, like obesity, can lead to lower testosterone and diminished sperm count.

During preconception, lowering inflammation is critically important. When both you and your partner lower inflammation, you improve your chances of turning on your positive epigenetics. By doing so, you are optimizing your sperm and ova and are passing on your healthiest genes, leading to the best health potential for your children.

Luckily, there are many ways we can lower inflammation, and all of the tips in this chapter are recommended for you and your partner. A functional medicine approach takes a holistic view of every aspect of life and looking for ways we can lower inflammation naturally. First, let's make sure that there are no health concerns that would affect fertility or conception for you and your partner. Then, you can begin to lower inflammation naturally in just three easy steps.

Indicators of Chronic Inflammation

Do you or your partner have any of these chronic, or ongoing, signs of inflammation?

- Brittle fingernails
- Carbohydrate cravings
- Daylong fatigue
- Digestive issues, stomach pain, reflux
- Groggy upon waking, vs. waking refreshed
- Headaches and migraines
- Joint aches and pains
- PMS (for women) or other hormonal disorders
- Poor sleep
- Runny, stuffy nose
- Weight gain

Common Causes of Chronic Inflammation

Lifestyle choices are closely linked and contribute to inflammation:

- Alcohol
- Caffeine
- Environmental toxins
- Lack of sleep
- Mold exposure
- Participating in extreme sports
- Poor diet
- Prescription medications
- Recreational drugs
- Steroid use
- Stress
- Tobacco

Have Your Primary Care Physician Run These Tests

As soon as you decide that you want to have a baby, the preconception clock begins. It's a good idea for you and your partner to start by getting a physical with your regular physician at the beginning of preconception. A medical doctor can identify if there are any health concerns that may influence your ability to conceive, as well as identify any medical causes of chronic inflammation.

If you want to dig a little deeper, you may want to consider a functional medicine evaluation, particularly if you think you are suffering from symptoms of chronic inflammation or if your lifestyle is one that may lead to chronic inflammation. A functional medicine checkup analyzes every detail about your health, starting with your mother's health history during her pregnancy. It's meant to uncover the *why* of illness: why someone has a health problem, instead of simply treating the symptoms. For instance, if you have a headache that won't go away, a conventional doctor might order an MRI of your head, but that's only looking for a structural problem. A functional medicine practitioner will examine all of your systems, and your lifestyle, in order to find the underlying cause of your headache.

A functional medicine checkup includes a comprehensive set of medical lab work to determine current health status. Functional tests go far beyond conventional medical testing. Besides testing your blood and urine, there is in-depth stool testing. What's more, traditional medicine testing pegs your lab results to a reference range of what is considered to be "normal," or how 90 percent of the population responds to those tests, and typically holds off treatment until lab results are very far out of the normal range. This is simply not good enough to ensure that you have a healthy pregnancy and a healthy baby.

Many times, the women we see come in with traditional lab results that are considered to be on the very edge of normal, and their doctor has told them that they are "fine." Yet we believe that being on the very edge of normal is never a good thing. In functional medicine, the goal is not to reach a normal level of health—we are looking to achieve an *optimal* level of health. We don't want to wait until symptoms are debilitating or lead to disease. Think about it; if you see rotting wood on your roof but it hasn't started leaking water into your house, is that roof "healthy"? You want to fix that roof *before* it starts to leak and ruin your furniture and possibly your entire home.

The following is an overview of typical functional medicine testing. If your doctor isn't a functional medicine practitioner and you want these tests, you'll need to find a doctor who will provide them. To find a functional medicine practitioner, go to the Institute for Functional Medicine website, or contact the labs we list directly, and they can point you to providers in your area.

Men and women should be testing their hormone levels during preconception. We recommend that everyone have an adrenal stress hormone evaluation, such as the Dried Urine Test for Comprehensive Hormones (DUTCH) Complete test from Precision Analytics. This test looks at the rhythm of cortisol production as well as the total amount of cortisol in the body. It also will look at how other hormones are processed, to make sure they are being utilized effectively and safely.

Men and women should also have a sex hormone evaluation. For women, pregnancy will be a time of incredible nutrient and metabolic demand. Preconception is then a time to focus on restoring, nourishing, and rebalancing hormones. Women should talk to a doctor about past reproductive history—if you have been pregnant before, did it take a long time to conceive? Did you need fertility treatment? Do you have a history of miscarriages?

Your doctor can test your hormone levels with

- Serum prolactin
- Luteinizing hormone
- Complete thyroid panel
- Sex hormone binding globulin (SHBG)
- Follicle stimulating hormone (FSH)
- Estradiol
- Testosterone (total and free)
- (DHEAS) Dehydroepiandrosterone sulfate

To check for egg quality

- AMH (anti-müllerian hormone) level
- Day 3 FSH and estradiol levels
- An ultrasound to check your follicle count

Men should test for testosterone levels, as low testosterone is a sign of inflammation. Low T is also associated with high insulin levels, which causes systemic inflammation that in and of itself can lead to low testosterone.

Men should test for testosterone and other hormones, including

- Testosterone (total and free)
- Estradiol
- Follicle stimulating hormone (FSH)
- Leuteinizing hormone (LH)
- Sex hormone binding globulin (SHBG)
- Thyroid panel

A second group of foundational tests would be a gut evaluation, which is beneficial for both men and women, even in the absence of symptoms. A normal, healthy, and balanced gut will improve and optimize hormone balance and reduce inflammation. Gut health is the biggest foundation of excellent health. This testing includes the SIBO-lactulose or glucose breath test that identifies intestinal bacterial overgrowth. We also recommend a stool test, which can provide a broad look at intestinal health, digestive health, beneficial bacteria, an overgrowth of bad bacteria, and outright infections, parasites, and yeast. It also can look at inflammatory markers. Stool testing from a conventional medicine lab doesn't quantify or qualify intestinal health the way functional medicine tests do. Ask your doctor to use one of the following three labs that provide more comprehensive testing:

- Diagnostics Solutions—GI-MAP
- Doctor's Data stool test
- Genova Diagnostics—GI Effects

We also recommend a nutrient assessment for men and women: companies like Integrated Genetic Solutions use blood samples to determine the levels of twenty-five different nutrients, vitamins, minerals, and hormones and will give you individualized recommendations for dosing of deficient nutrients needed to optimize your health. Another test, called Nutreval from

Genova Diagnostics, can give you very comprehensive information about nutrient and amino acid deficiencies, with some recommendations for dosing in general. Egg quality may also benefit from certain supplements that improve nutrient ratios, like myo-inositol, d-chiro-inositol, DHEA, omega 3 fatty acids (EPA and DHA), and melatonin.

Lastly, men and women can identify the source of their inflammation prior to conception through bloodwork. In addition to the standard bloodwork your doctor may run to assess health, consider the following tests that look a little deeper. These tests need to be asked for specifically because a conventional practitioner will not routinely order them:

- Anti-nucleic acid (ANA) test: screening test for autoimmune disease
- Anti-TPO (thyroid peroxidase antibody) and anti-thyroglobulin antibodies
- Celiac panel
- Complete chemistry panel for electrolytes, kidney, and liver functions
- Erythrocyte sedimentation rate (ESR)
- Fasting glucose and insulin
- Ferritin
- Fibrinogen levels
- Food allergy testing (IgG) — Cyrex or FIT testing
- Heavy metals: aluminum, cadmium, lead, mercury
- Hemoglobin A1c
- Hidden infections (H. pylori, EBV, CMV, HSV 1 and 2, and Lyme if indicated)
- Homocysteine
- hs CRP (high-sensitivity reactive protein)
- Omega-3 index
- Rheumatoid factor
- Serum glutathione
- Vitamins and minerals: B12, 25-OH, vitamin D, zinc, folate, magnesium
- White blood cell count with differential (CBC, diff)

> ## What You Need to Know About Sperm Donors
>
> If you will be utilizing a sperm bank, it is important to get as much information about the donor as possible. The information provided by sperm banks can vary. Choose a sperm bank that is the most transparent about the donor's mental and physical health: his physical characteristics are not as important as his health and lifestyle. The gold standard should include a mental health evaluation and a wide range of bloodwork panels. See what you can infer from the profile, and contact the medical director if you have specific questions.

Special Health Considerations

Testing may reveal that you or your partner is suffering from one of the following conditions that may affect the viability of germ cells or your ability to conceive. Discuss these with your doctor and create a plan that works for preconception and will cover your needs throughout pregnancy.

If You Have an Autoimmune Disease

Autoimmune diseases are classified as those that occur when the immune system attacks the organs and tissues in the body and brain, causing symptoms, illness, and inflammation. There are more than 70 autoimmune diseases and over 300 different autoimmune conditions. For women, the ability to keep an autoimmune disease in control for six months prior to pregnancy will predict complications during pregnancy: if your autoimmune disease is very well controlled in the six months prior to getting pregnant, then you are less likely to have problems like preterm birth, preeclampsia, or small-for-gestational-age babies.

Conventional medicine practitioners often try to control autoimmune diseases with medications, which may be necessary. However, many of these prescription drugs are not safe to take during pregnancy. Functional medicine looks to first address the underlying cause of the autoimmune disease. Most of the time, those causes are related to problems in the intestines that are related to food sensitivities that lead to inflammation. Toxins and stress, including psychological, emotional, social, and physical stressors, are correlated to autoimmune flaring. By following these guidelines, you may be able to avoid or at least reduce the need for these medications during pregnancy.

All of the modifications that we will discuss to generally lower inflammation and prepare for pregnancy will reduce autoimmune activity and can help you manage your autoimmune disease now and during pregnancy. For instance, if we remove inflammatory foods from the diet and increase anti-inflammatory, nutrient-dense foods, this one change will help calm autoimmune flares. If you rebalance the gut and prevent or reduce the presence of leaky gut syndrome, also known as intestinal permeability, you address one of the main pathways that lead to autoimmune diseases and will help prevent them from flaring during pregnancy. Stress control is also important because, if you don't have your stress hormones like cortisol balanced, then it can be very difficult to control autoimmune disease and may lead to autoimmune flaring.

It's also important to note that many women will develop thyroid issues or other autoimmune issues after pregnancy, seemingly "all of a sudden." However, nothing in the body happens instantaneously. By lowering inflammation beginning in preconception—by removing inflammatory foods, preventing leaky gut, and eliminating any intestinal infections and bacterial imbalances—and then continuing to keep inflammation in check throughout pregnancy, you are proactively addressing these concerns.

Common Autoimmune Inflammatory Conditions

Not all inflammatory conditions are autoimmune in nature, however, all autoimmune diseases have an inflammatory component. The following conditions need to be addressed during preconception (autoimmune diseases are marked with *):

- Allergies
- Arthritis (rheumatoid arthritis* is autoimmune)
- Asthma
- Bronchitis
- Cancer
- Cardiovascular disease
- Celiac disease*
- Diabetes (type 1* is autoimmune)
- Eczema
- Endometriosis* (women)
- Interstitial cystitis
- Gastritis
- Gingivitis
- Graves' disease*
- Hashimoto's thyroiditis*
- Inflammatory bowel disease (Crohn's, ulcerative colitis)*
- Low testosterone (men)
- Lupus*
- Multiple sclerosis*
- Obesity
- Periodontitis
- Polycystic ovarian syndrome*
- Prostatitis (men)
- Psoriasis*
- Sinusitis
- Sjögren's syndrome*

If You Have a Mood Disorder: Depression/Anxiety

Inflammation can compromise brain function, leading to a wide variety of symptoms including headaches, memory loss, anxiety, irritability, insomnia, and depression. If you or your partner is suffering from any of these symptoms, it may be related to your diet, infections, hormone imbalances, intestinal issues, nutrient deficiencies, toxic exposures, or even poor breathing habits. Proper testing will help you determine the cause. The lifestyle modifications in this chapter may be more effective in reversing these symptoms than medication. In fact, the lessons in the Restorative Breathing section, which will teach you how to adjust your breathing, may make all the difference.

We also recommend finding a therapeutic modality that works for you. Knowing where to start is half the battle. Beyond seeing a therapist, like a social worker or psychologist, life coaches can be particularly well suited to help you figure out how to handle a problem that's causing stress. There are also cognitive behavioral techniques that can teach you how to release trauma very quickly. These include EMDR (eye movement desensitization and reprocessing), EFT (emotional freedom technique), or DNRS (dynamic neural retraining system).

If You Have Hypertension/High Blood Pressure

Many people of childbearing age have high blood pressure, especially men. During preconception, testing is critical to determine the root cause. The five biggest causes of hypertension are imbalanced sugar levels, stress, toxins (heavy metals like lead and mercury), inflammation, and nutrient deficiencies. Sometimes just making a small nutrient shift can make a big difference.

Preconception is the perfect time to try lifestyle changes that can help control blood pressure, and may help you address why you have high blood pressure in the first place. Blood pressure medications can affect germ cells and are often not safe to take during pregnancy, so identifying alternative ways to control it now is ideal. For men, blood pressure medications can reduce sperm number and quality, which negatively affects fertility. Talk to your doctor during preconception so that you can switch your medications to a safer alternative. For instance, micronutrient supplementation with potassium, magnesium, and vitamin K can help to lower high blood pressure. Using these supplements may help reduce your need for prescription medications.

Supplements that can improve the quality of your germ cells are often ones that improve the function of your mitochondria, the energy powerhouse of each individual cell, which is critical for maintaining optimum blood pressure. For example, the supplement CoQ10 can help your mitochondria work more efficiently and is considered safe for both men and women during preconception and later, during pregnancy. You are going to need a lot of energy to create cells and to grow a baby! It is thought that CoQ10 improves sperm motility and quality as well as overall egg quality.

Getting your blood sugar levels under control makes a huge difference when it comes to lowering high blood pressure and total body inflammation. In fact, you don't have to lose a ton of weight to make a difference in your blood pressure. Use the Body Mass Index (BMI) as a general guideline for how much you should weigh.

If You Have Pre-Diabetes/Metabolic Syndrome/Polycystic Ovarian Syndrome (PCOS)

These three conditions are all mediated by abnormal sugar-insulin balance. High insulin levels occur with high blood sugar levels, which then causes inflammation. Hemoglobin A1C is a marker of what your blood sugar levels have been on average over the last three months, which is the life span of a red blood cell. If your hemoglobin A1C levels are above normal, using the typical reference range of 5.6 or greater, any decimal point above that increases the risk of having a baby with severe birth defects. Higher hemoglobin A1c levels also increase your risk for complications during pregnancy, so it's important to have a normal hemoglobin A1C in preconception.

PCOS does not affect men, but prediabetes and metabolic syndrome affect men and women equally. The same treatments can address all three concerns and involve normalizing the hormones responsible for blood sugar balance: insulin and cortisol. You can normalize insulin levels by reducing the amount of processed carbohydrates you eat and by increasing anti-inflammatory, nutrient-dense foods. Cortisol levels are related to any type of stress (physical, psychological, social, and emotional), so dealing with stress appropriately will help. Exercise, weight loss, and getting restorative sleep will also address cortisol issues.

If You Have Thyroid Issues

The thyroid hormone is responsible for how every cell in your body functions. The thyroid gland is particularly sensitive to environmental toxins. Many times when people develop thyroid nodules, it's actually the thyroid's attempt to try to isolate toxicity in the thyroid and prevent it from spreading throughout the body. The most noticeable symptoms that are related to poor thyroid health include weight gain or inability to lose weight, fatigue, feeling low energy, hair loss, cold intolerance, constipation, depression, puffy face, hoarseness, muscle weakness, high cholesterol levels, slowed heart rate, heavier than normal or irregular periods, brain fog, and infertility.

If testing confirms that you or your partner do not have optimal thyroid hormone levels, your doctor can help you determine the cause. In the United States, most thyroid health issues are autoimmune, including Hashimoto's thyroiditis and Graves' disease. Thyroid issues can also occur with certain nutrient deficiencies. Supplementing with iodine, selenium, zinc, B vitamins, vitamin A, vitamin D, and iron may help.

Addressing Inflammation Step #1: Balance the Gut's Microbiome

A microbiome is a community of bacteria, yeast, and viruses that we carry on or inside the body. These communities live in all of our hollow surfaces (intestines, mouth, nose, ears, eyes, bladder, lungs, and genitals) as well as on our skin surface. Your vaginal microbiome can be affected by many factors, including your partner's genital microbiome. This is why both you and your partner need to pay attention to your individual microbiomes during preconception. You are establishing good habits now because there will be natural changes that will occur during pregnancy that affect your vaginal flora, and you want to make sure your baby will be exposed to and become colonized with a diversity of beneficial microbes as they exit the vaginal canal.

An even more important microbiome to consider is in your gut. The gut's microbiome can weigh up to 5 pounds and is comprised of trillions of microbes that fall into two families. *Bacteroides* are supposed to be the dominant family that we are hosting. *Firmicutes* are the gate crashers, and when they take over the gut's microbiome, the imbalance they cause creates inflammation and potential autoimmune diseases. The goal of maintaining a healthy microbiome is to have a diversity of beneficial bacteria that is well balanced to keep "bad" bacteria and other unsavory microorganisms in check.

One of the best ways to lower inflammation and amplify your and your partner's epigenetics is to optimize the intestinal microbiome. Seventy percent of the entire immune system resides in the gut, and this microbiome comprises the majority of that immune system. This is why an imbalanced gut microbiome can lead to systemic inflammation and disease: they affect multiple systems in the body from working efficiently. For instance, if you tend to have yeast infections, this may be a result of a gut bacterial imbalance. At the same time, gut health issues are also related to this microbiome. Symptoms like heartburn, chronic constipation, or frequent diarrhea are all caused by chronic inflammation that starts with imbalances in the gut. For men, these gut issues are signs that their sperm health may be compromised.

Sometimes, your best intentions can create problems with your gut's microbiome. For instance, every time you take antibiotics, you are killing off some of the beneficial bacteria in the microbiome along with the infections they are supposed to attack. In extreme cases following many rounds of antibiotics, you may not be able to repopulate certain positive bacterial strains. This doesn't mean that we want you to disregard infections; we want you to take care of them. During preconception, make sure that both you and your partner inform your doctor that you are trying to improve your microbiome, and if you have an infection that isn't resolving, see if there are alternatives to taking antibiotics. There are several herbal combinations that are helpful to control pathogenic bacteria and can serve as natural immune boosters.

Men and women need to get to the root cause of gut health issues, and then treat appropriately. For instance, gut issues can arise when your diet is high in inflammatory foods like sugar. Luckily, your gut's microbiome will change when you change what you eat. In the Nourishment section, you will learn about foods and supplements that support a healthier microbiome. Many are the same foods that lower inflammation. And the right exercise program can have a positive impact on the microbiome as it aids in detoxification and can lower inflammation.

A good place to start is with a home stool testing kit from the company Viome. This product identifies and quantifies your gut's microbiome and then creates a personalized diet and supplement plan to address any imbalance. Finally, consider your oral microbiome. If you have dental issues like multiple root canals or cavities, this may be an indicator of an unhealthy oral microbiome that can impact the rest of your intestinal flora and be a significant source of chronic inflammation. Mercury fillings or inflammation of the gums (gingivitis) are also warning signs. A biological dentist can make sure that there aren't underlying, undetected oral infections present. Oftentimes, these cannot be found on standard dental X-ray imaging. We recommend brushing your teeth with non-fluorinated toothpaste (Biocidin is a great brand) and floss twice daily. The more you brush and floss, the lower the amount of unhealthy oral bacteria are present. Better oral health is associated with decreased risks of preterm delivery and poor perinatal outcomes.

Addressing Inflammation Step #2:
Lower Stress

Being resilient and managing stress effectively is critical for establishing wellness during preconception. A 2016 study published by the National Institutes of Health shows that exposure to stress can induce stable epigenetic changes in gene expression, which can be passed to offspring and subsequent generations.[3] That means the stress you are living with before pregnancy can not only affect you, it also affects the next two generations through epigenetic inheritance.

There are so many micro-stresses that we're faced with every day that we don't realize how impacted we are. Your lifestyle, work deadlines, a hectic schedule, travel, emotional burdens, or even your relationship can all be stressful. Then there are the stressful thoughts that arise when you start thinking about having a baby. We call them *thought viruses* because they infect and take over your thinking. *Can I get pregnant? Will my baby be okay? Am I going to miscarry? Are we going to be the couple that has problems once the baby arrives?* All of these worries can stress us out.

A little bit of stress is fine and inevitable. However, while you can shrug some of these worries off, they can build up and, when they do, can influence your health. When we are stressed, we produce the hormone cortisol in the adrenal glands. Cortisol is linked directly to the body's fight, flight, or freeze response. When it is released, the response is activated, and suddenly, our body has exquisite focus on only the most crucial activities that keep us alive. Your body doesn't know the difference between your boss coming down on you because you missed a deadline or if a bear is on the attack and you're about to be eaten. So when you're stressed, you might not feel hungry because you're not going to stop and eat a sandwich while a bear is chasing you. You might not feel like having sex or any sort of pleasurable experience. You might be unable to think clearly because now your body is only primed to run for your life.

Your body may prevent you from getting pregnant if you are under an inordinate amount of stress. This mechanism—the body's wisdom of recognizing that you are not in the best place to become pregnant—is the underlying reason why stress can lead to irregular cycles.

If the stressful event is a short-lived experience, your cortisol levels go up, you feel that adrenaline rush, and then your body rests and recovers, and nothing detrimental happens. But when you have chronic stress, you create an elevated hormone level that's supposed to be temporary. Your body is not supposed to be on an adrenaline rush all day. Consequently, your body never gets back to doing all the different operations it's supposed to be taking care of, like proper digestion. High levels of cortisol keep you from getting proper sleep. Your body is less likely to produce a feel-good hormone like serotonin, which can lead to developing anxiety. And if cortisol levels stay elevated for too long, it leads to systemic inflammation. Over time, if you stay in that inflammatory state, the gut's microbiome is affected, causing an imbalance. That's why chronically stressed people often have indigestion.

Finding a strategy that relieves stress daily is the best way to avoid experiencing its long-lasting effects. It's when we don't deal with it, when it lingers, that we create an inflammatory state. The antidote is choosing something that you enjoy that also makes you feel good so that your brain creates the hormone oxytocin, which naturally helps calm the mind so that you can relax. Women naturally produce oxytocin when they are breastfeeding, and both men and women produce it when they are having an orgasm or generally expressing love. It is also thought to reduce inflammation. This is why having fun and doing things that bring you joy during preconception is critical! By doing so, you will be creating the optimal stress-free environment before you become pregnant.

The best way to get the brain to make oxytocin will be different for everyone. Some might want to listen to music. Others might want to cook or bake, get creative, or sit down and read a book. Another person might want to go see a movie or spend time with a friend. Whatever it is that helps you rest and relax will stop the fight or flight cortisol response. Interestingly, the most thoroughly examined male behavior involves stress and elevated cortisol levels, which have been shown to change the health of sperm in a manner that relates to the offspring's predisposition for brain disorders and psychiatric illness. This is why it's equally important for men to find their fun and relax.

For instance, when Patricia was preparing to get pregnant, she found that listening to her favorite music during her commute was the perfect stress-buster. Instead of doing work, checking emails, or scrolling through social media, listening to her favorite music not only relieved her stress but avoided the opportunity for her to create more. Over time she noticed that it helped her transition to home life after a busy day at work.

When stressful events happen, deal with them as quickly as possible and make sure you're taking the time to do something to get you out of the stress state. Here are some suggestions that are known to enhance the production of oxytocin. Choose the ones that resonate with you. We're not saying that you have to start getting massages if you don't enjoy them. Just because we have something on the list doesn't mean you have to do it.

- **Aromatherapy/essential oils.** These oils are sourced from plants that can help the body resist stressors and lower cortisol.
- **Declutter.** By cleaning your home/office/car and putting things away, you are relieving anxiety and creating a calm environment.
- **Get outside.** Spending time outdoors promotes a calmness much like meditation.
- **Laughter.** Whether it's spending time with friends or watching a comedy alone, laughing out loud can reduce stress. In fact, just thinking about having a good laugh can lower cortisol production.
- **Massage.** Research has shown that fifty minutes of massage delivers the same stress-relieving benefits as four-and-a-half hours of nourishing sleep. You can get a massage by a professional, or you can bond with your partner by massaging each other.
- **Meditation.** A meditation practice cultivates nonjudgmental awareness, discipline, attention control, emotional regulation, and the right brain state for rest and relaxation.
- **Movement/Dancing.** Any kind of physical activity is hugely stress-reducing, and dancing encompasses both music and meditation. So you get the benefits of all three: meditation, music, and movement.
- **Music.** Singing, playing an instrument, or simply listening to your

favorite music is enormously effective. It doesn't matter what type of music you're into, just enjoy!

- ◆ **Sex.** Having an orgasm not only creates oxytocin, it resets the nervous system and reboots the body and brain to break the stress cycle. For optimal health, and the most anti-inflammatory benefits, men and women should orgasm two to three times a week.

- ◆ **Sleep.** You and your partner need between seven and nine hours of sleep every night in order to de-stress, reset your brain for the next day, heal and repair your body, and lower inflammation.

- ◆ **Socializing.** Spend time with the people you love and enjoy hanging out with. It doesn't matter if you are watching a movie together or chatting over a meal.

- ◆ **Traveling.** Some people de-stress by taking a day trip, visiting a place in their own neighborhood they've never been before, or learning something new about a different part of the world.

- ◆ **Volunteering.** When we give back to others, it makes us feel good. It helps us forget our problems and puts life into context. When we are helping or help someone who is in need, it not only makes us feel more human in the moment, it really does have long-lasting effects.

Avoidance Is an Excellent Stress-Reducing Strategy

And as much as you can, avoid the things that could potentially stress you out. You're not running away; you're making good decisions to keep your mood up and your inflammation down. During preconception, we can all follow some basic rules to avoid stress:

- ◆ Don't hang around that friend who leaves you feeling drained instead of uplifted. You need to keep your positive energy going and not be around someone who's constantly bringing you down. Now is the time to distance yourself from toxic relationships and focus on the friends and family who shower you with love.

- Don't do things you don't like to do. It sounds simple, but we sometimes do things we really don't want to do in order to please others or because we feel obligated. If you don't like to throw parties, now is not the time to plan a celebration no matter how well-intended. Focus on the things that make you feel good.

- Often, stress and money go hand in hand. You don't have to be rich, but you do need to feel financially safe. What this looks like will be different for everyone. Many people are totally fine carrying a lot of debt. But if you're stressed about your finances, try to get them in order as you get ready to have a baby. Work with a professional or come up with a plan that you are comfortable with so that you can feel like you're in a good place financially.

- Social media and the totality of online life really does cause stress. Limit your exposure to websites and influencers that actually make you happy.

- Consider enlisting a life coach to help you work on more complicated psycho-social-emotional situations that require change.

Lastly, try not to be stressed about being stressed, or worrying about getting pregnant. You're a wise woman: you're reading this book, you're being proactive, you're going to do great! Instead of worrying, let's get excited. Think about what pregnancy is going to be like. Imagine all of what's going to happen and focus on changing your day now to make time for the things that you love to do.

Other Cultures Proactively Address Mental Health

In Japan, a typical physical exam includes an extensive stress questionnaire that includes many questions about the status of one's various relationships. The payoff: the current generation of Japanese children is expected to live to 107!

Addressing Inflammation Step #3:
Reduce Your Toxic Load

Toxic chemicals are entering our bodies every day. We are inhaling them, swallowing them in our food or water, and even absorbing them through our skin. Scientists estimate that everyone carries at least 700 contaminants, regardless of where we live. Some chemicals are quickly processed out of the body through the digestive process or when we sweat. Others cannot be automatically removed and settle in our blood, fat tissue, muscles, bones, brain tissues, and other organs.

We can also only process so many toxins at one time, depending on how many toxins we are dealing with. As Jeffrey Morrison, MD, writes in his book *Cleanse Your Body, Clear Your Mind,* the body deals with toxins like a barrel that is being continuously filled with water. Once the barrel (your body) is completely full, the water (toxins) has nowhere to go and starts pouring over the sides: that's poor health. If toxic exposure is limited before the barrel is full, we won't notice that it is causing health problems. But once the body reaches that tipping point where it can't handle another drop, illness results. These illnesses can then cause inflammation, which lowers the body's ability to detoxify itself even more. What's more, when we cross that threshold of exposure, then the toxins that we are exposed to will cause excessive inflammation.

Men and women can lower their body burden, remove dangerous chemicals, and reduce inflammation by enhancing the body's natural detoxification pathways, including the skin and lymphatic system, nose and lungs, the kidneys and digestive system (including urination and elimination), and the liver. Women have an additional detoxification advantage: menstruation is another form of detoxification. Men are hampered because they have higher levels of the hormone testosterone, which is known to inhibit the detoxification pathways. This is another reason why men need a full six months to lower inflammation. At the same time, reducing your exposure to toxins through the choices you make helps further reduce inflammation.

Avoidance Is an Excellent Detoxification Strategy

Reducing environmental exposures will reduce your body burden and make conception easier. The message of this book is better safe than sorry. Adopting simple changes during preconception to your home, your food choices, and self-care can help you avoid many toxins:

- Choose organic produce, grains, eggs, meats, poultry, and fish whenever possible. Organic products are grown/raised without pesticides and other toxic chemicals. Ingesting weed killers like glyphosate, which is not only found on fruits and vegetables but in wheat and other grains—that both we and the animals we eat feed on—may interfere with how our hormones work and may be linked to birth defects and cancers.

- Avoid fish that are high in heavy metals, like mercury-laden tuna. Most doctors will tell you to avoid sushi and high-mercury fish when you are pregnant, but you and your partner need to be doing this in preconception, not just during pregnancy.

- Food Storage. Avoid storing food, especially warm food or liquids, in aluminum or plastic because they are toxins that can leach into foods. Even BPA-free plastic can contain other chemicals that will probably soon be on the "naughty" list, so the sooner you can break your plastic habits, the better. Reusable stainless steel or glass containers are the best options. You can even bring them with you when you eat out if you like to take home leftovers. Carry a stainless steel thermos for picking up your morning coffee, or a glass, ceramic, or stainless steel water bottle. Bring stainless steel or bamboo utensils from home and keep them at work.

- Cooking. Choose glass, porcelain bakeware, cast iron, or stainless steel. Avoid chemically treated, Teflon nonstick pots and pans because when heated, they release chemicals that get into the food you're cooking and into the air that you're breathing.

- **Home cleaners.** The various chemicals that you might be cleaning with or putting on your lawn contain weed killers, pesticides, and other noxious substances that disrupt the endocrine system. They cause inflammation and reduce the quality and quantity of sperm. Instead, use organic cleaning products or vinegar-based ones you can make yourself. Avoid all commercially prepared air fresheners, antibacterial products, fabric softeners, and dryer sheets; there are no safe alternatives for them. Consider using more natural cleaning products. Find alternatives on the Environmental Working Group site for product recommendations.

- **Water purifier.** Tap water can contain microorganisms, radioactive substances, medication residue, and other toxins like lead. If you are concerned about lead or other chemical exposures, have your water tested, and follow public health guidelines about avoiding drinking, cleaning, or bathing with water that contains any lead. Then, simple carbon filters can remove other trace elements to provide you with better drinking water. The added bonus is that your water often tastes better. Reverse osmosis water filtrations systems are the most effective and can be hooked up as a whole-house filtration system or can be used in "point of use" areas like the kitchen and bathroom. It is important to consider the water you shower and bathe in beyond what you drink, as chlorine and other chemicals typically found in tap water readily absorb into the body through the skin. Check out Aquasana, AquaTru, and Berkey tabletop water filtrations systems.

- **Improve indoor air.** Indoor air can be two to five times more polluted than outdoor air. It can contain mold, toxic gases like carbon monoxide or radon, harsh chemicals found in household products like air fresheners and cleaners, or toxins like lead and formaldehyde. Opening windows (for as little as twenty minutes) and using fans can make a big difference toward reducing indoor air pollution, especially when you are cleaning your home. An air filtration system can effectively improve the air quality in your home and office. We recommend the IntelliPure Ultrafine 468, AirDoctor, or iQAir.

- Check your home and office for mold. While there are no medical studies on the effects of mold in pregnancy, we do know that mold is a toxin, and if you are sensitive to mold, your overall health will suffer. Mold can grow in damp, hot, humid areas of the home. ERMI testing is the gold standard for identifying a mold problem. Our friend Jill Carnahan, MD, is a functional medicine expert on mold, and her website provides comprehensive information on how to detect and remove mold from your home and the objects in it. If you notice a musty, damp smell, or have experienced water damage or water leaking in your home or workplace and feel better away from those environments, mold may be an issue for you.

- Personal-care products. Consider the creams, cleaners, deodorants, and body soaps you and your partner use. Whatever you're putting on your skin ultimately gets absorbed into the rest of the body. We recommend using only natural, organic ingredients for creams and body products and aluminum-free deodorants (we like the Magnesium Deodorant from Violets Are Blue or Native brands). Perfume can be replaced by essential oils because perfumes are not FDA regulated and often contain toxic ingredients that are only listed as "fragrance" on the packaging. In this situation, think of the word "fragrance" as code for "tons of chemicals." In contrast, pure essential oils have been used for centuries in Chinese and Ayurvedic healing traditions and are safe and *adaptogenic*: they respond to and support the body's needs. Skincare products that have SPF are meant to be sunscreens. However, that term "sunscreen" has become another catch-all for all types of chemicals. Oxybenzone and avobenzone are both endocrine-disrupting chemicals and should be avoided at all costs. Instead, look for the word "sun block" on the label with zinc oxide as the active ingredient. However, it's important to get vitamin D from sun exposure every day, and using sunblock will prevent you from getting the benefit you need. Turning a light pink on your skin is a way of noticing that you've gotten enough UV radiation to activate vitamin D. That usually happens within fifteen to twenty minutes. This amount is far from harmful and should not have a negative cumulative effect. It doesn't matter where the sun is hitting your skin in order to produce vitamin D, so you can protect your face with zinc oxide to prevent wrinkling.

Ramp Up Your Body's Internal Detox Abilities

The best way to remove toxins is to address each of the detoxification pathways gently. For instance, dry brushing is a technique to gently detoxify the skin and lymphatic system. Humidifiers, saline sprays, and neti pots keep the nose clear, moist, and lubricated so that it can filter toxins as you breathe. Drinking lots of clean water assists the kidneys and your digestive system to work optimally.

The liver is particularly important because it filters our blood, stores vitamins, and processes toxins. The liver is also primarily where your reproductive hormones are produced and helps keep your menstrual cycle regular. So when you are trying to become pregnant, you want your liver to be optimally functioning. Constipation is a sign that your liver isn't optimally working. Drinking lots of alcohol and caffeinated beverages along with taking recreational drugs make the liver work harder, which is why you want to avoid these habits during preconception.

Many of our patients ask for a "pre-pregnancy detox" to implement just before they plan to conceive. However, you'll need as much as twelve months preconception to actually remove all the toxins from your body and amplify the health of your germ cells. Detox is not advised once you are pregnant. An effective detox will send toxins into the bloodstream before they are removed, which could potentially concentrate their exposure to the developing baby. A dedicated detoxification is only appropriate when your stress hormones and gut are balanced and healthy. Mobilizing toxins into your system prematurely can lead to more health problems if done too early in your health optimization process.

What's more, there is no one-size-fits-all approach to detoxification: you need to know what toxins are affecting your health and which approach is safest for you. A functional medicine practitioner can do the appropriate testing and create an individualized detoxification program that addresses your specific needs. Then, start a program after you've addressed your diet, your stress, your exercise, and your microbiome. You have to make sure that your gut function is really optimized before you start dumping more toxicity into it because, if your intestines are troubled, the gut will not be able to handle more toxicity coming out of the liver during a detox.

When you are cleared by your physician and ready to begin, start with supplements that help clean the liver and increase its ability to get toxins out of the body. These supplements are safe for men and women to take throughout preconception:

- ◆ **Milk thistle.** One of the most studied of all medicinal herbs, milk thistle can be used to protect and regenerate liver cells. It aids the liver in clearing toxins and boosts the antioxidant activity of liver cells.
- ◆ **Dandelion root.** Dandelion has a gentle, protective ability to increase the production and flow of bile, helping to clear excess hormones from the body.
- ◆ **Calcium d-glucarate.** This supplement helps the liver remove fat-soluble toxins.
- ◆ **N-acetyl-cysteine, L-glycine, and L-glutamine.** Any of these amino acids are important for the synthesis of glutathione, a powerful antioxidant that plays an important role in the liver's detoxification pathways.
- ◆ **Vitamin B6, vitamin B12, and folic acid (or methylated folate).** These vitamins are compounds that have a decongesting effect on the liver.

These supplements can be taken individually, or look for a supplement blend like

- Apex Energetics: Liver detox collagen powder called ClearVite
- XYMOGEN: Liver Cleanse (add their S-acetyl glutathione)
- Thorne Research: Liver Cleanse

DIY Home and Garden

This all-purpose cleaner can safely be used everywhere in your home/office/car. Simply mix together in a glass spray bottle:

¼ teaspoon baking soda

1 tablespoon white vinegar

¼ teaspoon organic, vegetable oil—based dishwashing soap

1 cup hot water

10 drops of tea tree essential oil

For the garden, you can use compost as a fertilizer. Rake an inch of compost into your lawn each spring and fall. This promotes good bacteria entering your soil, which are essential for growing healthy grass. Leaving grass clippings on the lawn as you mow provides beneficial nitrogen. Spraying your garden with compost liquid or "tea" can be used to rid your plants of unwanted pests. Dr. Zach Bush's website is a great resource for creating healthy soil.

A Word of Caution: Wireless Radiation

While radio frequency waves have been used for more than a hundred years to transmit signals, our reliance on this technology has changed, and receivers are much closer to users than ever before. The consequence is that wireless radiation is all around us. We now know that close proximity and constant exposure to wireless radiation can cause damage on the cellular level, including germ cells. If you wear a Fitbit, Apple Watch, or some other kind of tracking device for exercise or health, we highly recommend that you stop using it.

Here are a few simple tips that can keep you safe during preconception, and later, when you are pregnant:

- Avoid carrying your phone directly on your body. Do not tuck your phone into exercise pants or a bra or wear it around your arm during exercise.
- Men should not keep their phone in their front pants pocket because it is linked to lower sperm count and infertility.
- Do not have your phone near you when you sleep. It should be at least 5 feet away from you, and set on airplane mode.
- Turn off your router at night to limit nighttime exposure.
- Pay attention to your home's proximity to existing cell phone towers and future construction.

RESTORATIVE BREATHING

Breathing is an involuntary function. We typically don't think about our breathing every day because the body knows how much air to breath in and it knows how much to blow out. However, sometimes our breathing can become compromised. If we are adapting to some type of stressor or pain, or something is irritating our environment, we can shift our breathing as a coping mechanism. And when the cause of that shift is extended over time, we end up creating long-term, poor breathing habits.

Some people compensate and reduce the smoothness of their breath, making it stop and start jaggedly or hold their breath. Either is detrimental because any form of poor breathing means that you're not getting the right balance of oxygen and carbon dioxide flowing through your body. When we breathe poorly, we actually become less present in the environment, which doesn't allow us to cope as well as we could. People with poor breathing habits will report memory loss or fatigue, not seeing colors vividly, having a delayed or dulled response to certain stimuli, and may get nausea or headaches. What's more, if you aren't breathing properly during exercise, you may not receive all the health benefits from your workout, and you may develop lactic acid buildup, which leads to muscle spasms or poor recovery.

Proper breathing calms the nervous system. For example, both yoga and tai chi put emphasis on the flow of breath through the body as a means to reduce stress. This type of breathing activates the vagus nerve, which turns down the stress-inducing activity of the fight, flight, freeze response that affects the rest of your organs. During preconception, restoring proper breathing for men and women may increase the likelihood of conception as it helps you to stay calm and relaxed.

For women, we want you to practice proper, efficient breathing during preconception because later in pregnancy, the added girth of the baby will affect your ability to breathe well. This happens to 100 percent of pregnant women: as the baby grows, they push their way into the space under the mother's lungs where the diaphragm is located, making it hard to access the diaphragm for proper breathing. This leads to *hypocapnia*, a condition where you blow off too much carbon dioxide on each exhale, depleting your lung reserves and causing a reaction to suck more oxygen in.

Symptoms Associated with Poor Breathing Habits

While some of these symptoms sound completely unrelated to poor breathing habits, the truth is these symptoms are connected, and if you have had poor breathing for an extended period of time, some of these symptoms may not be apparent to you because they are either mild or part of your daily life.

- Anxiety, apprehension, emotional outbursts
- Attention deficit, poor thinking, poor memory, poor concentration, impaired judgment, problem-solving deficit
- Blackout, blurred vision, confusion, disorientation
- Dry mouth, nausea, lightheadedness, dizziness, fainting
- Feelings of suffocation, sweaty palms, cold hands, tingling skin
- Numbness, heart palpitations, irregular heartbeat
- Reduced pain threshold, headache, trembling, twitching, shivering, muscle tension, spasm, stiffness, abdominal cramps, bloating
- Shortness of breath, breathlessness, chest tightness/pressure, chest pain
- Stress, fatigue, weakness, exhaustion

The Right Way to Breathe

Normal breathing for life's basic activities should be through the nose, utilizing the diaphragm.

When you breathe through your nose you are able to produce nitric oxide, which is integral for oxygenating muscle tissues and reducing blood clots.

The diaphragm is a dome-shaped muscle located toward the bottom of the rib cage (see shaded gray area below). It sits underneath the lungs and above the abdominal organs. It contracts and expands depending on whether we're inhaling or exhaling.

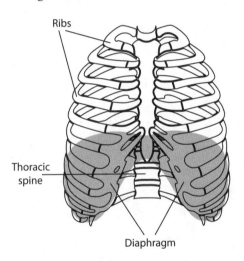

Ribs

Thoracic spine

Diaphragm

Think of your abdomen as a canister. The diaphragm sits on top of the abdominal canister while the pelvic floor sits at the bottom, the deep transversus abdominis muscle is at the front, and the deep lumbar multifidus is at the back. Interestingly, they work together creating a pressurized, supportive system. When urinating, if you stop your urine stream, you are lifting your pelvic floor. In order to do that, the diaphragm has to open to allow for that lift. If the pressure isn't right, then you can have dysfunction, like leaking urine, constipation, or painful sex.

During preconception, we want to strengthen the muscle fibers in the diaphragm and pelvic floor to be working synchronously as you breathe. This sets the stage for pregnancy, when you don't want to develop pelvic floor problems; you'll want the pelvic floor to fully lift in order to support a growing uterus and abdomen and then be able to expand when you're ready to give birth.

Proper diaphragmatic breathing expands and deflates the sides and back of the lower ribs. The belly should fill up and rise on inhalation and fall on exhalation. You are inhaling followed by a smooth exhale, pause, and then there's an involuntary reflex that kicks in to take the next inhale.

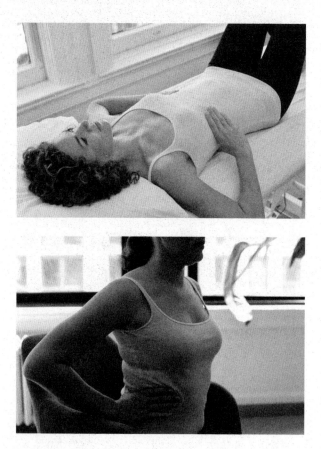

The following are cues to improve your breathing mechanics to help you achieve optimal breathing in preconception before it becomes more difficult during pregnancy. Try each one of these strategies once, sitting comfortably in a chair for three to five minutes, and see if it feels good. Use the one that helps the most throughout the day, at least once an hour if you are having symptoms. As you investigate your breathing, it's common to feel a little bit stressed out about it. Just be patient with yourself and go through the exercise. Think of something you love to do, or someone you love to be with, or even imagine a baby in your belly as you try each of the breathing cues that follow.

If these breathing cues work, continue; if they don't, you might need to modify the exercise by lying down on your back. This may be easier because you are in a position that allows the diaphragm to work more easily.

If you are still having difficulty, add a few pillows under your pelvis so that your head is lower than your pelvis. This inverted position is a larger modification that provides further access to your diaphragm.

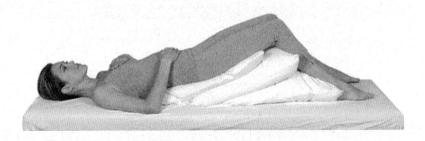

1. **Position your tongue properly.** Your tongue should be resting at the roof of your mouth with the tip of the tongue touching the back of the front upper teeth, and your mouth completely closed. This tongue position brings your jaw into the most ideal position and opens up the back of the airway so that you can sustain nasal breathing. When we speak, we breathe a little bit through our mouth, but generally we should breathe through the nose with the tongue in this neutral position.

    If you find yourself mouth breathing, it may be that your nose isn't working properly. Use the neti pot or saline nasal spray to keep your sinuses clean, clear, and moist. If you can't breathe through your nose with your mouth closed, then you may need to see an otolaryngologist, or ear/nose/throat specialist, known as an ENT.

2. **Pay attention to your breath, making it as soft and quiet as possible.** If you just close your eyes and think about making your breathing quiet, you may very well be able to change how you're breathing. The biggest misnomer is that many people think that they have to breathe deeply in order to breathe efficiently. For your everyday life, what we are really looking for is involuntary breathing through your diaphragm in a nice, rhythmical way that doesn't require deep breaths. Some people can concentrate on shifting their breathing more easily while wearing earplugs. Listen for the change as you employ the cues listed in this section.

3. **Gently breathe in through your nose and feel your lower ribs expand outward on your inhale and then come back down and in gently on your exhale.** Try to focus on your exhale and let yourself get to the very end of your exhale, pause for a moment, and allow the body's innate breathing reflex to take over for the next inhale. Some people don't feel the reflex but most do if they allow themselves to be more of an observer of their breath.

   The only way to truly know that you are breathing efficiently is to be hooked up to a capnometer, which produces a report in real time, similar to an EKG. If you practice these techniques, and they feel good, that is a sign that you are on the right track. Your body will adopt them, and slowly the efficient breathing reflex will be energized to do the work for you—we just need to get out of our own way and let the reflex do the work. If you are having difficulty with the exercise or experiencing symptoms, you may need to see a behavioral breathing analyst.

What Kind of Breather Are You?

Since many people have a breathing dysfunction that they've been carrying for years, symptoms may not be drastic, but when you correct the dysfunctional mechanics, you'll notice a huge difference in energy level, mood, and more. Refer to the chart below to see if you are breathing optimally.

Question	Your Response	Proper Breathing
Are you a mouth breather?		Breathe through your nose, with mouth closed and lips touching.
Where do you feel the position of your tongue?		Your tongue should be resting at the top of the mouth, with the tip of the tongue touching the inner side of the top front teeth.
Are you breathing from your chest or is your belly or ribs moving?		We should always be breathing from the diaphragm—the sides and back of the lower ribs and the belly will move. No neck breathing, chest breathing, or shoulder breathing. Your body should not be moving up and down.
Do you notice any breath holding?		You should never hold your breath; you should breathe regularly at a comfortable pace.
Can you hear your breathing? Is it loud?		Breathing should be quiet where no one notices it for low exertion tasks.
How's your posture?		Good posture—with a neutral spine, your head in line with your spine, and your chest open, shoulders floating up and back—also supports good breathing habits. (See posture section of First Trimester.)

Breathing: An Alkaline Response

One hot topic in Functional Medicine circles is the importance of following an alkaline diet. The most recent research shows that when an internal alkaline environment is maintained, the body is able to have better metabolism, an enhanced immune system, and the ability to boost its repair mechanisms so that you can function at your best. Dark, leafy greens and berries are often recommended to create "mineral buffering reserves" and maintain an alkaline state.

However, proper breathing is also a pH balancer: when you're breathing correctly, you're actually adjusting your acidity without needing to drastically change your diet. As Patricia's mentor and behavioral breathing analyst teacher Dr. Peter Litchfield says, the best way to balance your pH is to breathe efficiently. You are able to blow off excess lactic acid, restoring a more alkaline internal chemistry and lowering inflammation.

MOVEMENT

The most powerful anti-inflammatory drug is doing the right type of physical exercise. Lack of exercise, or leading a sedentary lifestyle, leads to inflammation. Engaging in an exercise routine can help you normalize glucose intolerance and reverse the earliest warning signs of diabetes. We also know that certain exercises, like aerobic exercises that get your heart pumping, help the brain and body to overcome depression, anxiety, and chronic stress.

Both men and women need to reevaluate their relationship with exercise during preconception in order to positively alter the genetic expression of the sperm and ova, increase fertility, as well as shed pounds and reduce stress. Researchers have shown that if a woman exercises before getting pregnant, genetic reprogramming can occur to reduce the risk of congenital heart disease and other cardiovascular outcomes in their offspring.[4]

However, exercise can be inflammatory if it is aggressive to the point where you can't breathe, feel extreme strain, or vomit. These are signs that the exercise is stressful on your system, and you are likely producing excessive cortisol, which leads to inflammation. This is particularly important for men to keep in mind during preconception. Men who currently exercise intensely—training for competitions like marathons, triathlons, tough mudders, ninja warriors, or intense boot camps—will need to lower their exertion to a more moderate level during preconception, and can resume intense exercise after conception. Women can continue moderate exercise exertion, or at the very least, start an exercise program. Moderate exercise is defined as achieving a 60 percent exertion, where you can still say a few words as you exercise.

The exercise program we recommend for women during preconception begins to strengthen some of the key stabilizing muscles of the body that will help you feel supported and maintain good posture as your belly grows. These exercises lay the foundation for connecting with the deep stabilizing muscles like *the transversus abdominis, lumbar multifidi, diaphragm, pelvic floor, gluteus medius,* and *serratus anterior.* By engaging these muscles now, you can begin to create muscle memory and have less chance for *diastasis*, the stretching of the central seam of the abdominal muscles.

Diastasis can happen during pregnancy and often leads to a bloated-belly look or a decreased ability to create supportive abdominal tension after childbirth. The *linea alba* (central seam of the abdominal muscles) stretches in all pregnant women, but for as much as 30 percent, the original tension is difficult to restore after pregnancy. We have found that women who usually exercise intensely have very tight abdominal muscles, or those on the other end of the spectrum who never exercise before pregnancy, are the most likely to experience diastasis. If you have a six-pack, or very tight abdominals, now is the time to limit abdominal shortening exercises (like crunches) and begin stabilizing the deeper abs with these exercises that always include proper breathing.

Try Mayan Abdominal Massage

We have included many tools to help bring functional tension back to the linea alba in the postpartum section of the book. However, if you have very tight abdominals, or previous abdominal surgery, including C-section, appendectomy, hernia surgery, or suffer from gastrointestinal issues or severe bloating, you may benefit from Mayan abdominal massage. This technique helps to guide the abdominal organs, like the uterus, bladder, and intestines, into their proper position so that their functions are supported and enhanced, which may improve fertility and relieve painful menstrual periods. It may also help the abdominal muscle tissues stretch appropriately to reduce the likelihood of diastasis. Abdominal massage also releases restrictions due to scars and improves the mobility of the abdominal muscles, fascia, and connective tissue.

Do not perform deep strokes over your lower abdomen during your period; during this time your organs are inflamed and may shift positions as they contract during menstrual flow. Instead, use smoothing, light strokes with warm hands that can be comforting, and deeper work on the upper abdomen is fine. If you have an IUD, do not perform deep work over your lower abdomen—just use smoothing, warm hands instead of deep penetrating strokes.

The following Mayan massage is based on Maya Abdominal Therapy®. It can take up to ten minutes to complete. First, empty your bladder. You can perform the massage through loose clothing, a sheet, or on bare skin with or without oil. Lie on your back with pillows under your head and knees—whatever is comfortable for you. Perform the strokes on the exhale. All circles are clockwise.

Upper Abdomen Sequence

Start with the upper abdomen in order to stretch the diaphragm. This is the area below the sternum down to the navel:

- **Find the solar plexus at the bottom of the sternum.** Using your first and second fingers of one hand, perform nine small clockwise circles about the size of a coin directly on your solar plexus. Use light pressure to stimulate the group of lymph nodes located there.
- **Cup your hands and bring the nail beds together to form an M for Maya.** Starting at the solar plexus, press at a comfortable depth with your fingertips and wrist, and move straight down to the navel, stroking slowly and firmly on an exhale. Perform three strokes, then move your hands to the right side of the solar plexus at the bottom of the ribs, and stroke diagonally to the navel, three times. Repeat on the left side three times. Repeat this sequence of nine strokes three times (total

twenty-seven), and then finish with an additional three strokes down the center, for a total of thirty strokes.

- **Return to the solar plexus.** You may feel a subtle, ropy line extending to the navel, which is what we're massaging, *the linea alba*. Using the fingers of one hand and applying comfortable pressure, gently and slowly massage along the line moving a half inch to either side with a zigzag stroke. Follow the line down to just above your navel. Perform this movement for a minimum of three times or up to nine times.

- **Working clockwise around the edge of the navel, perform small spirals with one finger.** Start at the top of the navel and draw tiny circles with your finger around the navel, applying light pressure. Repeat three times, concentrating on the areas around the navel that may be more tender.

- **With legs relaxed, reach down as far as you comfortably can.** Use your fingers to stroke the insides of your thighs with a light touch, moving from the tops of your thighs toward your belly, crossing the bikini line. This motion helps take excess lymphatic fluids out of the legs, moving it toward the pelvis. Perform nine strokes on each leg.

Lower Abdomen Sequence

The lower abdomen is the region from your navel to the pubic bone.

- Bring your hands together with index fingers touching, thumbs crossed on palms. Put your index fingers at the top of the pubic bone with them meeting in the middle. The palm of your hand is resting gently on the lower abdomen; fingertips are slightly curved and relaxed.

- Slowly slide your hands off the top of your pubic bone. Applying comfortable and consistent pressure into the soft tissue of the lower abdomen, on the exhale slowly move your hands up toward your navel, stopping halfway between the pubic bone and navel. Perform this short stroke three times.

- Move to your right side, find your hip bone, and sink your hands into the soft tissue. Stroke diagonally toward the center, stopping short of the center. Perform this stroke three times. Repeat on the left side three times.

- Repeat this sequence three times (total twenty-seven) and finish with an additional three strokes up the center, for a total of thirty strokes.
- To finish, use both hands flat on your abdomen, make a clockwise spiral lightly around the navel, moving outward into bigger and bigger spirals until you reach the bony borders of the abdominal cavity. Then, slowly spiral back toward your navel, finishing with both hands on the center of your abdomen.

Wise Women Are Spartan Women

Did you know that the Spartan women of ancient Greece trained to be warriors? They put a huge emphasis on being fit and strong. This was not only to protect themselves but to ensure that they would have strong and healthy babies!

Every time you exercise, think of these Spartan women. Even in ancient times, the wisdom of movement, exercise, and staying physically fit was a priority for women of childbearing years.

The Preconception Exercise Routine

Performing the preconception routine should take less than twenty minutes to complete, can be done every day at home, and requires minimal equipment. The aim of these exercises is to strengthen and stabilize your pelvic girdle muscles as well as the muscles in the core, diaphragm, and lower back. Many parts of the routine are considered *eccentric strengthening* exercises. The purpose is to strengthen the muscles when the muscle tissue is lengthening.

During eccentric strengthening, you will be focusing on the "negative" of the exercise. For example, if you were working your bicep, you bend your elbow. The bicep muscle shortens as you pull your hand toward your shoulder.

When you come out of the position, you extend the elbow, and the muscle elongates. By focusing on the second part of the exercise, you are firming the muscle as it elongates. These exercises will lengthen your trunk by working your muscles in this elongated fashion, turning on the stabilizing muscles that support your growing belly without compromising your posture or putting added pressure on your hips, knees, and ankles.

However, none of these exercises will feel like a bicep curl, where you work the muscle, it gets tired, and then you stop. The goal is to engage with these muscles so that you're actually firing them up and keeping them sharp and primed for daily activities. In this routine, you are simply getting comfortable with recruiting them. We're going to be using visuals and cues to try to get you to do these subtle contractions well. Be patient when you do these exercises because they are not as simple as they may seem. You are not going to be working up a sweat, but you will feel that you are connecting with these deep muscles, possibly for the first time.

Once you've completed the routine, continue to exercise for at least thirty minutes a day, every day, doing whatever type of exercise you love to do. This can be taking a class at the gym, taking a walk in nature, weight training, or some combination of exercises. Choosing an activity because you "have to" is not helpful because you won't stick with the program and will lose out on the opportunity to positively affect your germ cells.

If you have not exercised before, consult with your physician to make sure you do not have any health concerns that would interfere with an exercise program. Once you are cleared, the key is starting off slow. You can walk outdoors, indoors, or on a treadmill. Walking in nature has a multitude of stress-relieving benefits. For instance, Dr. Zach Bush teaches that we receive positive microbes from nature from breathing clean, fresh air, which makes for a more diverse microbiome, ultimately improving mood and lowering inflammation.

Start with continuously walking for at least twenty minutes on Day 1. Keep up a pace where you can comfortably speak, and walk as fast as you can. By day three or five, increase to thirty minutes a day. By day eight or ten, you can ramp up your pace to where it's more difficult to talk. You can break this walk up into two fifteen-minute sessions, and feel free to walk longer if you are comfortable and enjoying the activity.

We have found that people receive the most health benefits when they exercise after work, or later in the afternoon. This is because it is the time of day most closely linked to your natural circadian rhythm, when your body has the most energy to put toward exercise.

Exercise Equipment You'll Need:

- Firm chair
- Pillow
- Tennis ball
- Yoga mat or large towel

Exercise : Transversus Abdominis Activation and Marching

EQUIPMENT: Towel or yoga mat.

PURPOSE: To isolate a contraction of the deepest abdominal muscle, the transversus abdominis (TrA) muscle. This muscle acts like a corset around the tummy and lower back and protects the spine when you lift, bend, and push. As the belly grows, you want this muscle active as it provides good abdominal and back support. This is a very deep muscle, and it's supposed to be working involuntarily in conjunction with your diaphragm. You're only supposed to feel like you are giving 20 percent effort during the exercise.

START POSITION: Place a towel or yoga mat on the floor and lie down on your back with knees bent, with or without a pillow under your head. Place your fingers on your lower abdomen just inside the prominent bones of the pelvis. If lying on your back is uncomfortable, try a modification in an alternate position: lying on stomach, lying on side, on hands and knees, sitting, or standing; do whatever works best for you. Then, choose *one* of these cues below for isolating the TrA:

1. Draw the area above your pubic bone toward your spine.
2. Imagine bringing your hip bones together or apart.
3. Lift the pelvic floor (imagine that you are stopping the flow of urine, lifting the vagina, or drawing your pubic bone to your coccyx, or tailbone).
4. Count out loud (slurring numbers continuously) as you exhale. This activates the TrA involuntarily.
5. Breathe in and hold the rib cage up, exhale half the air out while drawing the lower belly in and up.

SEQUENCE:

STEP 1. Breathe in and out, activating the diaphragm (the belly should rise on inhalation and fall on exhalation) as outlined in the breathing section.

STEP 2. Using a cue from above that best isolates your TrA, create a TrA contraction on your exhale. Use your fingers to feel the deep, subtle tension as you slowly maintain the cue while breathing. There should be no movement or tilting of the pelvis, and you should be relaxed without bracing any of the abdominal muscles. You should not be feeling any sort of quick contraction or outward bulging pressure. Engage this muscle and keep the cue going for 10 seconds as you inhale and exhale.

STEP 3. Rest and repeat 5 times.

STEP 4. Engage your TrA cue again on your exhale, maintain that contraction, and slowly lift and lower one knee toward your chest, followed by the other. Keep breathing the whole time and keep the cue engaged throughout. Make sure your pelvis stays level and doesn't tip as the leg lifts and that your low back doesn't lift up as you lower the leg. Your lower back and pelvis should remain neutral.

STEP 5. Rest, reset, and repeat for a total of 10 sets.

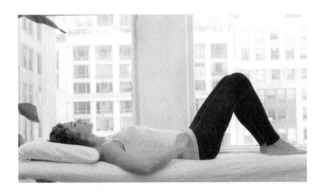

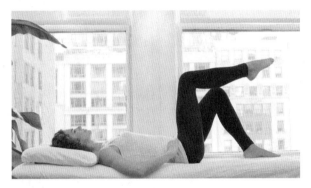

Exercise: Transversus Abdominis Toe Taps and Knee Extensions

EQUIPMENT: Towel or yoga mat.

PURPOSE: To challenge the transversus abdominis (TrA) muscle for improved core support.

START POSITION: Place a towel or yoga mat on the floor and lie on top of it on your back with knees bent, with or without a pillow under your head.

SEQUENCE:

STEP 1. Engage your TrA as you did with Exercise #1 on your exhale. Maintain that contraction and slowly lift one knee up toward your chest. Keeping your knee lifted, lift the other knee toward your chest. This position is referred to as the 90–90 position.

STEP 2. Make sure your lower back doesn't lift off the ground and that your pelvis stays level and still. Exhale and lower one foot toward the floor, and tap your toes on the floor. Inhale and return the leg to the 90–90 position. Repeat with the other foot, coordinating the breath each time. Perform 10 reps on each leg. Take a 2 to 3 breath break before the next step.

STEP 3. To challenge yourself further: maintaining the 90–90 position, inhale and extend one knee out at roughly a 45-degree angle. The higher you lift the leg, the easier it will be on your abdominals and the lower you extend it, the harder it will be. Bring your leg back to starting position on your inhale. Extend the opposite knee on the exhale, then inhale and bring it back in. Make sure your pelvis stays level and that your low back doesn't lift up off the towel/ mat as your leg extends. Your lower back and pelvis should remain neutral the whole time.

STEP 4. Rest, then repeat for a total of ten reps (one rep is extending both sides once). You can do 1 to 2 sets of this, as tolerated. If the 90–90/tabletop position doesn't feel supported or you have pain, try doing each leg movement with the opposite foot still on the floor (see final photo).

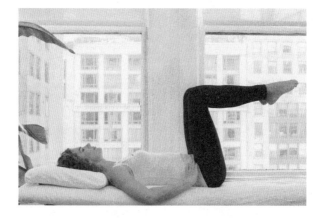

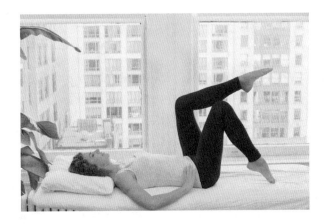

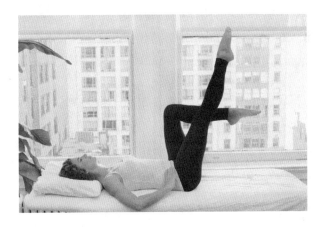

Modification

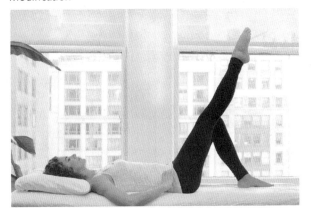

Exercise: Kegels with Resting Squats

PURPOSE: To engage and strengthen the pelvic floor to help support the pelvis, abdomen, and diaphragm. Rising from the resting squat allows for an involuntary contraction of the pelvic floor to keep it strong.

START POSITION: Stand with your feet shoulder width apart and feet pointing straight ahead or slightly toed out.

SEQUENCE:

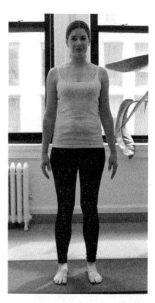

STEP 1. Inhale, draw your pelvic floor muscles up, imagining all four points of the pelvic floor (from pubic bone to tailbone, and from sitz bone across to other sitz bone) ascending up the center into the abdomen. Gently draw your pelvic floor muscles up as if they were traveling 3 to 5 floors of an elevator without gripping in your hip or buttocks muscles. Hold the contraction for 3 breaths (gentle inhales and exhales) and release slowly. Repeat this 10 times.

STEP 2. Inhale, slowly bend your knees, and lower your pelvis close to the ground, allowing your back to relax. Hold the squat position for 5 seconds and then press into feet firmly as you exhale and rise up. Repeat this 5 times.

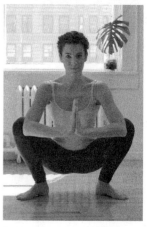

Modification for Step 2. If you are having difficulty, hold onto something sturdy for balance (like a locked doorknob). You can widen your feet farther apart or toe out a little more as needed, as long as your knees are in line with your second toes.

Exercise: Airplane

EQUIPMENT: A heavy chair or countertop that you can hold onto (optional).

PURPOSE: To strengthen the glute muscles that stabilize the hips and pelvis.

START POSITION: Stand with your feet hip width apart.

SEQUENCE:

STEP 1. Hold onto the back of the chair or a countertop, transfer your weight to your left leg with a soft knee, and let the right leg float up behind you. Your body will tip forward slightly; maintain a neutral spine alignment where the midback and low back are straight, not rounded.

STEP 2. While keeping your left knee slightly bent so that the center of your knee is aligned with your second toe, exhale and gently rotate your pelvis so it faces to the right, utilizing the deep muscles of the side of the left hip (the side of your buttocks, the *gluteus medius* muscle). You should feel these muscles at the side of the hip working to support the whole movement. Keep breathing naturally throughout.

STEP 3. Keep the tempo slow and repeat 10 to 15 times on each leg, or until fatigued.

Modification: Once you get the hang of this exercise, you can let go of the chair and extend your arms out, shoulder height, for balance.

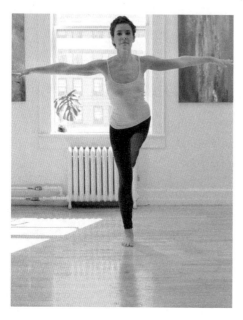 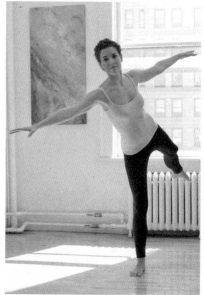

Exercise: Glute Bridges

PURPOSE: To support the hips and pelvis by strengthening the buttocks, or gluteal muscles.

START POSITION: Lie down on your back with your feet on the floor and knees bent. You may use a pillow for your head. Your arms should be at your side with your palms down.

SEQUENCE:

STEP 1. As you exhale, press your heels firmly into the ground, and with your toes on the ground, raise your pelvis off the floor as high as comfortable, anywhere from 2 to 8 inches, keeping low back relaxed. Breathe normally and hold this position for 5 to 10 seconds, then lower.

STEP 2. Repeat 10 to 15 times, 1 to 2 sets.

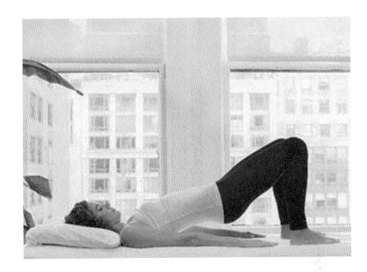

Progression #1: If this exercise is not challenging, in Step 2 lift one heel off the floor while keeping toes on the floor as the pelvis remains level and the spine is still neutral. Hold for 3 to 5 seconds, then lower. Repeat with the other leg. Lower the pelvis and rest. Repeat 10 to 15 times, 1–2 sets.

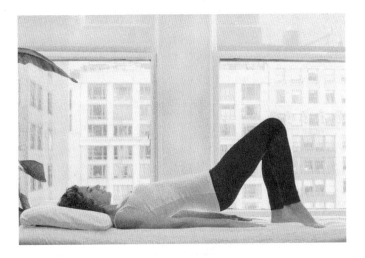

Progression #2: For an even greater challenge, lift the whole foot off the floor while the pelvis remains level and your spine is still and elongated. Hold 3 to 5 seconds, then lower. Repeat with the other leg. Lower the pelvis and rest. Repeat 10 to 15 times, 1 to 2 sets.

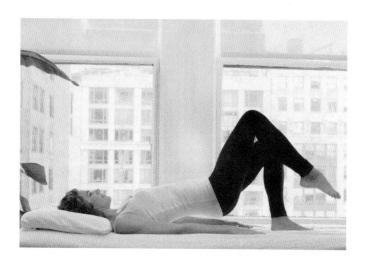

Exercise: Deep Neck Flexors

PURPOSE: Strengthen the muscles that elongate and support the neck. This exercise keeps your head and neck aligned with your spine, decreasing the chances of developing a "dowager's hump" after pregnancy. This rounded posture often happens in the third trimester or postpartum, due to excess girth of the belly and breastfeeding, which pulls on the base of the neck, creating a hump if you aren't strong enough to support a neutral neck posture.

START POSITION: Lie on your stomach in bed, with your head hanging off the edge of the bed. You can use a pillow under your belly for extra spinal support. Your body should be fully supported, and resting on the bed, through your shoulders.

SEQUENCE:

STEP 1. Relax your neck, inhale, and gently bring your head in-line with the rest of your spine, lifting it up and back, while keeping your chin tucked in to your chest. Your ear will line up with your shoulder, but your chin remains tucked in. Your low back should be relaxed. You may feel some work in your upper back or diffusely across the neck.

Hold this position for 10 to 20 seconds while continuously breathing.

STEP 2. Relax the head down.

STEP 3. Repeat 3 to 5 times.

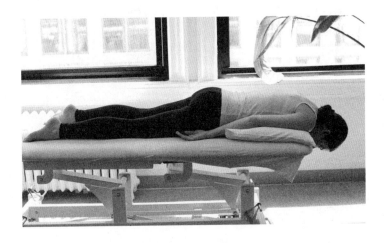

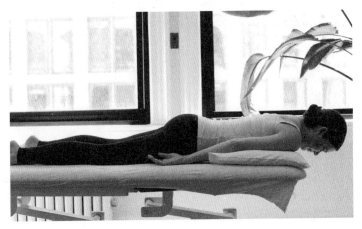

Exercise: Downward Dog Piked Pushup

EQUIPMENT: Towel or yoga mat.

PURPOSE: Strengthen the serratus anterior muscle to support your shoulders and upper body. It also lengthens the muscles of the lower body and opens up the diaphragm to improve its functionality with breathing.

START POSITION: Gently bring your hands and knees onto the floor, towel, or mat. Extend both elbows and knees in a comfortable range without locking them, and go into an inverted "V" position. Keep your hands under your shoulders or slightly narrower. Your inner elbows should face each other. Your heels will be lifted depending on how flexible your calves and legs are.

SEQUENCE:

STEP 1. Keep your neck relaxed, exhale, and gently let your body weight fall through your shoulder blades. The blades will come together, and the body will be a little more forward than the starting position.

STEP 2. Press through the heels of your hands, inhale, and lift your body weight off your shoulder blades, allowing for the shoulder blades to separate. Your body will move slightly up and back. Elbows stay relatively straight and still, as does your lower body. Do not round in your midback; try to isolate the movement to just your shoulder blades.

STEP 3. Repeat 10 times, slow, 1 to 2 sets.

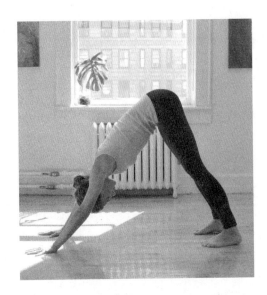

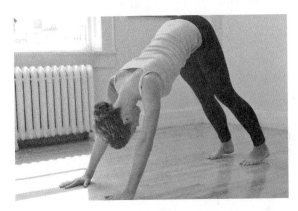

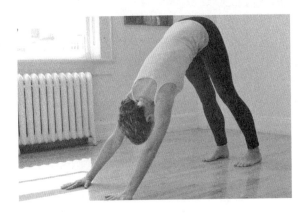

Exercise: Foot Doming

EQUIPMENT: A firm chair.

PURPOSE: To strengthen the arches of the feet. The arches tend to flatten during pregnancy primarily because the deep muscles of the feet are not strong enough to support the change in body mass/position. If the arches flatten a decent amount, your foot will "grow" as you will not be able to maintain an arch that shortens the foot.

START POSITION: Sit down at the edge of a chair with both feet flat on the floor pointing straight ahead.

SEQUENCE:

STEP 1. Pull one arch up from the floor, keeping your toes straight and firm, and heel still. The tiny movement will feel like you are sucking your arch away from the floor. You are activating the deep muscles of the foot with this small motion.

STEP 2. Hold the "dome" position and breathe normally for 5 seconds. Try to keep your thigh and hip muscles relaxed, keeping your focus on the small, deep muscles of the foot/arch. Perform 10–15 repetitions on each foot, 1–2 sets.

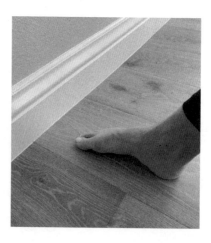

Agnes Created Lasting Habits During Preconception

Agnes came to see Patricia because she was worried about getting pregnant and being able to deliver a baby vaginally. She had been diagnosed with hip dysplasia (a malformation of the hip socket) as a child and always had a feeling of tightness and limited mobility in her hips, with more pain in her right side than the left. She was planning to start trying to get pregnant in a few months and wanted to improve her range of motion and reduce her pain before pregnancy.

Patricia showed Agnes how to work on her hip muscles with the Airplane sequence, which helped her increase her hip stability and support, and increased the mobility in her hips. She learned to strengthen her pelvic floor with Kegels and connect with her abdominal muscles with TrA Marching to support her core. She also worked on improving her breathing so that she could practice it during these exercises and throughout her day.

As they addressed Agnes's needs, she was able to let go of her anxiety about getting pregnant. Once she understood the importance of the preconception period, Agnes decided to put off conceiving until she and her husband could clean up their environment. Soon after the preconception period was over, Agnes called to let Patricia know that she was pregnant and still mobile and pain free.

NOURISHMENT

The goal during preconception is for men and women to completely clean up their diet and lose weight, if necessary. According to a 2018 study published in *The Lancet*, a child's health can be compromised by the weight and diet of both parents before conception: obesity in one or both parents increases a child's chance of having a heart attack, stroke, immune disease, and diabetes later in life.[5]

Further, maintaining high levels of the stress hormone cortisol causes us to hold on to belly fat. The more belly fat you have, the more inflammation you have. Lowering stress, balancing the microbiome, removing toxins, and exercising are all effective strategies to lower inflammation and lose weight. By combining these activities with following an anti-inflammatory diet, you and your partner are completing a comprehensive preconception program.

Reduce Inflammatory Grains and Gluten

The foods we choose have an important role in affecting inflammation. We suggest that during preconception you and your partner follow a limited grain diet, with the goal being a reduction or elimination of gluten-containing grains like wheat, rye, and barley. Gluten is generally a very inflammatory food for most people. Inflammatory foods, like gluten and grains, can increase the chances for developing intestinal permeability, leading to increased food sensitivities and immune activation. We also advise avoiding processed foods with added sugars. Limiting grains, processed foods, and added sugars is the best anti-inflammatory approach that helps to optimize the gut's microbiome and improves sugar and insulin balance. These basic guidelines will stay in place throughout preconception and into pregnancy and postpartum stages, with specific modifications made along the way.

Focus on Fresh, Organic, One-Ingredient Foods

While it's important to pay attention to the foods you need to avoid, it's more important—and enjoyable—to focus on the delicious foods you can add into your diet. Choose fresh, whole foods that are organic, wild caught, and locally grown in season. The organic designation is important: conventionally grown and raised foods are often genetically modified, which poses a health risk. Genetically modified organisms (GMOs) are designed to help the genetically modified plants withstand pesticide spraying. This means that often GMOs have high levels of pesticide exposure contained in the food itself. In the years since GMOs first made their way into the marketplace, it's become harder and harder to know where they are hiding—in fact, 70 percent or more of the foods you'll find in the grocery store are made with GMO ingredients. Labeling laws do not currently require disclosure of these ingredients, so it's important to choose organic produce whenever possible. Animal proteins should be lean and organic; then look for grass-fed meats and free-range poultry and eggs.

You can have plenty of low-mercury wild fish and seafood. You can also have dairy products if you aren't allergic/sensitive, or choose nondairy sources. Each day, add lots of bright-colored fresh fruits and vegetables to your plate, aiming for seven to twelve servings a day. You may also include beans, seeds, nuts, and legumes (unless you have medical issues or allergies that require avoidance). Lastly, gradually lower your caffeine intake. You shouldn't have too much caffeine when you are pregnant or breastfeeding: one cup of a caffeinated beverage a day is acceptable. Switching to green tea or matcha instead of coffee during preconception will make this transition even easier.

Focus on Foods That Naturally Lower Inflammation

Make sure to include at least one anti-inflammatory food in every meal:

Vegetables

+ Bok choy
+ Broccoli
+ Brussel sprouts
+ Cabbage
+ Cauliflower
+ Collard greens
+ Fennel
+ Garlic
+ Kale
+ Onions
+ Spinach
+ Sweet potatoes
+ Turnip greens

Fruits

+ Apples
+ Avocados
+ Blackcurrants
+ Blueberries
+ Cherries
+ Cranberries
+ Kiwi
+ Grapefruit
+ Lemon
+ Lime
+ Papaya
+ Pineapple
+ Pomegranate
+ Strawberries

Gluten-Free Grains

Look for gluten-free breads made with these ingredients, or prepare them yourself as part of a meal:

+ Buckwheat
+ Oats
+ Rice (organic, grown in U.S. is preferred)
+ Quinoa (although it looks and acts like a grain, quinoa is actually a sprout that contains a healthy dose of protein)

Fish

Smaller-sized fish that are low in mercury are ideal choices.

- Anchovies
- Halibut
- Herring
- North Atlantic mackerel
- Pollock
- Rainbow trout
- Sardines
- Wild Alaska salmon

Nuts, Seeds, and Oils

- Monounsaturated fats such as avocado and olive oil are the best choices for cooking.
- Almonds
- Brazil nuts
- Coconut oil
- Extra-virgin olive oil
- Flaxseed
- Hazelnuts
- Sesame oil
- Sunflower seeds

Spices and Herbs

- Basil
- Cayenne/Chili peppers
- Cinnamon
- Cocoa (at least 70 percent)
- Ginger
- Mint
- Oregano
- Parsley
- Rosemary
- Thyme
- Turmeric/curcumin

Best Anti-Inflammatory Bets

Broccoli sprouts, sea vegetables (seaweed), and dark leafy greens (spinach, mustard greens, dandelion greens, kale) are all powerful anti-inflammatory foods that are also very efficient detoxifiers. Eat these as often as possible, at least once a week.

Inflammatory Foods

Avoid the following inflammatory foods

- Breakfast bars
- Fruit juices
- Processed flour products, like cookies, pastries, and chips
- Sweetened teas, soda
- White bread
- White rice
- White sugar

Follow a Seed-Cycling Protocol

Seeds are good sources of essential fatty acids and can provide a simple and natural way to balance hormones. These seeds support the creation of estrogen and progesterone and support a healthy menstrual cycle. If your cycle is irregular, adding pumpkin seeds, sunflower seeds, flax seeds,[6] and chia seeds to meals every day may help to keep your menstrual cycle regular and robust and provide some of the nutrients needed to optimize fertility.

Following your next period, begin a seed protocol that will last throughout preconception. Every two weeks you will be changing your choice of seeds. For the first fourteen days of the month, you can add up to one quarter cup of ground flax seeds, or a tablespoon of chia seeds, which you can add to salads, gluten-free steel-cut oatmeal, or yogurt each day. For the last two weeks of the month, use up to one quarter cup of pumpkin or sunflower seeds, which can be eaten by the handful or added whole to foods and smoothies.

Supplements to Consider

There are specific micronutrients you and your partner need to supplement during preconception:

- **CoQ10.** This powerful antioxidant has been shown to improve egg and sperm quality and pregnancy rates in women over thirty-five. CoQ10 supports energy production in the mitochondria. Egg quality is dependent on having enough energy to build a healthy mature egg and sperm.

- **DHEA.** DHEA is an adrenal hormone that acts as a precursor to testosterone and estrogen. Recent studies show that DHEA can help a woman's eggs grow and develop. DHEA used in higher doses has been used in ART (assisted reproductive technology) to treat decreased ovarian reserve and premature ovarian failure.

- **Glutathione.** This helps protect the eggs from damage throughout the developmental process. Eggs with greater levels of glutathione have been shown to produce healthier, stronger embryos.

- **Inositol.** Inositol reduces anxiety/depression, improves insulin balance, and boosts fertility.

- **L-arginine.** This is an amino acid that may help improve pregnancy rates by improving blood circulation to the uterus and ovaries. This improves the implantation site for a fertilized egg.

- **L-carnitine.** Men with low sperm counts and women undergoing in-vitro fertilization can supplement with L-carnitine; we have seen fertility rates increase by 25 percent by taking L-carnitine for a minimum of six months.

- **Maca.** Maca's effect on fertility is perhaps its most documented health property. Many studies have confirmed that couples who regularly consume tablets or powder made from maca have increased chances of conception by increasing sperm count in men,[7] and increased fertility in women when taken with methylated folate (see below).[8]

- **Magnesium.** Stress depletes magnesium, which we need in order to relax. Magnesium also helps digestion.

- **Methylated folate.** A more absorbable form of folic acid, this is preferable to folic acid, which may not be bioavailable to those with methylation issues. Almost half the population has genetic variants that don't allow the use of folic acid, the synthetic version of folate. If you are one of these people, then folic acid will actually block your ability to use folate itself.

- **Myo-inositol.** An essential B vitamin that has been shown to improve egg quality in women with PCOS (polycystic ovarian syndrome). Clinical studies have demonstrated that inositol can restore normal ovulation, and improve egg quality and fertilization rates in women with ovulatory dysfunction. In addition, inositol also reduces anxiety/depression and improves insulin balance.

- **N-acetyl cysteine (NAC).** This helps to increase glutathione, the master liver detoxifier. NAC can help women with ovulation disorders and can prevent damage to the end of the egg's DNA.

- **Omega-3 fatty acids.** These have been shown to regulate hormones and help fertility. They help reduce inflammation and promote ovulation and implantation.

- **Prenatal vitamins.** Look for a prenatal vitamin with zinc, selenium, iodine, iron, bioavailable folate, and fat soluble vitamins. While prenatal vitamins can correct important nutrient deficiencies, it is not sufficient on its own to fundamentally improve the baby's health. Some other options to consider mentioning: treatment of nausea and vomiting of pregnancy begins with prevention. Two studies found that women who were taking a multivitamin at the time of fertilization were less likely to need medical attention for vomiting.[9]

- **Probiotics.** A broad-range probiotic can help balance the microbes in your gut. They can help increase the healthy gut bacteria, improve digestion to increase nutrient absorption, and strengthen the immune system. Klaire Labs Therbiotic Complete is a great one. If you are prone to yeast infections, take probiotics plus a yeast supplement like *saccaromyces boulardii.*

- **Tumeric (curcumin).** This decreases inflammation.

◆ **Vitamin B6.** Studies show that individuals with the highest vitamin B6 intake had the lowest levels of inflammation.

◆ **Vitamin C.** Vitamin C lowers inflammation and boosts the immune system.

Or look for a very high-quality multivitamin that contains these nutrients and pair it with an Omega-3 supplement like Nordic Naturals. Willner Chemists, Metagenics, Thorne Research, and Standard Process are good quality choices for a multivitamin.

Supplementing for Dietary Restrictions

If you or your partner follow a restricted diet, it's very possible that you are not getting all the vitamins needed to support good health from the foods you eat. The blood work we discussed earlier in the chapter can show nutrient deficiencies, which can be made up through proper supplementation.

Vegan/vegetarian: You may need to supplement for a lack of protein with B vitamins, especially B12, iron, and zinc. Omega-3s are necessary if you are not eating fish, and vitamins A and D if you limit or avoid dairy products.

Keto: High-protein diets like keto may require that you supplement with a prebiotic blend or powder as well as both soluble and insoluble fiber, as you are limiting carbohydrates. One of the dangers with following a keto diet is that you're not getting a ton of vegetables and fruits, so you may be low on antioxidants, B vitamins, vitamin A, and vitamin C.

Conception

Preconception is also the ideal time to start thinking about providing the optimal environment for conception. As you are cleansing your body of stress and toxins, eating nourishing foods, improving your breathing, and exercising daily, one added bonus is that you're priming your body to align with its natural circadian rhythm. Every cell in our body operates on its own clock, and by orchestrating their timing, you are allowing each of your organs to work at their highest potential. This is important because a healthy circadian rhythm can influence the quality of your germ cells and enhance your ability to conceive.

One of the ways we can best restore proper circadian rhythm is by getting good sleep at night and using the daytime to accomplish our tasks, like work and exercise. For example we know that women who are night shift workers, who live in opposition to their circadian clock, have a harder time conceiving.

Great Things Take Time

Getting to pregnancy is a journey. Your idea of when it will occur may not be aligned with when it will *actually* occur. Great things take time: focus on yourself and know that the timing will be perfect. Trust that your body is intelligent, your body knows when the best time for conception will be, and you may even be pleasantly surprised at what comes your way when your baby is born.

Getting Off Birth Control

Whether you started using birth control for contraceptive or medical reasons, they have provided a very effective method of regulating your hormonal output. However, its very effectiveness means that you have a limited idea about your reproductive capability, since the pill completely suppresses your body's innate hormone mechanism. What's more, birth control pills contain high doses of hormones that have been taxing your liver.

In order to figure out what your inherent hormone situation is, we recommend that you take yourself off of the birth control pill for at least three or four months before conceiving. This will also help your body start flushing out the unique toxicity of the pill itself and allows your liver to better address other toxins that it might not have been able to handle while you were on a daily high dose hormone medication. What's more, by reestablishing your own menstrual cycle, you can time conception appropriately or determine if there is anything you need to address if your cycles are erratic or irregular.

If you have an IUD, talk to your doctor about removing it. There are two different types of IUDs, and each requires a different timing. The copper IUD doesn't impact your hormone production. However, it does create an inflammatory process in the lining of your uterus; that's actually one of the ways that it prevents pregnancy. The IUD creates a hostile environment against sperm by creating inflammation. Removing a copper IUD at least three months before you plan on conceiving will allow your uterine lining to shed a few times and reduce the amount of inflammation that it was exposed to with the device.

The second type of IUD is one that is coated with progesterone. This creates an environment that is not at all hospitable to accepting a fertilized egg for implantation. Because of the hormonal component, it may take longer for you to return to your normal cycle, by as much as six to twelve months. If you are using a progesterone-coated IUD and you're still getting periods, then you don't have to worry that your cycle's not returning. If you're in the group of not getting a period with these IUDs, remove it at the beginning of preconception to give your body a little more time to start cycling on its own.

Other popular birth control options include hormone-containing silicone rings that fit inside the vagina, like the NuvaRing. There are patches like Ortho Evra and subdermal hormone implants. Any of these can cause a delay in the return of your natural menstrual cycle. Give your body at least three to six months to reset by removing these early during preconception.

Conception Traditions

In the Sephardic Jewish tradition, men and women are taught not to drink alcohol before conceiving.

In Norway, women in the preconception period often "borrow a baby": taking care of a friend's baby for a day. This is thought to prepare the woman to open her heart and mind for her future baby.

Aligning Conception with Your Natural Cycle

The best advice for conception is to have sex a day or two before you ovulate. Conception is most likely to occur within the first seven days of your menstrual cycle, up to the day of ovulation, with the highest likelihood happening twenty-four to forty-eight hours prior to ovulation.

What does this mean for you and your partner? First, you need to know when you are ovulating. Preconception is an ideal time to try using an app or an ovulation predictor to help chart your cycle. However, when you're ready to conceive, take the app off your phone: just monitoring it can be stressful. Instead, have sex frequently—every other day after your period and for a week or two—and you don't have to worry about your timing.

Then, you need to make sure that you and your partner are not exposed to stressful events during that time so that you don't create an opportunity for increased cortisol, which can affect both germs cells and the timing of ovulation. Changes in cortisol can impact timing of ovulation.

Last, but not least, be quiet afterward; the rest of the day needs to be spent in a relaxing way. The period of time immediately following conception—the first two hours—is the most sensitive time to environmental behaviors. Couples should plan those days to be as stress-free and relaxing as possible. You're not supposed to conceive and then run off to a heavy day of meetings. If you think about how people have evolved, we used to live in tribes, and often multiple people shared the same home or shelter. We can imagine that when early couples engaged in sexual activity, they remained very quiet so they wouldn't call attention to themselves. Biologically, the benefits of orgasm increase when you remain quiet, calm, and peaceful following intercourse.

Painful Intercourse?

Consensual sex should be pleasurable. If you have recurrent pain during intercourse, you may have a pelvic floor dysfunction. Millions of women suffer from this, and the good news is that can be fixed. Typical symptoms include painful intercourse, urinary urgency, frequent constipation, or pain around the anus or vaginal region.

A certified pelvic floor physical therapist will be able to help you restore balance to your pelvic floor and surrounding tissues to restore sexual pleasure and resolve the associated symptoms. By addressing pelvic floor dysfunction now, not only will you be able to amplify conception and make it more enjoyable, you will feel better throughout your pregnancy, delivery, and postpartum recovery.

Consider Feng Shui

Feng shui is a traditional practice dating back over 4,000 years. It optimizes energy flow to harmonize individuals with their environment. The Chinese term *feng shui* literally translates as "wind-water" in English. Although it is most commonly identified with ancient China, it actually originated in a combination of places: aspects of it come from India as well as other parts of Asia, including Tibet.

According to feng shui expert and author Andie SantoPietro, modern-day feng shui way is based on many of the same principles as acupuncture. Just as an acupuncturist follows the body's meridian lines and looks for blockages, in feng shui, the same meridians that run through the physical body also run through your home or office. Instead of needles, feng shui specialists like Andie use crystals, wind chimes, mirrors, and plants to help activate, slow down, or augment the feel of *chi*—or energy—flow that moves through the surrounding environment and in turn, affects all the individuals who live or work there. Andie practices a particular form of feng shui that comes from Tibetan tantric Buddhism (founded by the late Grand Master Prof. Thomas Lin Yun Rinpoche). She shared the following tips so that you can give your home a quick feng shui makeover before you try to conceive. She's used these techniques with her clients who were having difficulty getting pregnant, and once she assessed and reorganized the chi flow in their homes, many were able to conceive.

◆ Check all your doors to make sure they fully open, are completely unobstructed, and are not being used as a hanger for your clothes. Doors should open and close freely because doors are where the energy comes into the home, and the energy flow is going to be a determining factor in your life circumstances and the quality of your pregnancy.

◆ The quality of energy in your bedroom, or the room you are planning to conceive in, is key. Ask yourself these questions: *Do I like this bedroom? Does it nurture me? Am I excited to jump into bed at night? Do I like the feeling of the mattress?* The curtains, rugs, and general décor don't have to be fancy; they just have to be pleasing to you.

◆ Make sure the colors in your bedroom are aligned with a *yin* energy, or a nocturnal energy state. Your bedroom should be calming and relaxing: choose soft, pastel colors and subdued patterns, especially with the covers or sheets that you are putting over your body at night. In terms of feng shui, there are only two things we should be doing in the bedroom: sleeping and lovemaking. Not reading, not watching TV, not looking at our phones.

◆ Keep your home neat and free of clutter. In the bedroom, keep the nightstands organized and the area under the bed clear.

WISDOM

All of the suggestions we've discussed in this chapter are meant to amplify your wellness and that of your partner. Our goal is to help you achieve a life in balance. You may not be perfect in every category right now, and we don't expect you to be. However, as you address each of these areas to the best of your ability, you will naturally come into balance and achieve wellness.

The best way to keep track of your progress is with a journal. Besides making notes on the foods you've been enjoying, or how certain supplements make you feel, record how you are getting closer to balance in every area. Write down exactly how you want to feel and what you're going to do to make the changes you need so that you can achieve this wonderful goal. You might need to make some significant changes to your lifestyle. Maybe you're already exercising, but you're not doing so great on the stress-relieving activities. Or maybe you aren't eating as cleanly as you should be. Keeping yourself accountable is the best way to create long-term habits.

Then, we encourage you to set your intentions about becoming pregnant in your journal. But be very clear on your vision, including every detail of all the wonderful things that are going to come. Focus on what you want your pregnancy to look like, and how you want to feel. When you write it out, you can plan for it, and make it happen. Remember, you are a wise woman, and a wise woman would align everything in her life so that the outcome she desires will occur. The universe will align with your desires because you've set that intention.

And because every cell in your being is going to work in favor of that intention, you can rest easy. We are helping you to have all the tools you need to have a wonderful pregnancy ahead of you, but you need to set that intention and remind yourself of what you want every single day.

You don't want—or need—to spend your time in preconception worrying. You don't have to compare yourself to that one friend who got pregnant on her first try, or someone who looked fantastic and glowing her whole pregnancy. You don't have to dwell on bad news that a friend or family member has told you that would make you nervous. Instead, find the balance. Think about how much everything around you will change, and then focus on being present in each of the stages of change and helping each stage build on the next, so that your life just keeps getting better. Because it will.

Matrescence is the birth of a mother. It's a relatively new term and a new way to talk about the upcoming and ongoing transitions of body and mind women face during pregnancy. The truth is, you will be going through a lot of transitions. We're here specifically to prepare you for these changes, so that you can take on matrescence as a wise woman. We want you to be calm and excited, not frantic and worried. Because matrescence is a long haul, in many ways, it's the rest of your life. Once you're pregnant, you're always going to be a mother.

The best advice we can share, as mothers, is to continue to focus on regaining a sense of balance. When you know what you need to be healthy inside and out, and when you get to know yourself better and understand what resonates for you, then you're able to maintain balance no matter what happens.

A Matrescence Meditative Prayer

By Agapi Stassinopoulos, bestselling author, international speaker, and Thrive Global Facilitator.

Dear Beloved,

For this gift of bearing life in me and preparing my womb and body in giving birth, I ask that the blessing of this miracle of life bless every part of my body and the life that is forming in me.

I ask that any thoughts that are out of fear, anxiety, or worry be transmuted into the trust and acceptance of what is to be; and I ask that I may be moved into the deepest, calmest place in my heart to allow this child to grow and flourish in my womb.

I see it filled with health and with a radiant light that helps it grow in perfection, and I flood my womb and my body with so much love, awe, respect, and reverence for that which is happening is so beyond me.

I let the joy of the prospect of becoming a mother fill my whole being.

I ask that any support that can come my way — whether it is from friends, family, information that I need to know as I am preparing to become a mother —I ask that I'm open to receive it.

Most of all, I ask to listen inside to the soul of this child and what it needs every day. I ask, and I receive, and I allow moments of stillness and presence to know that beyond this body that's being formed in my womb, the soul is waiting patiently to enter the body and come into this earth. May I know this soul, and may I connect with it and listen to its presence, and may it become a love affair that will materialize and develop as this child is born.

Give me patience, give me understanding, give me respect and love for myself for what my body and self are going through in this transformation. Let my tenderness for myself be equal to the tenderness that I have for this child that's being created right now, and let this tenderness lead my way to its birth, and then on.

Although I cannot predict what this journey will be about as this child is born, let me delight in the unknown and surprise of each day, watching the miracle of life in the form of this child become a human being.

I ask for your blessing, and any spiritual support on any level that can come and assist me on all new levels and own progressions that I'm open to receive.

I am so grateful. I am so thankful. I am filled with thankfulness, gratitude, peace, and bliss for this gift of life.

Amen!

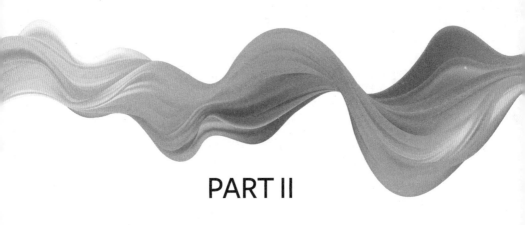

PART II

The First Trimester: Three Months of New Beginnings

Congratulations, you're pregnant! It's an exciting time, and we want you to bask in the wonderful expectations of new beginnings. As a wise woman, be present with all of the exhilarating changes that are happening to your body, and begin to deeply connect with your new baby to create a lasting, joyful bond.

The moment your fertilized egg implanted itself on a well-prepared *endometrium*—the mucous membrane lining the uterus—it began the process of producing an interface between you and your baby. This connection becomes the *placenta*, an organ that truly belongs to the baby, and from which it will receive from you the blood flow, oxygen, and nutrients it needs to develop. It is, in fact, the baby's first organ to form and can be both positively and negatively impacted by your environment, which then can affect the course of your baby's development.

One of the main goals of pregnancy is to maintain and enhance the placenta instead of harm it. Luckily, you may already be off to a great start. All the healthy habits that you adopted in preconception that lower inflammation—dealing with stress, exercising appropriately, avoiding toxins, and eating well—are the same practices that amplify the health of the placenta. If you're just starting our program, you still have plenty of time. You can't undo the past, but you can enhance the present, and you can certainly prepare for the future. And if you did the work of preconception, just because you started off well, it doesn't mean that your work is done.

Think of this section as another way that we are extending our arms around you, keeping you safe and supported during your first trimester. You will have everything you need to know, and you're going to do great.

YOUR BODY

The first three months of pregnancy are a time of massive change.
The single-celled egg has been fertilized and begins the process of cellular division and specialization. This growing cellular mass becomes an embryo, with its own beating heart, and by the eighth week, it officially turns into a fetus. By the end of the first trimester, your fetus will have arms, legs, and a face and is tens of thousands times larger than the original fertilized egg.

At the same time, your own body is changing to accommodate this new life, and it's very likely that you won't feel like yourself. Interestingly, the reason has everything to do with your hormones, and the different ways your body is coping with the hormonal surge necessary to support your baby. From the moment you conceive, what used to be your normal levels of estrogen and progesterone rise significantly and abruptly. These are the same hormones that ebb and flow as part of your normal menstrual cycle. But in pregnancy, they rise and remain high. Your body needs higher levels of these hormones because they are important for creating the best environment to nurture your pregnancy as they aid the growth and development of the placenta. These hormones are then transferred to your baby, who needs them for development.

A rise in the hormones estrogen and progesterone will enlarge your breasts, and the added weight can subtly change your posture: pregnant women often round their shoulders forward to compensate. The belly may begin to feel fuller, especially in the afternoon/evenings, decreasing your abdominal muscles' ability to function and support you through your activities. Reducing the abdominal muscles' automatic firing mechanism can lead to an injury like pelvic misalignment/shifts, back strains, or upper back pain.

Choosing Your Birthing Professional(s)

Now that you're pregnant, you will need to decide who is going to deliver your baby. Most women continue to use an obstetrician. However, you can have other birthing professionals be there for you along your journey, including a midwife or a doula/birth coach.

The best part about having a baby right now is that there are so many safe options for where to have your birth. You are a wise woman, and you will know what's best for you. Just make sure you do the research before you make a final decision about having a hospital birth, a home birth, or delivering at a birthing center (see page 327 for more information on each of these options).

You may already have an ob-gyn you are happy with, or you may want to choose a different practice based on the doctor's location, relationship with a specific hospital, philosophy, and openness to the birth that you are envisioning. You will want to interview ob-gyns and get a feel for how the relationship with them will go. This doctor should be there to support you, work as a team, and respect that you know your body. You don't want to feel intimidated, put down, or dismissed.

Midwives are certified birthing professionals who may work at hospitals, birthing centers, or are available for home births. They work with you throughout labor and delivery and are trained to handle normal, uncomplicated births. They do not perform cesarean sections or epidurals but will refer you to other medical professionals for these.

Doulas are birthing professionals and labor coaches. The word *doula* is Greek and means "women's servant." Doulas have been serving women in childbirth for centuries. They provide an additional layer of support and advocacy that can positively impact the labor experience. Doulas will coach you throughout your pregnancy and labor and continue to work with you postpartum. Often doulas will work together with midwives or ob-gyns.

Common First Trimester Complaints

Discovering that you're pregnant can be one of the most exciting times in a woman's life. Yet it's hard to be enthusiastic if you don't feel great. The same hormones that affect the way your body looks are also affecting the way you feel and can cause a variety of unpleasant symptoms. Every part of your body—from the brain to your intestines to your reproductive organs—has estrogen and progesterone receptors, and they are all very sensitive to increased levels, which is why first trimester symptoms can be so varied. The good news is that once your hormonal spike stabilizes, you may no longer feel symptoms as severely, if at all.

Not every woman will experience all of these complaints. Studies indicate that the severity of some symptoms, like nausea, is related to a genetic variance.[1] This means that women who experience extreme nausea may have certain genetics that create a much more exuberant hormonal response during pregnancy compared to women who don't get that reaction.

Discuss any of these issues with your obstetrician/gynecologist: the first trimester is the exact time to line one up and begin to have monthly checkups.

Acne and Skin Changes

Hormonal changes can lead to a variety of skin issues including pigmentation change, breakouts, oily skin, dry skin, etc. Increased hormones can stimulate oil production in the skin, causing acne. What's more, your liver is more focused on processing the surge in hormones, so its ability to generally detoxify is hampered. Problems with your skin just might be the unfortunate outcome.

To deal with changing skin, you might want to create an entirely new skin-care regimen. We like the Immunocologie brand because it is formulated with a mineral-rich clay or clay water from France that lowers the skin's inflammation and can reduce or eliminate blemishes with one application. We also like the Aimee Raupp Beauty line of products that is specially formulated for pregnant women and new mothers.

Pregnancy Kit for the Face

Your skin routine should include the following and can be used throughout your pregnancy:

- **Exfoliating Cleanser** (three nights per week): this is a very gentle way to removed dry, dehydrated skin cells without causing a reaction.
- **Moisturizing Cream:** use a light day cream for both day and night applications.
- **Facial Mask** (one night per week): treats pesky breakouts by absorbing excess oil.

Constipation

An increase in progesterone actually causes a reduction in *peristalsis*, the rhythmic contractions of the intestine that move food through the digestive process to elimination. The additional progesterone causes the intestines to relax, which leads to less efficient movement that keeps you feeling somewhat blocked.

Staying well hydrated is the best way to combat constipation. However, some women develop liquid aversions and may feel more nauseous after drinking water. The following are some of our favorite tips for getting more water into your diet and addressing constipation:

- Add lemon slices or other citrus to your water to make it more appealing.
- Some fruits have a high water content, like watermelon. Others have a high fiber content, like berries. We suggest that you eat a variety of fruits that are in season.
- Eat cooked, high-fiber vegetables like dark leafy greens, artichokes, carrots, beets, and broccoli.
- Reduce your consumption of processed foods.
- Stay away from binding foods like bananas and rice.

Proper Breathing Prevents Constipation

Proper diaphragm breathing—the practice we endorse in this book—not only optimally oxygenates the body, it massages the intestines, keeping digestive motility going and preventing constipation.

Digestive Issues: Heartburn, Gas, and Bloating

Increased estrogen and progesterone can relax your lower *esophageal sphincter*, a muscle that acts as a door between the esophagus and the stomach. When this happens, it loosens an otherwise tight seal: the stomach remains a little bit open, or less able to withstand the pressure of stomach fluid or stomach gas, and you can develop acid reflux, heartburn, gas, and bloating. What's more, digestive issues are also related to a shifting blood flow from your organs to the placenta. This causes your digestive system to work slower, allowing for more gas buildup and, again, constipation.

Here are some tips for preventing these digestive complaints:

- Avoid food triggers: the most common acid reflux triggers include spicy foods, high fat foods, fried foods, tomatoes and tomato products (such as ketchup or spaghetti sauce), citrus fruits and juices, chocolate, and peppermint (which can cause acid reflux).

* Avoid wearing constricting clothing.
* Chew gum between meals.
* Chew your food thoroughly, twenty to thirty times for each bite.
* Eat smaller, more frequent meals throughout the day: it's easier to digest food when your stomach is not completely full. Shoot for five to seven small meals, with the last meal being at least three hours before bedtime.
* Get plenty of sleep: the production of the hormone melatonin rises at night and is necessary for improved sphincter tone in the esophagus.
* Practice appropriate diaphragm breathing: this will help reduce acid reflux and keep your bowels moving.
* Skip high-fat meals at night.
* Try slippery elm: this supplement is known for treating heartburn and acid reflux.

Ancient Wisdom and Digestive Health

One tenet of traditional Chinese medicine is that you should chew each bite of your food as many times as your age. The reason is that as we age, the digestive process slows down, so we require extra chewing to break down food in our mouth, making digestion easier. In pregnancy, the digestive system also slows down, especially when the baby begins to take up more space. Taking the time to chew your food more thoroughly now will set you up for better digestion as the baby grows.

Sensory Issues: Strong Sense of Smell, Excessive Salivation, Metallic Taste

Hormones enhance our sensory abilities, so when you have more hormones coursing through your system, you will be more sensitive to odors and tastes. For example, the perfume you always wear becomes unappealingly strong. You may also want to replace scented soaps, cleaners, candles, and skin products with fragance-free, organic varieties.

Excessive saliva production could be related to counteracting a metallic taste you now sense. If you are missing micronutrients like selenium (which is found in protein like beef, turkey, and chicken), iron, or iodine, you may find that certain foods taste metallic. By increasing these nutrients, the metallic taste might go away, and with it, the extra saliva.

Frequent Urination

Hormonal changes increase blood and urine flow, creating this very common first trimester complaint. Your kidneys are also primed to be more efficient: they need to be effective enough to eliminate waste produced by both you and your baby.

Reducing your liquid intake is not the way to treat frequent urination. In fact, there's not much you can do. When you have the urge to pee, embrace it because your body is doing its job, cleansing you from the inside out. Some of the exercises in this section, like Kegels, support bladder functionality, so you can control your urge to pee even when you're not near a restroom.

Nausea

Nausea, or morning sickness, is the most common complaint of early pregnancy, yet it can actually occur at any time of the day or night. If you are experiencing strong bouts of nausea, there is good news: it has been associated with a reduced risk of miscarriage and a greater chance that your pregnancy will have a healthy outcome.[2] The not-so-great news is that we are still not entirely sure why it develops. Some researchers believe that it is a holdover evolutionary strategy that keeps women from ingesting toxins by lowering their desire to eat at all.[3] Nausea may also be a reaction to peristalsis: when food sits in your stomach, it can create nausea. Some research suggests it is also associated with the presence of H-pylori, a bacterial infection in the stomach,[4] which can be easily identified and treated by your doctor.

Non-food therapies are known to help, including diaphragm breathing, acupuncture and acupressure, or electrical nerve stimulation (acustimulation), as long as the treatment is ongoing; it's not a "one-and-done" fix. Hypnotherapy may also help because it allows pregnant women to access a more relaxed state, which can help with the management of nausea.

Spotting

Spotting or staining in the first trimester is very common and should be taken seriously. It is often caused by hormone shifts that lead to an inflammation of the cervix. It can also happen during the embryo's implantation.

Talk with your doctor if you are spotting. He or she can make sure that your bleeding isn't caused by an infection, polyp, or other issue with the pregnancy.

Tender Breasts and Darkening Nipples

You may notice that your breasts are feeling fuller, your bra size may change, and the area around your nipples, the *aureola*, is getting darker. These are natural changes that are also linked to an increased hormone production.

If you find that your breasts are very tender, a warm compress may be soothing. An Epsom salt bath with warm water, not hot, might make you feel better. You may need to wear less form-fitting clothes, and ditch the underwire bra. We recommend that you wear a wireless, supportive bra that is soft and made of a uniform material for extra support. If you are large-breasted, try a sports bra that is not constricting or compressing. Maternity stores are a great resource. A racer-back style is recommended for large-breasted women.

Urinary Tract Infections (UTIs)/Yeast Infections

Urinary tract infections can occur because progesterone relaxes the muscles in the bladder, which decreases the bladder's ability to fully empty. When this happens, bacteria can grow, creating a UTI. At the same time, the microbiomes of the vagina and intestines can become out of balance if you're resolving nausea with glutinous crackers or snacks with lots of processed sugars, which then can cause a urinary tract infection.

To combat UTIs, we recommend supplementing with vitamin C, or cranberry juice extract, and staying well hydrated. Good hygiene, including allowing yourself to pee when you have the urge and peeing after intercourse, is also helpful.

There are many natural remedies for yeast infection prevention and treatment that are safe and effective during pregnancy. Improving the vaginal and bladder bacteria with probiotics or prebiotics, such as a yeast-based probiotic like *saccharomyces boulardii*, can be very beneficial. A probiotic that can be inserted directly into the vagina can start to work immediately in the area. And as you've learned, cleaning up your gut's microbiome by eating foods that are supportive of a more beneficial bacterial balance is very helpful. Eliminating starchy foods and adding dairy or nondairy yogurts can also help control yeast overgrowth.

Tired of Feeling Tired?

Many first trimester moms complain of ongoing fatigue. We believe that there are two primary causes of this complaint: first, there is a huge amount of cellular activity going on in both your body and in the baby's, both of which require an enormous amount of energy. Secondly, your body is ramping up its production of the hormone melatonin to support placental development. Melatonin is secreted by the pineal gland when you are sleeping and surrounded by darkness. This is why we sleep so well at night—because the melatonin we are naturally producing helps us sleep. When you are pregnant, the extra melatonin production may be causing you to feel more sleepy. So if you fight the urge to sleep just as you need to create more melatonin, you will not be making enough melatonin to help you sleep, and you are not supporting the placenta.

All this is to say that your body is perfectly calibrated to do the right things at the right time, so go with it. During the first trimester, you will be tired, and you need to listen to your body and sleep. This is one area where the tried-and-true advice reigns: honor your body (rest when you feel like resting, whenever possible) and get eight or more consecutive hours of sleep each night. Even closing your eyes for five minutes during the workday can provide the rest you need.

One of the best ways to ensure that you are getting the right amount of sleep is to change your habits at night. According to Satchin Panda, PhD, author of *The Circadian Code*, reducing the amount of overhead light at night, limiting screen time—television, phones, tablets, etc.—before bed, sticking with an eating schedule where you finish your last meal at least three hours before you go to sleep, and creating a sleeping schedule will help restore the body's natural rhythm. The added benefit once again is increased melatonin production.

Lastly, restrict your evening commitments so that you can get the rest you need. You'll have your energy back again in the second trimester when you will feel more like your old self and can enjoy being more social.

Amplify Your Baby's Health by Controlling Stressors

You and your baby are connected for the duration of your pregnancy, so everything you eat and put on your skin is transferred to the baby via the placenta. But did you know that your stress is transferrable as well? Your ability to handle stress is a more critical influence over your baby's long-term health than what you eat during pregnancy. Maternal stress can disrupt vital aspects of placental growth and function. This is why you want to continue to lower your environmental stressors by living as cleanly as possible. The combination of cleaning up your environment and ramping up different ways you can feel supported will reduce stress and amplify the health of the placenta.

Recent studies show that the adversity a mother experiences during the first trimester is a predictor of a baby's lifetime physical and mental health. In fact, extreme maternal stress during pregnancy predisposes offspring to neurodevelopmental disorders including schizophrenia, attention deficit/hyperactivity disorder, and autism spectrum disorders.[5] Chronic, ongoing stress can manipulate your baby's physical health by influencing the length of your baby's telomeres—the protective ends of DNA strands that influence life span. We want to keep your baby's telomeres as long as possible. However, your baby's telomeres can get shorter when you are experiencing the kinds of stress that increase cortisol production and lead to chronic inflammation, and this shortening is related to chronic disease and premature aging.[6] This is why one of the key takeaways for this book is to try to keep calm and find the support you need throughout your pregnancy.

During the first trimester you may find that you are more sensitive to stress in general, which might throw you off. You may even feel frustrated at yourself that you are so easily rattled, more anxious, or more stressed. Women often experience mood swings with the ebb and flow of hormones during a menstrual cycle, so it's not surprising that you could have more mood swings during the first trimester when your hormone production is peaking. Huge shifts in these hormones impact the production of brain chemicals that influence mood. You may also be tired and nauseated, which, in and of itself, is going to affect your resiliency to stressors.

In Patricia's Greek culture, the partner's role during the first trimester is to keep a newly pregnant woman stress-free, which means avoiding discussing bad news as well as providing needed support. While these traditions may seem quaint, the fact is that during the first trimester, pregnant women are not as resilient, and you need to honor this reality by taking life more slowly and creating a stress-free environment at home and at work. A little bit of daily stress is expected, yet being stressed about being stressed is actually a double whammy! If you are feeling burdened by feeling stress in your work or at home, you may need to learn how to just let some things go. The first trimester is a time when you need to be a little more respectful of your need for self-care. If something or someone is ticking you off, just literally let it go because carrying that stress around and letting it build up inside you is not worth it.

The truth is, we cannot control what happens to us—our external circumstances—all the time, but we can control our response. Resilience is a skill that can be learned, and if you master it in your first trimester, it can serve you well throughout your pregnancy.

Dr. Dan Siegel and Dr. Elissa Epel promote two basic ways to handle stress and create resiliency: *top down* refers to training your mind, and *bottom up* includes lifestyle changes that affect the mind and body. Try any one of the following techniques when you're sensing a shift toward stress, whether it's feeling anxious, or when you're tightening up muscles or scrunching your face. Be cognizant of the cues that your body is sending you, and then implement these strategies, so you feel like you're on a vacation on a beautiful beach rather than stewing in your worries.

Top-Down Stress-Relieving Techniques:

- **Mindfulness.** The hard part of remaining calm is being aware in the moment that you have actually experienced a stressor. Too often, people have become numb to the various things that stress them out and choose not to deal with them. However, this strategy doesn't really serve you, or your baby. Instead, we want you to practice mindfulness: becoming aware of your feelings as they arise, and seeing if they are appropriate to the stressor you are experiencing. When you are stressed, label your experience. For instance, think about how you are feeling: what are you focusing on? Practicing mindfulness also means trying to slow down, do one thing at a time, and take control of your schedule. It's perfectly reasonable to say "not now" to others, or even to your own thoughts.
- **Focus on your breath to break the cycle of negative thinking.** When you are sensing a stress feeling, or an anxious wave of emotion, use the breathing techniques in this chapter. Taking a few quiet, controlled breaths in private after a stressor comes on can be so impactful.
- **Focus on how you are feeling when you first wake up and right before you go to sleep.** Instead of dropping off to sleep or jumping out of bed and into your to-do list, take five minutes to concentrate on joyful thoughts. What are you most looking forward to today? Tomorrow? Elissa Epel, PhD, coauthor of *The Telomere Effect*, reports that starting or ending your day with joy has been linked to maintaining your telomere length.

- **Avoid negativity.** Limit watching, listening to, or reading the news; limit negative social media exposure, and tell your family and friends that they shouldn't be calling you with devastating news. Relax with uplifting and calming movies, and avoid violence or thrillers. On a personal level, limit your exposure to knowingly stressful situations: if you're having problems with a coworker, don't go to lunch with a group where he or she is present.

- **Give yourself permission to take a break.** Listen to your favorite music, or go out and take a thirty-minute walk in nature. Meditate, pray, or try new things that bring you calm. The meditative prayer from pre-conception (page 87) is something that you can return to when you're feeling stressed.

- **Visualize the entirety of the ocean, and use it as a metaphor.** There will always be changes in our lives, and these changes can create either a small ripple or big wave. When you are in the thick of an emotional situation, think of yourself swimming leisurely at the bottom of the deep ocean floor. Even though you can see the waves crashing on the top, you are in the calmness.

First Trimester Mantra

If you find that you're worrying about your pregnancy, take a mindful walk to the restroom, honor your new, growing belly, and shift your focus to joy. If you need a little more encouragement, try the following mantra whenever life becomes overwhelming:

I am beautiful, I am wise, I am safe.
My body is miraculous.
Everything is progressing as it should.
And I am happy.

Bottom-Up Stress-Relieving Techniques:

Following the same advice as in preconception, some of the best ways to manage stress are with easy and commonsense lifestyle interventions:

- **Get plenty of good sleep.** During deep sleep your body and brain experience a complete biological reset to prepare you for the next day. Yet poor sleep is correlated with inflammation, which can shorten telomeres for your baby. The quality of your night's sleep is determined by what happens the day before, so if you go to sleep stressed, you may continue to produce higher levels of cortisol through the night, which creates wakefulness.

- **Movement.** Movement helps your mental state, and movement in nature is even better. Go for a walk in the park, or out in the woods, or by the sea, whatever you have access to that calms you the most. You can also listen to the music you love and make sure you do some exercise that brings you joy every day, as long as you're keeping your phone on airplane mode.

- **Have sex.** It's perfectly safe to continue to have sex with your partner in the first trimester and throughout the majority of your pregnancy. During pleasurable sexual activity, the hormone oxytocin is released, which as you learned in preconception, lowers your stress response. Achieving orgasm two to three times a week is considered optimal for achieving both mental and physical health benefits throughout your life.

Develop Multi-System Resiliency

Getting good, restful sleep at night, and exercising, practicing proper breathing, mindfulness, and meditation during the day work together and create *multisystem resiliency*. There is an additive effect when you do all these daily protective behaviors together, making you more resilient to stress.

The Difference Between Stressed Out and Depressed

Many women are surprised when they feel blue within eight weeks of their pregnancy test, and you may feel a range of emotions that you weren't expecting. These feelings are perfectly normal and may be due to severe fatigue, which often accompanies feelings of frustration and lack of energy. These feelings can be interpreted as feeling sad or not oneself. Chronic stress can also increase the risk of feeling sad or apathetic.

Yet these emotions are not the same as depression, which is a mental disorder that has an overpowering effect on many parts of a person's life. True depression is diagnosed when an individual is experiencing five or more of the following symptoms during a two-week period, and at least one of the symptoms should be either (1) depressed mood or (2) loss of interest or pleasure:

- Depressed mood most of the day, nearly every day
- Markedly diminished interest or pleasure in all, or almost all, activities most of the day, nearly every day
- Significant weight loss when not dieting or weight gain, or decrease or increase in appetite nearly every day
- A slowing down of thought and a reduction of physical movement (observable by others, not merely subjective feelings of restlessness or being slowed down)
- Fatigue or loss of energy nearly every day

If you are currently taking medication to treat anxiety or depression, or any mental illness, discuss continuing or discontinuing these medications with your doctor. But if living with a low mood is new and accompanies pregnancy, these feelings may resolve on their own in as little as a few days, especially if you can get the sleep you need. To help you move out of a low mood, you can try increasing exercise. In the same way that movement is linked to combating stress, new studies are clearly showing that exercise is a powerful tool for alleviating depression. A large 2018 study from Yale University showed that people who exercise regularly have half as many incidents of depression each month.[7] Researchers have also found that aerobic exercising for thirty to sixty minutes, three to five times a week showed the biggest benefits. This is just one of the many reasons why we recommend at least thirty minutes of walking each day throughout your pregnancy. You can also try soothing activities that can lift your mood, like meditation, tai chi, yoga, dance, and prayer, as well as improve your indoor air quality (see below) and get good sleep.

There are some essential oils that are helpful for reversing low mood. We love doTERRA's Cheer Uplifting Blend, as well as essential oil concentrations of ylang ylang, rose, lavender, peppermint oil, and Melissa (lemon balm).

Environmental Stressors

Just as everything you are eating and feeling affects your baby, your environment—everything that surrounds you—is also influencing your baby's development. Environmental pollutants have been shown to affect fetal gene expression and immune function. Exposures can prompt epigenetic changes in gene expression, which can be passed not only to your baby but to subsequent generations.

Creating new habits and making good decisions over the next three months set the stage for limiting your environmental exposures throughout your pregnancy. For instance, indoor air pollution is a stressor that you need to avoid. As we learned in preconception, indoor air can be two to five times more polluted than outdoor air: it can contain mold or pollen, toxic gases like carbon monoxide or radon, the off-gassing of chemicals in household products like air fresheners and cleaners, and even fire retardants used in furniture fabrics. We also know that a mother's exposure to air pollution can increase the risk of respiratory diseases, like asthma and bronchitis, for babies still in the womb.[8] The indoor filtration systems we discussed in the preconception chapter are just as important now. Another easy fix is to bring the outdoors in, and fill your home or office with indoor plants. Choose ones you know you're not allergic to or that emit strong odors.

We also want you to be mindful about chemicals that may be in your home.

For example, phthalates are a type of chemical family that are often found in plastic products, including toys, vinyl flooring and wall covering, nail polish, and perfumes. They are used to make plastics more durable and are often used in the packaging of personal care products, supermarket food, water bottles, and other household items. Unfortunately, exposure to them may be linked to delays in your baby's language development, as shown in one recent study published by *JAMA Pediatrics*.[9] You can significantly reduce your exposure to phthalates by buying products that are labeled *phthalate free*, using alternatives to plastic when microwaving food or beverages (such as glass or porcelain), and avoiding packaged foods.

A second chemical family you need to avoid are PFOA or PFAS. These chemicals can be contaminating your drinking water if you live close to a chemical plant, and they can also be found in carpets, some seafood,[10] microwave popcorn packaging, and other takeout food packaging that is meant to be grease-resistant, like pizza boxes.[11] The problem is that these chemicals from the packaging can leech into your food

We also want you to continue to be vigilant with your exposure to electromagnetic fields (EMFs). In 2008, UCLA researchers found that prenatal exposure to cell phones was associated with a higher risk for behavioral problems and hyperactivity in children.[12] Therefore, a few simple tips can keep you and your baby safe when you are pregnant. There are products you can use at home, including bed-shielding tents, special paint that blocks EMF transmissions, and installing covers on smart electrical meters.

When it comes to your cellular phone or your laptop, we recommend that you shut off the wireless feature whenever possible; it may sound old-fashioned, but you are more protected this way. The following guidelines are a good start:

- At home, wired options are better than wireless ones. Unplug your home Wi-Fi when not in use.
- Avoid carrying your phone directly on your body. Avoid placing a phone or laptop directly on your abdomen.

- Streaming a movie or video game creates higher levels of wireless radiation exposure than downloading and viewing the same game on a device in airplane mode.
- Switch your phone to airplane mode at night and when you are not using it, even when it's in your purse or bag.
- Use the speaker setting or headphones when you are making a phone call, instead of holding your phone to your head for long periods of time. Look for an "air tube headset" that delivers sound through hollow tubes rather than traditional wires and limits EMF exposure.

The Importance of Keeping to a Healthy Weight Gain

Excessive weight gain during pregnancy is associated with poor health outcomes for both you and your baby. We believe that the average pregnant woman needs only about 300 additional calories more a day than she did before she was pregnant. This guideline will help you gain the right amount of weight during pregnancy.

There's actually no recommendation really for weight gain during the first trimester. In fact, if you are following our suggestions, you may even lose weight now that you are eating healthier. We believe that keeping first trimester weight gain down is linked to having a healthier pregnancy because excess body fat in and of itself is very inflammatory.

In an ideal situation, distribution of weight gain would follow these guidelines if you are only carrying one baby and if you were considered normal weight before pregnancy. Talk to your doctor for a more personalized weight gaining approach.

- Zero to five pounds in the first trimester
- Five to ten pounds in the second trimester
- Ten to fifteen pounds in the third trimester

RESTORATIVE BREATHING

We have found that some of first trimester nausea can be related to breathing issues. Your internal organs are beginning to shift, and there will be some changes to the abdominal cavity that can promote a little bit of pressure to the diaphragm, which then reduces your breathing efficiency and could amplify nausea. This is especially true if this isn't your first pregnancy, as your body can automatically revert to old habits.

Review the basic diaphragm breathing instructions that follow. You can continue this practice throughout your pregnancy. Ultimately, it will become your natural, preferred way to breathe.

- Place the tongue at the roof of your mouth, relax your facial muscles, and breathe through your nose. Your body is relaxed, and you're breathing gently and quietly. Focus on the breath that is expanding through the back and sides of your lower ribs as you inhale, and deflating your lungs from the back and sides of your lower ribs as you exhale.

Breathing to Combat Nausea

Whenever you start to feel nauseous, you can adjust your breathing to quell this queasiness. Cupping your hands around your mouth and breathing in and out will provide an additional boost of carbon dioxide from your outbreath, which will make you feel less nauseous. Typically, we blow off too much carbon dioxide with each exhale, which depletes the reserves in our lungs. When we inhale extra carbon dioxide (CO_2) by using this method, it restores our reserves and the internal system balances, which then alleviates the nausea. Deep breathing during this time is not going to be helpful, and can actually make you feel a little more nauseous, if not lightheaded.

The technique is simple. You can try this breathing whenever you feel the need, as often as once an hour, if not more.

- Place the tongue at the roof of your mouth, relax your facial muscles, and breathe through your nose. Your body is relaxed, and you're breathing gently and quietly. Focus on the breath that is expanding through the back and sides of your lower ribs as you inhale, and deflating your lungs from the back and sides of your lower ribs as you exhale.
- Then, place your hands together by putting your fingers and your thumb close together, then curve your hands to form a cup, or a mask, and cover your nose and mouth. This will create a little space to breathe into. Breathe in and out into your hand, and as you do so, you are going to be reinhaling some of the blown-off carbon dioxide.

Break Out the Earplugs

One way to hear your breathing is to block out noise from the rest of the world. Put in some earplugs and listen to your breathing. Make it as quiet as possible. Then, extend the transition time between exhale and inhale to longer times: pause for two, four, then eight seconds. As you pause, see if you can hear the silence in between breaths.

Jane Improved Her Breathing to Prevent Nausea

Patricia's client Jane is a perfect example of how the right breathing can make all the difference during pregnancy. Jane came to see her when she

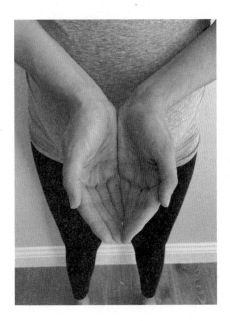 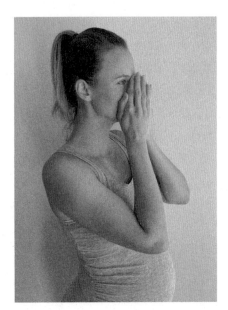

was newly pregnant because she wanted to make sure she wouldn't get the diastasis her sister experienced. Jane was in good physical health but already had intermittent nausea that was affecting her ability to work and complained of pain in her neck and shoulders when she sat at her desk. Patricia quickly realized that Jane was not properly breathing, even when she was sitting still, and that her breathing was likely connected to her nausea. She frequently shifted to chest/shoulder breathing instead of the more efficient diaphragm breathing, which caused her neck and shoulder muscles to be tense. When Patricia hooked Jane up to a capnography machine that measures carbon dioxide flow, she noticed that Jane was blowing off too much carbon dioxide and breathing too heavily.

Patricia taught Jane how she could optimize her breathing using the same directions that are in this book. They developed a cue so that whenever she was breathing incorrectly, Jane would realize her mistake and practice proper breathing instead. The cue was to monitor her breathing after fifteen minutes of sitting. If she started to feel her shoulders rise to her ears, she would stop, then place her hands on the sides of her lower ribs, and move her breath toward her hands, expanding the rib cage outward. Her next cue was to get to the end of each exhale gently, allowing for a slight pause before the next inhale. By learning this technique, Jane was also able to stay connected with her deep muscles—the transversus abdominis—the part of the abdomen that prevents diastasis and provides deep lumbopelvic support. Then Patricia explained how activating these muscles would also help her release tension in her neck and shoulders. Jane was grateful to have the right tools to correct her breathing and prevent nausea and diastasis for the remainder of her pregnancy.

MOVEMENT

*It wasn't that long ago that doctors believed exercise during preg-*nancy could harm you or your baby. Prior to 2002, the American College of Obstetricians and Gynecologists recommended only minimal exercise, and that pregnant women should never elevate their heart rate. Then, James F. Clapp III, MD, published the results of decades of his research, and with that information, the American College of Obstetrics and Gynecology officially revised its guidelines. Unfortunately, it's hard to change a doctor's opinion, even when science is on our side. Most doctors have still not adopted these new guidelines or best practices.

Clapp's research clearly showed that not only is exercise during pregnancy recommended, it's encouraged. The reasons are many: the baby literally exercises with the mother, and benefits not only in the womb, but during delivery, and for the entire life span. Clapp's research[13] proved the following:

- Pregnant women who exercised in the first trimester had improved placental function, where more oxygen and nutrients can get across to the baby.
- Exercising during pregnancy means that there is a decreased chance for premature labor or the birth of an underweight baby and a very low incidence of obstetrical complications at the start of labor.
- After birth, women who exercise have healthier babies who are not overweight, their mental performance is better, and their physical

performance is better as well. Babies who were lean at birth grew normally and stayed lean, leading to long-term benefits in health over the course of their lives.

Exercise is also the absolute best way to prevent and reverse a multitude of discomforts and ailments during pregnancy, including lowering stress and improving mood. As we learned in preconception, it's the number one way for women to reduce inflammation. Clapp also outlined how women who exercise enjoy easier pregnancies in these ways:

* Exercise offsets the effects of ligament laxity, improves strength, maintains muscle tone, and reduces the incidence of low-back pain, leg and pelvic discomfort, and other musculoskeletal complaints.
* Reduces stress.
* Improves balance.
* Less weight gain—women who exercised gained an average of seven fewer pounds and 3 percent less body fat.
* Lower risk of gestational diabetes.[14]
* Lower risk of preeclampsia (pregnancy-induced hypertension).
* Improved outcomes for labor and delivery: exercise is the single largest determining factor in the outcome of labor, including, among other benefits, a 75 percent decrease in the need for an operative intervention (either a forceps delivery or cesarean section).

These are the reasons why we want you to exercise. But not any program will do.

The Benefits of Balletic Training

Your body, with all of its curves, is made to support this baby. However, if you've had a history of injury or poor postural habits, you may be predisposed towards not carrying the baby as gracefully as you should. The type of exercise we recommend during pregnancy is not an aggressive physical activity that bulks up your muscles. Instead, it's based on Patricia's ballet background and physical therapy approach. In many places throughout the world, physical therapists are involved in the care of a pregnant woman because they know how to properly support the female body, the joints that are going to be stressed during pregnancy, and the injuries that may occur. A physical therapist wants to keep a pregnant woman successfully moving, exercising, and feeling good. This program is therefore completely preventative: the goal is to optimize body mechanics, alignment, muscle tone, strength, and flexibility so that your body can support you throughout your pregnancy.

Before Patricia was a physical therapist, she was a professional ballet and modern dancer. The muscles that you work in balletic movements are the same muscles that you need to maintain good postural alignment despite a growing belly. You may already be familiar with some of these exercises, as some yoga poses use the same principles. We have incorporated some yoga postures in the routines. Maintaining this alignment is the secret to having a pain-free pregnancy.

These exercises will also help you develop a long, lean balletic look as you start to engage the exact muscles that are going to be tested as your baby grows—the deep, muscular system of the spine and each of your joints. By activating the deep muscles that support your spinal column, you will appear taller, longer, and move with stability and control. This is what sets this program apart from others. Not only will you feel fit and strong, you will be graceful and feel like you are walking on air, even when you have your biggest belly.

This program combines the best of both parts of Patricia's training and will keep you at the right amount of activity throughout your pregnancy. We have found that women who did not exercise at all, or women who exercise intensely and have very tight abdominal muscles before pregnancy, are those most likely to experience diastasis.

When Patricia was putting her program into practice during her own pregnancies, she did not have any pain and carried pretty heavy babies as well.

The muscles she developed as a dancer were the exact ones that allowed her to carry her babies without compromising her posture. Her feet didn't grow during pregnancy because she continued to activate the deep muscles of the lower leg and feet, which kept her arches from flattening.

Understanding Body Mechanics

We are supposed to have a slight curve that goes in the same direction for the neck and low back, and a curve that goes in the opposite direction at the midback. Maintaining all three curves is the key to supporting the head and the rest of the body properly against the pull of gravity. When these curves are reduced or flattened, you will place more load onto the spine, which can cause pain and improper posture, which then leads to a lack of support throughout the entire body.

As Carolyn Richardson outlines in her GravityFit program, each curve is supported by its own set of core muscles. This program focuses on stabilizing these three cores—the neck, the midback, and the abdomen/lumbopelvic core—and getting the muscles of each core to work together in unison. If one area is off, it shuts down the effectiveness of the others. In this program, we're working the core muscles that get stressed when you're pregnant:

- **The cervical core.** This is comprised of the deep muscle system in the neck, including the *longus colli* and *longus capitis*. When these muscles are activated, they align your neck to your deep abdominal core and improve their connection. The neck and the abdominal/lumbar core mirror each other and need to work well together in order to keep your whole muscular system energized.
- **The thoracic core.** The thoracic core contains the muscles of the diaphragm and the serratus anterior, which supports the midback (thorax), ribs, and chest. This core needs to be in proper alignment to provide good shock absorption and freedom of movement for the other parts of the body.

- **The abdominal/lumbar core.** These muscles, the *transversus abdominis, lumbar multifidi,* pelvic floor, and *gluteus medius,* support the abdomen, lumbar, and pelvis and keep them in a stable position. The lumbar core is the most compromised area of the body during pregnancy. When your lumbar core is balanced and energized, you have less likelihood of experiencing pain or strain.

You will also be working the deep muscular systems of each joint of the body that stabilizes and supports it, along with the superficial system that moves the joint.

Maintaining Good Posture

Balletic training begins by working on your posture. Good posture keeps your lymph system, your circulatory system, and nervous system flowing so that your organ systems can function optimally. It keeps your spine from getting tweaked so that you can avoid injury. It also keeps your arms and legs supported. All of these attributes are important during pregnancy.

The goal is to develop a neutral posture. The minute we flex our spine into a rounded low back position or allow our head to drift forward (like when we are looking at a laptop or device), the deep core muscles immediately shut off, and we start compensating with the shorter, superficial muscles. In the long term, poor posture that relies on these muscles usually leads to a weakened core, tension in various muscles, increased risk for injury, and even pain.

These three photos show various ways that we typically stand with poor posture:

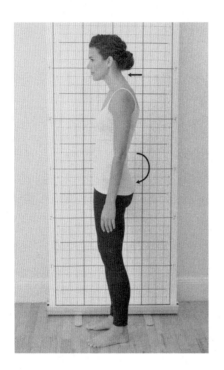

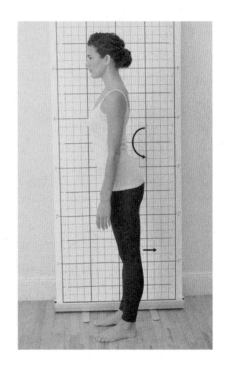

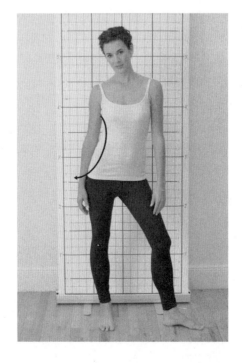

Find Your Neutral Standing Posture

To find the best, neutral posture, try moving in and out of the two extremes of movement at each joint:

Feet: Roll your arches away from each other and toward each other without moving your foot. Try to find the midpoint between the two extremes of this movement. Your arch should be mildly lifted. Center your body weight between your heels and your toes at the midpoint of the foot, keeping all toes on the floor.

Knees: Tighten your quadriceps muscles at the front of your thighs. This will make your knees extend back. Then let the contraction go and relax the knees. That is technically neutral for the knee—unlocked, not hyperextended, and not very bent either.

Hips/Pelvis: Tuck your pelvis under, bringing your pubic bone forward, then reverse the movement by sticking out your buttocks. Rock between these two extremes of movement and find the exact center. Your low back should be in a neutral lordosis—slightly curved, like a C.

Midback: Focus on only moving your chest and midback. Push your chest forward, then collapse the chest back and down. Find the center point, which should technically be slightly rounded in the midback (thoracic spine) with your chest lining up over your belly.

Shoulders: With your arms at your sides, lift your shoulders up, rotate your palms and pinkies forward, and gently lower your shoulders. Keep both shoulders open in the front as you relax your arms. Do *not* push shoulder blades down. Shoulder blades should feel like they are floating and like your shoulders are lifted up and back slightly.

Head/Neck: Imagine that you are wearing goggles and someone is pulling the goggle strap back. Your head should glide back in-line with your spine. Relax your chin down, taking all the wrinkles out of the back of your neck.

Take this new standing posture and shift your body weight in one unit front and back. Find the center point and stand there. You're now in a centered posture. Breathe and pay attention to this stance. Then, shift your weight right and left and find the center point so that you are standing equally on both legs. Lastly, imagine someone pulling a string from the crown of your head. Lift up tall. Be patient as you correct tendencies and get familiar with the process. It may feel odd for upward of a month.

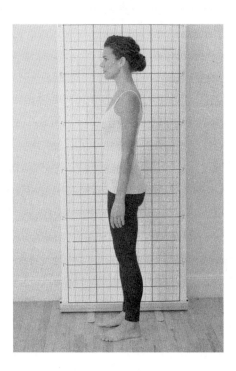

Sitting Tall Is Good Posture

When we sit well, we are also allowing for good spinal support and reducing compression on our diaphragm and internal organs. This is important for keeping oxygen circulating and good blood flow throughout the body during pregnancy.

Feet: Keep both feet on the floor. Avoid crossing your legs.

Hips/Pelvis: Rock pelvis forward and back over your sits bones (the two prominent bones at the bottom of your pelvis that you can feel by putting your hands under your buttocks). Find the center point of this pelvic motion, which should be toward the center, or slightly at the front half, of your sits bones. Your thigh-torso angle should be between 95 to 110 degrees (an obtuse angle when looking at yourself from the side).

Low Back: Maintain a C curve as described in standing section. You can use a sweater or pillow to support your spine if necessary.

Continue with same centering movements from Standing for the Midback, Shoulders, and Head/Neck: You can use a sweater or a pillow scrunched up against your back to support this position, with it extending down to support your lower back up to the shoulder blades. Always grow tall from the crown of the head and breathe through the diaphragm by expanding and deflating the back and sides of the lower ribs.

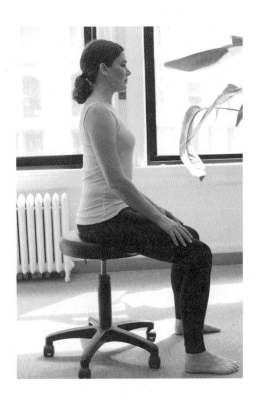

Posture and Your Devices

It is very important that we practice good posture when using electronic devices. Always bring devices like phones up to eye level, instead of looking down at them or holding them by your chest or stomach.

The First Trimester Exercise Routine

Thirty Minutes of Aerobics

You will be exercising aerobically every day at a moderate, comfortable level. You should be able to talk while exercising without losing your breath. In fact, we want you to exercise at a slightly lower intensity than during the preconception phase, especially if you live in a hot climate or during hot summer months. The goal is to maintain a normal body temperature. During early pregnancy, it's difficult to regulate your body temperature, and an elevated body temperature, known as *hyperthermia*, is not good for the baby. We want you to keep your core temperature below 38 degrees Celsius, or 100.4 degrees Fahrenheit at all times, including during exercise. Easy ways to keep your body heat down during exercise are to wear appropriate clothing and make sure that you continue to drink plenty of water. Choose cooler clothing and dress in layers that can be easily shed. If you like baths, warm or tepid water is fine; hot tubs, saunas, and even hot showers and tubs are not recommended.

Every day, you will be walking for at least thirty minutes. If you don't like walking, choose an aerobic activity that you enjoy, whether it's riding a bike or taking an exercise or dance class. Just make sure to keep the exertion at a moderate rate for between thirty to sixty minutes, and practice proper breathing using your diaphragm because you're likely to unconsciously shift the breath to your chest and shoulders. As you are getting your heart rate up, breathe through the sides and back of the lower ribs as much as possible.

Exercising aerobically for at least thirty minutes a day is not a random time commitment: this is the exact amount of time it takes to optimize *neuroplasticity*, the healthy development of new brain cells. With enhanced cellular turnover, pregnant women can reset their mind, improve mood, enhance learning, have more energy, and improve circulation, all of which benefit both you and your baby. Keep joyful thoughts and enjoy this special time that's meant to be just for you. Listen to your favorite music while you are exercising to lower stress and bring you joy.

Exercise Equipment You'll Need:

- Bed or bench
- Hardcover book (three inches thick) or yoga block
- Firm chair
- Physioball (optional)
- Large towel or yoga mat
- Medium resistance band
- Pillows (two)
- Small towel
- Tennis ball

Twenty Minutes of Eccentric Strengthening

The following exercises provide a comprehensive program that will take approximately twenty minutes a day to complete. These exercises can be done before your aerobic routine, or at a totally different time of day.

You may not feel tired or sore when you do these exercises. Instead, you'll feel lifted and, over time, toned. Stay mindful throughout the exercise: you will be asked to conjure an image in your mind that relates to the movement or a certain feeling in your body. This image alone will not produce a movement but will help you activate the targeted muscle group. For example, a common instruction is "grow tall from the crown of your head." Here, we're asking you to imagine that a string is pulling the crown of your head, and therefore your body, toward the ceiling. The result is that you will feel lengthened and supported with better posture. The deep abdominals, spinal stabilizers, and even the deep hip supportive muscle groups will all activate.

As you move through these exercises, pay attention to how your body reacts as you enter and exit different positions. When your body tells you to stop, stop. The joints of your lower back and pelvis should not click when you exercise (or move, for that matter!). If any of these exercises causes discomfort, stop and consult with your doctor or physical therapist.

Continue with these preconception exercises from Part I throughout the first trimester as well: Transversus Abdominis Activation and Marching, Transversus Abdominis Toe Taps and Knee Extensions (if you still can do this comfortably with no movement at your spine and pelvis), Kegels with Resting Squats, Glute Bridges, and Foot Doming (see pages 62–71).

How to Use Resistance Bands

Resistance bands are safer than weights, which can cause nerve pressure when you are pulling down on your upper body while holding them in your hands. Bands allow you to control the eccentric portion of an exercise because you control the resistance band coming back to the start position, so it doesn't snap back. This is an excellent way to strengthen through a greater range of motion and facilitate muscles that control movement (stabilizing muscles) together with the muscles that move (the superficial movers of the joints).

There are many companies that sell resistance bands, loops, and tubes. For more versatility, use a regular resistance band, but tubing or handle attachments are fine. If you purchase a set, get three: a light, medium, and heavy resistance and use the first three levels of resistance in the series, from lightest to heaviest.

Make sure you can complete each exercise's full range of movement with a sensation of a mild tug. You should feel your muscles working by the seventh rep. If you feel like the exercise is becoming difficult before seven reps, the band may be too taut, and you need to put some more length/slack in it, or you need an easier resistance band. If you don't feel much work by the seventh rep, it is too easy, and you may need to use a band with more resistance or shorten the band.

Exercise: Seated Trunk Rotations
[Thoracic Core]

EQUIPMENT: A firm chair, or for more challenge you can sit on a physioball.

PURPOSE: To strengthen the deep spinal muscles of the midback for improved posture and support throughout your body.

START POSITION: Sit tall on the edge of your chair. Keep your arms by your sides, with palms facing your legs or on your lap with palms facing up.

SEQUENCE:

STEP 1. Imagine a pole on your back from your head to your low back. Elongate your neck as if a string is pulling you up from the crown of your head, with your chin relaxed down so your eyes are level with the horizon. Smoothly rotate your head and chest to the right, as if you were rotating around this imaginary pole. You are simply rotating your body so that your chest faces to the right. Make sure you are keeping your body weight even on both buttocks, that you are tall through the sides of your body, and that you are not leaning or bending to the side.

STEP 2. Rotate back to center and repeat on your left. Maintain this lifting feeling from the crown of your head the whole time.

STEP 3. Perform 10 to 15 reps while breathing comfortably. Each rep is moving to the right, center and left, center.

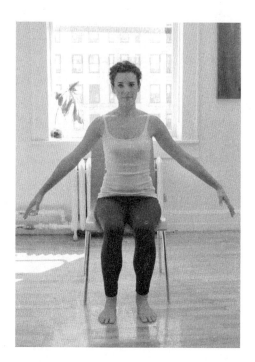 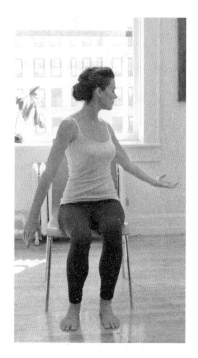

Exercise: Seated or Standing Ballet Arm Series

EQUIPMENT: A chair (optional).

PURPOSE: To strengthen arms, shoulders, and shoulder blades and to elongate the trunk [Thoracic Core].

START POSITION: Stand or sit tall on the edge of a firm chair, with heels together, toes slightly apart, and arms comfortably by your sides.

SEQUENCE:

STEP 1. Grow tall from the crown of your head, with chin relaxed down as you look straight ahead. Breathe in and gently lift your arms out in front of your chest.

STEP 2. Keep the left arm in this position, breathe in as you lift the right arm above your head, and then return to chest level on your exhale and repeat with other side. Do this until you fatigue, or perform 2 sets of 10 reps, at a slow tempo. You may look up at your lifted arm if it is comfortable; if it isn't, look straight ahead. Make sure your shoulder blades stay lifted up and back the whole time, the elbows are lifted, and that the sides of your body feel long. Take a few diaphragm breaths as a break before the next step.

STEP 3. Return to your tall, lifted, seated (or standing) posture. Slowly lift the arms with elbows higher than your hands through the middle of your trunk and continue to lift the arms so that both arms end with hands above the head.

STEP 4. Gently open the arms out to the side to make a right angle with palms facing up, then rotate the right arm by lifting the elbows upward so that your palms now face the floor. Gently pulse the arm in a lift (elbow up), and lower the arm slowly by your side. Repeat with left arm. You may do this sequence with one arm at a time or both together, if tolerated. Repeat this arm sequence 10 times or until you feel fatigue in shoulder and arm muscles.

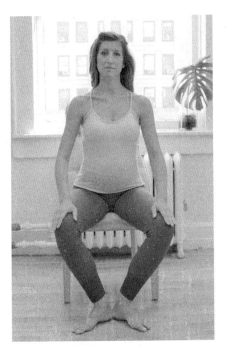
Step 1A

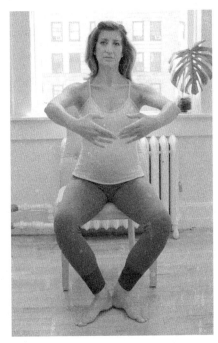
Step 1B

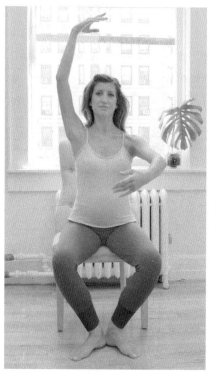

Step 2A

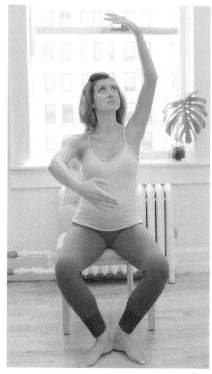

Step 2B

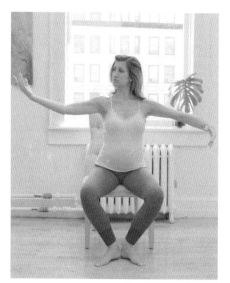

Step 4A

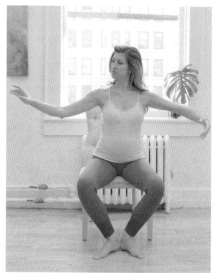

Step 4B

Exercise: Pelvic Rotation on Hands and Knees [Lumbar Core]

EQUIPMENT: A bed or a bench.

PURPOSE: This exercise activates and strengthens the deep muscles—*gluteus medius, lumbar multifidus*—that help support the hips and pelvis as the pelvis widens with pregnancy.

START POSITION: Start on hands and knees with your feet hanging over the end of your bed or bench. Move to the left edge and let your left leg dangle off the side. Use both hands and right knee to support you. If this position is uncomfortable, do the seated version below.

SEQUENCE:

STEP 1. Press your weight into your right knee and rotate your pelvis so that your belly button faces left, away from the right leg. Keep the left leg and pelvis relaxed; do not use the left side at all. Keep your belly/abdomen, low back, and front of right thigh relaxed. Feel the work in the deep muscle on the side of the right hip.

STEP 2. Slowly relax and return to the start position. Perform these slow pelvic rotations until you feel fatigue (at least 8 reps) in the side gluteal muscles while breathing continuously.

STEP 3. Move to the other side of the bed and repeat with the right leg hanging off the bed.

If you do NOT feel the side of the gluteals working, stop and move on to the next exercise instead.

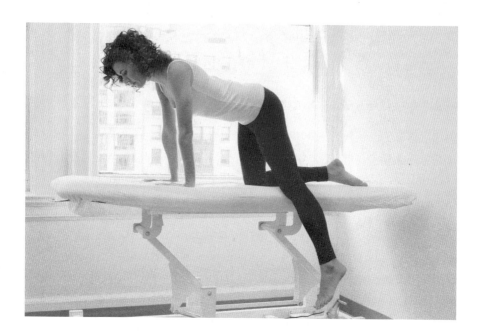

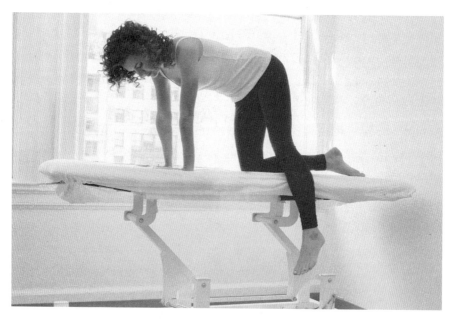

Exercise: Seated Hip Rotator Strengthening [Lumbar Core]

EQUIPMENT: A firm chair, a tennis ball, a medium resistance band.

PURPOSE: This exercise activates and strengthens the deep muscles (*gluteus medius, lumbar multifidus*) that help support the hips and pelvis as the pelvis widens with pregnancy. This exercise activates the muscle without movement, but a tiny bit of movement is okay. If you feel appropriate activation on the previous exercise (Pelvic Rotation on Hands and Knees), then you can skip this exercise and move on to the next.

START POSITION: Sit tall on the very edge of a chair with the resistance band around your thighs and a tennis ball between your heels. Toes should be pointed out and knees apart, about 12 inches.

SEQUENCE:

STEP 1. Gently squeeze both heels into the ball, feeling the work in the deep muscles under your buttocks. You should not feel anything at the front of your hips or thighs.

STEP 2. Exhale, keep the ball pressure between the heels, and gently rotate the thighs outward into the resistance band. Your effort meets the resistance of the band, so there will be no movement.

STEP 3. Perform a 10-second hold, then rest and repeat 10 times.

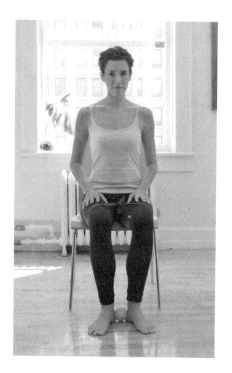
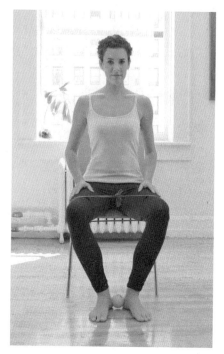

Exercise: Squat/Chair Pose
[All Cores]

PURPOSE: To strengthen legs, neck, and midback for more elongation in your body.

START POSITION: Stand tall with feet pointing straight ahead and close to one another.

SEQUENCE:

STEP 1. Gently bend your knees like you are sitting back into a chair and bow forward with a flat back. Keep your chin tucked into your chest (elongating the back of your neck) as you keep your gaze on the floor out about 2 to 3 feet in front of you. Raise both arms so that your arms are in-line with your ears. Reach your arms out away from your tailbone and your tailbone away from

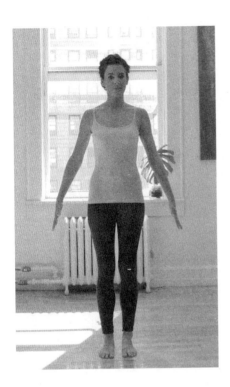
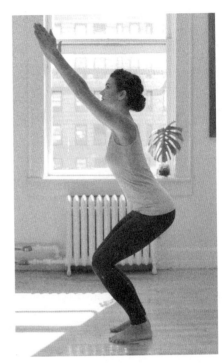

your arms. Feel an energy pulling the crown of your head up and out as well. This will activate multiple muscles that keep you elongated.

STEP 2. Hold this pose for 10 to 20 seconds as tolerated and perform 3 to 5 repetitions.

Exercise: Standing Rotator Cuff with Resistance Band [Thoracic Core]

EQUIPMENT: A medium resistance band, a chair.

PURPOSE: To strengthen the shoulders and shoulder blades.

START POSITION: Stand with softly bent knees, or sit tall in a chair. Hold the resistance band in both hands with your elbows bent 90 degrees.

SEQUENCE:

STEP 1. Keep your shoulders lifted up and back, elbows away from your sides. Pull band apart with both arms as you exhale, keeping your wrists still and straight. Shoulder blades will come together in the back.

STEP 2. Continue to breathe as you hold the position for 5 seconds, then control back to center and repeat 10 times, 2 sets.

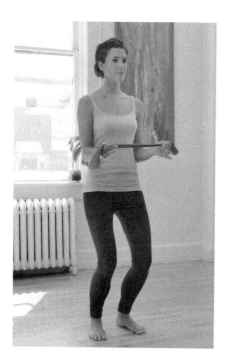 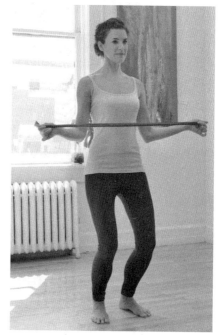

Exercise: Sling Squat (Heel Raises with Knees Bent)

EQUIPMENT: A sturdy chair (optional).

PURPOSE: To strengthen and gain control in the stabilizing muscles of the feet and ankles. The exercise will strengthen the calves to support good standing posture.

START POSITION: Stand tall with shoulders lifted up and back and neck elongated as if a string was pulling up through the crown of your head. You may hold onto a sturdy chair for help with your balance.

SEQUENCE:

STEP 1. Bend your knees 30 degrees, as if your back was up against a wall. Keep the knees tracking in front of your second toes.

STEP 2. Keeping knees bent the whole time, lift and lower your heels with control. Keep your arches over the center of the foot with your ankles in a neutral position. If you find that your arches or feet are rolling outward or that you are wobbling, hold the chair and don't come up as high. Lowering with control is the key part of this exercise.

STEP 3. Maintain good posture and breathe diaphragmatically and consistently throughout the exercise. Repeat 10 slow reps, 1 to 2 sets.

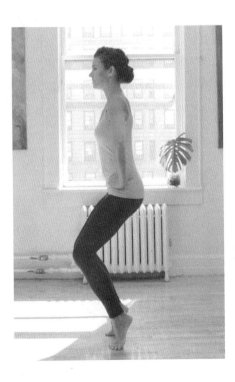

Exercise: Warrior II into Side Angle Pose

PURPOSE: To open the chest, lengthen the side of the body, and work the hip muscles [Thoracic and Lumbar Cores].

START POSITION: Stand tall and take a lunge forward with the right leg.

SEQUENCE:

STEP 1. Bend front knee so that the right knee is at a 90-degree angle over your right foot in-line with the second toe. Your back leg should be straight, and both heels should be in-line with each other with the back foot toes slightly pointing in, and the heel pointed out. Arms should be outstretched with one arm in front of you at shoulder level and the other out over your back leg. Both palms should be facedown to the floor.

STEP 2. Place your front hand in-line with your second finger. Reach outward with both arms and feel your feet pressing into the floor. You will feel the pressure of your front hip and thigh rotating outward and your legs coming toward one another, even though you are not moving. Pull up through the center of your body; your lumbar/abdominal core will naturally activate. You're going to feel the abdominal muscles working. Maintain this pose for 3 breaths and then release.

STEP 3. Slowly lean your right elbow and forearm on your right thigh. Extend your left arm to the sky with palm facing forward. Look up toward your left arm, but if your neck is uncomfortable, keep your neck in-line with your right thigh. Continue to engage the right thigh rotating outward. Activate the sensation of your feet coming together without actually moving. This will ground your lower body. Breathe into the left side of the body for 3 breaths.

STEP 4. Slowly come back up, straighten both legs for a break.

STEP 5. Repeat the sequence 2 more times on the right, and then perform the same sequence 3 times with the left leg.

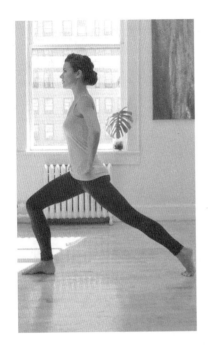

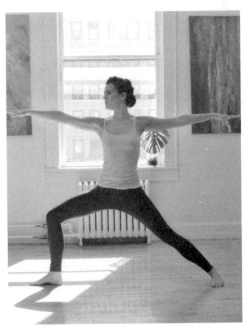

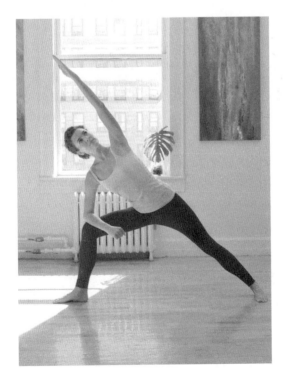

Exercise: Sun Salutation into Modified Half Moon Pose

PURPOSE: To improve balance and open the chest, lengthen leg muscles, strengthen the cores and hips [All Cores].

EQUIPMENT: A yoga block or 3-inch-thick hardcover book.

START POSITION: Place yoga block or book in front of you on the floor. Stand tall with feet close together and your arms by your sides.

SEQUENCE:

STEP 1. Inhale and reach arms up and over your head. Either touch them together or keep them apart above your head. You may gaze upward to follow your hands above your head. Exhale and release them back down by your sides. If this movement is restricted, only go as high as you feel comfortable. You can remain looking straight ahead if looking up is difficult.

STEP 2. On your exhale, bend your right knee and transfer your weight to place your right hand on the block/book in front of you. Slowly straighten the right knee in comfortable range, as you lift your left leg behind you, making a straight line. Open the left arm and reach to the ceiling. Tuck your chin slightly and look straight ahead, feeling the energetic pull from the crown of your head outward. As you hold this position, keep lengthening the left leg, reaching your heel out behind you. Your left arm reaches farther to the ceiling and your right shoulder is lifted away from the block. Hold for 3 breaths. Bend both knees and come back to center.

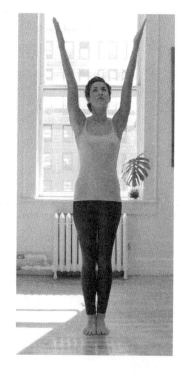

STEP 3. Repeat switching sides, going through this sequence 2 to 3 times on each side. Each time you repeat the Sun Salutation movement, reach higher up to the ceiling with energy flowing out your fingertips.

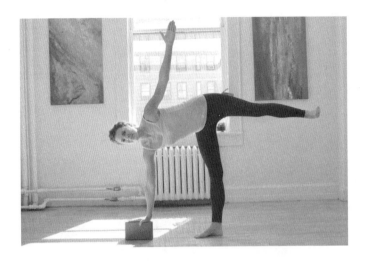

No More Sit-Ups

Stop doing sit-ups or double leg lifts while lying on your back. These exercises strain the central seam of the abdomen, which will get very stressed later in pregnancy. These exercises may actually leave you feeling unsupported or, worse, contribute to diastasis.

The Wise Woman's Pregnancy Stretching Program

Stretches keep good circulation and flow in the body, which allows us to feel more flexible throughout. Try each of these either as a sequence after you complete the previous exercises or before bed. You will be directed to come back to this specific stretching program section throughout your pregnancy. If any of the stretches do not feel good at any point, go into a smaller range of motion or just stop completely.

Quads Stretch

EQUIPMENT: A chair, a towel.

START POSITION: Stand tall with your left hand on the back of a chair (or wall). Bend your right knee, grab your shin with your right hand if comfortable, or wrap a hand towel around your shin and hold the ends of the towel with your right hand.

SEQUENCE:

STEP 1. Gently bend the right knee, bringing your heel closer to your buttocks by pulling on your shin. Keep both thighs in-line with each other throughout the stretch. Stop bending the knee when you feel the stretch at the front of your right thigh. You can intensify the stretch by tucking your pelvis under, which moves your tailbone forward. Breathe diaphragmatically and consistently throughout.

STEP 2. Hold for 30 seconds.

STEP 3. Repeat 1 to 2 sets and then switch to your left side.

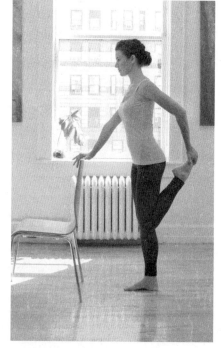

Calves Stretch

EQUIPMENT: A chair.

START POSITION: Stand tall and lunge forward with your left leg. Keep your left knee bent and your right leg straight with your heel down on the floor. Hold onto the wall or a sturdy chair in front of you.

SEQUENCE:

STEP 1. Slide your back heel so that your toes point slightly in and your heel points out. Bend the front knee as much as you can before your back heel lifts. You should feel the stretch in the right (back) calf.

STEP 2. Gently raise and lower your right (back) heel to go in and out of the stretch. Repeat 10 times, and hold the final stretch with heel down on the floor for 30 seconds. Breathe diaphragmatically and consistently throughout.

STEP 3. Repeat on the left.

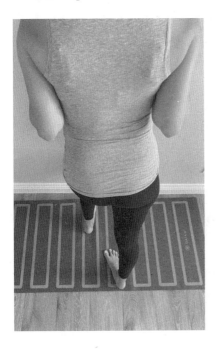
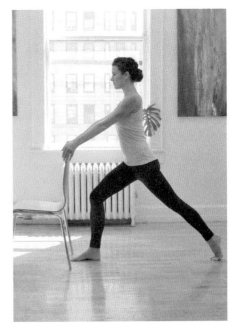

Hamstring Stretch

EQUIPMENT: A chair.

START POSITION: Stand tall and hold onto the wall, bannister, or a table for support with either hand.

SEQUENCE:

STEP 1. Place your right leg on a chair or step in front of you. Keeping your back flat, bow forward, creasing the front of your right hip as you lift your buttocks behind you. Stop stretching forward when you feel the stretch in the hamstring at the back of your right thigh.

STEP 2. Hold for 30 seconds and then release. Complete 1 to 2 sets and then switch to your left side. Breathe diaphragmatically and consistently throughout.

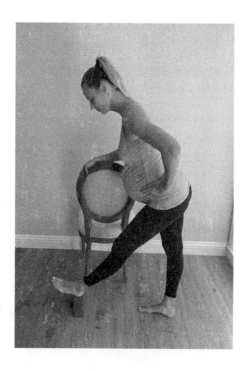

Plantar Fascia Stretch

EQUIPMENT: A wall.

START POSITION: Stand tall and hold onto the wall with both hands for support in front of you.

SEQUENCE:

STEP 1. Place your right toes on the wall with your heel on the floor. The left leg should be one foot width behind you, allowing you to stand comfortably.

STEP 2. You will feel a stretch under your foot. If you don't, lean your body toward the wall. Hold for 30 seconds and then release. Complete 1 to 2 sets and then switch to your left side. Breathe diaphragmatically and consistently throughout.

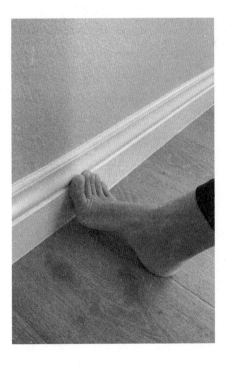

Back of the Shoulder and Triceps Stretch

START POSITION: Stand tall with feet shoulder width apart.

SEQUENCE:

STEP 1. Bring your right arm across your chest and support your upper arm with your left hand. Keep the right arm close to your body.

STEP 2. You will feel a stretch in the back of your shoulder and down to your tricep muscle (back of the arm muscle). Hold for 30 seconds and then release. Repeat on the other side. Complete 1 to 2 times on each side. Breathe diaphragmatically and consistently throughout.

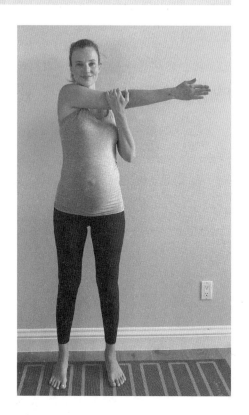

Pec Stretch

EQUIPMENT: A wall.

START POSITION: Stand tall and place left forearm and hand on the wall in a doorway.

SEQUENCE:

STEP 1. Take a comfortable lunge forward with your left leg through the doorway space in front of you. Let your body come forward so that the left elbow is slightly behind you now. *The further along in the pregnancy you are, the smaller the lunge and this body movement should be due to pelvic laxity and breast tenderness.* You will feel this stretch in the front of your chest. Hold for 30 seconds on each side. Breathe diaphragmatically throughout.

STEP 2. You can target another part of the pectoral muscle that tends to get very tight. Resume the same position as in Step 1, but this time angle your body away from the wall and still lean somewhat forward. Only stay in a tolerable range of motion. If this is not tolerable, just do another set of Step 1 instead. Hold for 30 seconds and then release and repeat with the other side. Breathe diaphragmatically and consistently throughout.

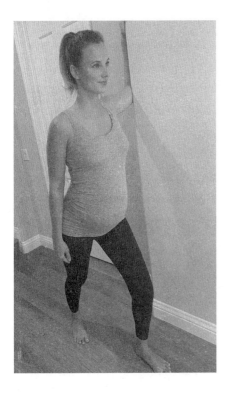
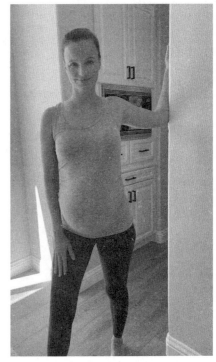

Leg Swings for Release

EQUIPMENT: A wall or sturdy chair and a step stool or step or yoga block.

START POSITION: Stand tall, hold a wall or chair, with one foot on a step and the other dangling off to the side, relaxed.

SEQUENCE:

STEP 1. Gently let your leg dangle and swing forward and backward freely. Similar to a regular swing, effortlessly let the hip and leg move as low or as high as they feel comfortable. Use momentum, but do not control the swinging leg.

STEP 2. Do this for 30 to 60 seconds and then take a break and repeat with the other side. Breathe diaphragmatically and consistently throughout.

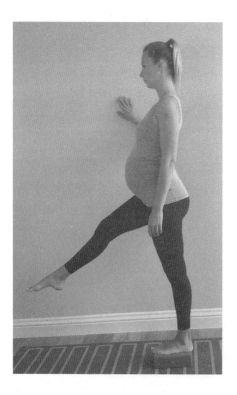
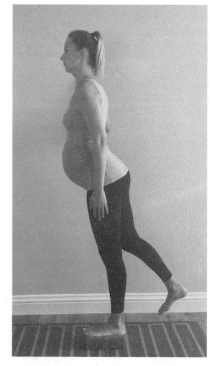

Hip Rotators/Piriformis Stretch

EQUIPMENT: A chair.

START POSITION: Sit tall at the edge of a chair. Lift your right ankle and bring it to the top of your left thigh, allowing your right knee to bend as you open your hip in an externally rotated position.

SEQUENCE:

STEP 1. Put your hands on your right ankle and right knee to stabilize them. Bow forward with a flat back over your thigh until you feel the stretch in your right buttock. Do not overstretch this area because you can make the nerves in the area sensitive.

STEP 2. Hold for 30 seconds and then release. Complete 1 to 2 sets and then switch to your left side. Breathe diaphragmatically and consistently throughout.

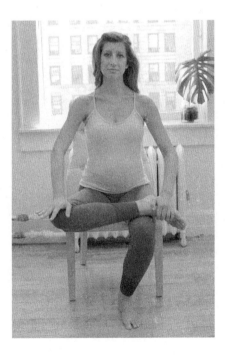

Hip Flexor Stretch

EQUIPMENT: A blanket or towel.

START POSITION: Get into a hands and knees position on a floor or mat.

SEQUENCE:

STEP 1. Keep your left knee and hands on the ground and extend your right leg behind you on the floor. Allow your pelvis to drop down to the floor and your body weight to shift backward as your left knee swings out into a turned-out L position in front of you. You may use a folded blanket or towel under your left hip for support.

STEP 2. You will feel a stretch in the front of your right thigh/hip. Hold for 30 seconds and then release. Repeat on the other side. Complete 1 to 2 sets, breathing diaphragmatically and consistently throughout.

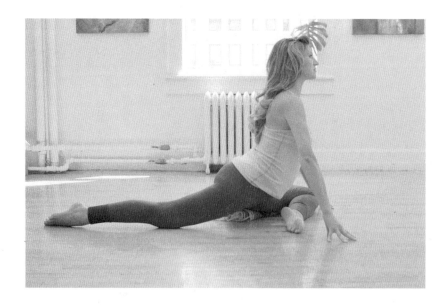

Inner Thigh Stretch

START POSITION: Bend down to put your hands on the floor, keeping toes on the floor and heels lifted, as in a crouched position.

SEQUENCE:

STEP 1. Keep your weight on your hands and extend your right knee out to the side. Your weight should be distributed evenly on your hands and your left toes.

STEP 2. You will feel a stretch along the inner part of the right thigh. Hold for 30 seconds and then release. Repeat on the other side. Complete 1 to 2 sets, breathing diaphragmatically throughout.

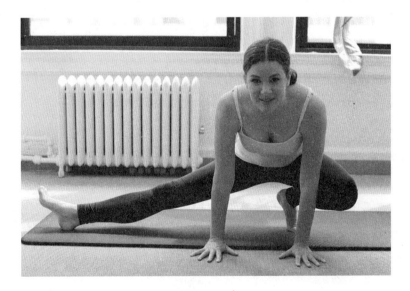

Exercise: Child's Pose

EQUIPMENT: A towel or mat, or your bed.

START POSITION: Get onto hands and knees on a towel/mat on the floor or on your bed.

SEQUENCE:

STEP 1. Gently sit back so your buttocks reach down to your heels with knees apart. Extend both arms forward resting on the surface in front of you. Place your forehead on the floor or bed. As your belly grows, you will need to separate your knees farther.

STEP 2. Breathe into the back and sides of your lower ribs, relax your body and hips, as you hold this position for 5 breaths.

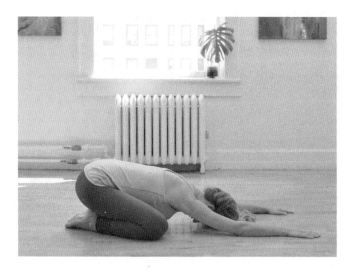

Exercise: Cat/Cow

EQUIPMENT: A towel or mat on the floor, or your bed.

START POSITION: Get onto hands and knees on a towel/mat on the floor or on your bed.

SEQUENCE:

STEP 1. Exhale and gently round your back, letting your head hang down in a relaxed fashion.

STEP 2. As you inhale, let your back sag downward as you lift your gaze, creating a C curve with your spine. Do this in a relaxed fashion; do not put tension in your spine.

STEP 3. Perform 10 reps slowly, coordinating your breath with the sequences.

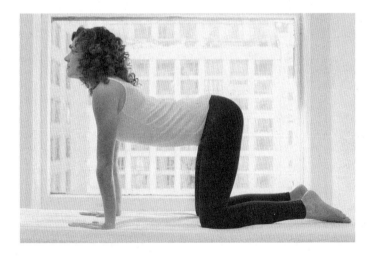

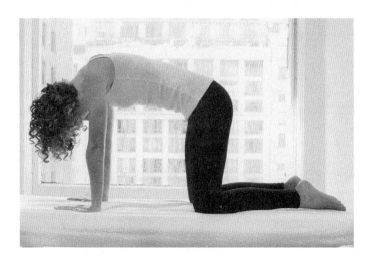

Exercise: Book Opening

EQUIPMENT: Bed, or on the floor with a towel or mat; 2 pillows.

START POSITION: Lie on your left side with a pillow under your head and the second one wedged between both knees. Place both arms straight in front of you with right hand over the left, in-line with your chest.

SEQUENCE:

STEP 1. Open right arm up and back and allow your head to turn to look at your right arm. Keep your right hip still, lined up over your left hip. Only your midback and head rotate as you open up the right arm behind you. Do not lift your head, and only turn it as far as it is comfortable. You will feel a stretch in the front of the chest and a release in your midback as you rotate.

STEP 2. Hold this position for 3 breaths and then return to the starting position. Repeat 5 times, then turn onto the other side and repeat.

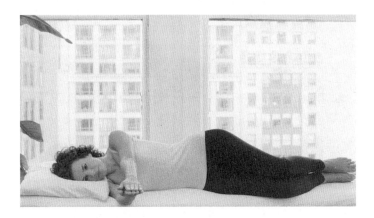

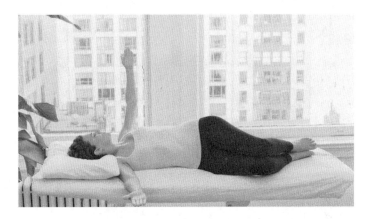

Exercise: Happy Baby

EQUIPMENT: A bed or a mat on the floor; a belt or towel.

PURPOSE: To relax the hips, lengthen the back and inner thighs, and provide support for the pelvis. The stable position of the pelvis is in a posterior rotation/tilt position where the bones "lock in place" better. This exercise helps guide the pelvis to relax into its supported position and often gets rid of muscular tension that prevents it from happening.

START POSITION: Lie on the floor or your bed with both knees bent, feet on the surface, and a small pillow under your head if you like.

SEQUENCE:

STEP 1. Exhale, hug your right knee toward your shoulder, and support it with your right hand, or forearm/elbow, followed by your left.

STEP 2. Grab hold of the outside of your feet with your hands, keeping both knees out wide so knees are in-line with the side of your body. Stay in a range of motion that feels comfortable. If this position is too extreme for you, you can use a towel or belt to help anchor your feet for pelvic and leg support.

STEP 3. Hold this position as you breathe into the diaphragm (back and sides of the lower ribs) for 5 breaths. With each breath, allow for the front of the hips to soften and fold as the pelvis resets in its stable position of rolling backward (posterior tilt). You can repeat this 2 times or more as you need.

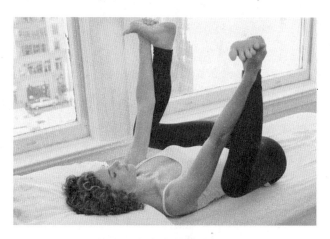

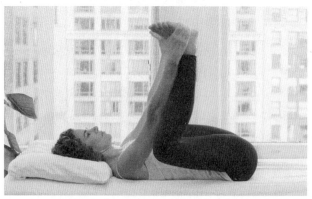

NOURISHMENT

We're not going to sugarcoat it: in the first trimester, eating may very well be challenging. Many wise women are tired or nauseous, or both. However, you can—and should—continue to make good food choices. Some of the foods we recommend for the next three months will be beneficial to you; others are going to amplify the health of your baby.

The easiest way to make good choices is to have the right foods on hand. In order to do that, have a plan. Stock up your home and place of work so that you don't have to scramble when you aren't feeling well. Meal prep for the week ahead, and get your partner involved. Nothing says support more than having someone else do the cooking!

What to Eat During the First Trimester

Your diet is the only source of nutrition for your developing baby. If you don't get a variety of key nutrients, your baby is at risk for developmental delays, birth defects, and cognitive deficits. For instance, protein is one of several essential nutritional requirements during pregnancy because amino acids are needed for your baby's bone, tissue, and musculoskeletal development. It also is important for placental growth and is needed for the increase in red blood cells you will be creating during pregnancy. If you are a vegan or vegetarian, you will have to supplement with vitamin B12 because you can only get this vitamin in your diet from animal proteins.

If you eat enough food high in protein, essential fats, and vitamins and minerals during pregnancy, you are more likely to give birth to a full-term baby who has a healthy birth weight, both of which are markers of future health and development.[15] However, an excess of nutrients can influence your baby's propensity to be overweight throughout their lifetime, possibly developing the chronic illnesses that are associated with it, like diabetes and heart disease. This is another important reason to maintain but not exceed a healthy weight gain.

Throughout your pregnancy, we want you to enjoy pro-immunity, anti-inflammatory foods, including all of the suggestions we outlined in the pre-conception section. You will be eating foods high in omega-3s, like olive oil and wild salmon, as they are packed with nutrients that are excellent for your baby's brain development. The fish has to be caught wild in order to get those benefits; conventionally farmed fish just doesn't have it.

We also we want you to focus on warming foods like soups and stews, which are easy to digest, instead of raw vegetables and salads. In fact, traditional Chinese medicine warns against eating cold or raw foods during the first trimester because of potential contamination. Plants that grow above ground can also have chemical residues that are unhealthy for the baby. Choose vegetables that are organic, thoroughly washed, and in season, and cook them—they could be steamed, sauteed, baked, or roasted. Because warming foods are easier to digest, you'll have less constipation.

Another principle of Chinese medicine is that there are times in the life cycle when you want heat in the body and times when you want to keep the body cool. Pregnancy is a time when you want to keep the body warm, which is why we recommend avoiding dairy products that cool the body, like a glass of milk or ice cream.

Choose organic fruits that are in season whenever possible. If buying conventionally grown, check out the Environmental Working Group's Dirty Dozen for the produce that is most contaminated (like strawberries), which you should avoid, and their Clean Fifteen that are the least contaminated (like avocadoes). We recommend cleaning your produce with an organic fruit/veggie wash.

At least twice, possibly three times a day, include proteins in a meal. It doesn't matter if you choose fish, meat, poultry, or vegetarian options like beans. Protein is necessary for all cellular development, and now it is essential as you are nourishing new cellular activity.

We also want you to choose foods that support a healthy gut microbiome, as outlined in the preconception section, as we now understand how your microbiome affects your baby's health. We used to believe that the mother's beneficial bacteria could only be transferred to the baby during a vaginal delivery, but the latest research shows that the mother's gut microbiome has an even greater influence during fetal life. Research beginning in 2008 shows that the beneficial bacteria in the mother's microbiome is transferred to the fetus via the placenta.[16] These findings turn one important theory of pregnancy and childbirth on its head. If the microbiome is transferred from mother to baby via the placenta as well as the vagina during birth, and the breasts during breastfeeding, babies delivered via C-section will still receive plenty of the beneficial bacteria. One less thing to worry about!

However, if your gut isn't functioning appropriately, then you're not going to be able to absorb the nutrition you're taking in to nourish your baby. That's another reason why we recommend that you continue to focus on gluten-free, anti-inflammatory foods and nutrients, just like in preconception.

Beat Nausea with Good Food

Doctors often recommend that the best way to alleviate nausea is to follow the same advice for avoiding digestive issues: eat small, frequent meals.[17] We agree with this idea. However, some doctors also advise women to "follow their cravings" and eat lots of carbs or sugary treats to alleviate nausea, but we do not support this recommendation.

The desire for these types of foods is inherent to pregnancy and has an evolutionary basis: women are driven to gain weight in the first trimester in order to develop the caloric reserves needed to feed and nourish their baby, and lots of carbs equals lots of calories. Newly pregnant women are also drawn to foods high in carbs rather than fat because fatty foods slow down digestion, which is making them feel nauseated in the first place. Before the Industrial Revolution, this strategy wouldn't have been terrible because women would have met their carb cravings with fruit. They didn't have access to the ultra-processed, high-glycemic, gluten-filled food options that are now readily available, like cookies, crackers, or chips. So while crackers seem like the right choice to alleviate nausea, all that gluten only exacerbates inflammation and negatively affects your gut's microbiome, which to some extent you are also sharing with your baby.

What's more, studies have shown that protein-rich meals are actually more likely to alleviate nausea as compared to carbohydrate-rich or high fat meals,[18] which is why we suggest adding more protein to your snacks or meals whenever possible. This alone may address your nausea. Try hummus, avocado, cooked fish, and animal protein sources that you can tolerate. If you find that you really do better with carbs, choose gluten-free choices that are not inflammatory, like fruits or vegetables. Dried fruit is also a reasonable option: even though it has a lot more sugar than regular fruit, it's better than eating a bag of chips. Nuts are not a good choice because they are high in fat and therefore difficult to digest.

The best way to beat nausea is to have the right foods on hand:

- Pack healthy snacks like fresh fruit, including bananas and oranges, gluten-free crackers, or pumpkin seeds.
- Ginger can block the sensation of nausea.[19] You can supplement with ginger tablets, add fresh ginger to your meals, or drink ginger teas.
- Sucking on a slice of lemon when you're feeling nauseous can suppress queasiness.

- Satisfy your carb cravings with nutrient-rich options. Trade rice for quinoa, which is less binding and easier to digest. If you are craving pasta, look for rice noodles, quinoa noodles, or red lentil noodles.
- Separate drinking fluids from when you are eating solid foods: sometimes, drinking and eating at the same time makes you feel full faster, which leads to nausea.

We Can't Say This Enough: Stay Hydrated

Create your own flavored, room-temperature water by adding fresh fruits to make staying hydrated more palatable. If that is not enough, add a splash of organic fruit juice without added sugar. Some women, like Patricia, have an aversion to water during pregnancy. However, Patricia found that one particular brand, Mountain Valley Spring, which is a pH balanced water that's high in minerals, didn't pose a problem. Keep trying different options (preferably not in plastic bottles) until you find one that works for you.

You can also enjoy an unlimited amount of warming decaffeinated liquids, like teas and broths. Herbal teas contain lots of important anti-inflammatory nutrients, and broths, including miso soup and chicken soup, are also immune system enhancers.

Keep the temperature of your beverages in the warm range. Avoid adding ice to beverages and drinking very hot liquids. This practice conserves your energy and keeps your body balanced.

Follow Your Hereditary Diet

We believe our bodies develop based on the foods we are introduced to early in life. In essence, we are wired to process certain foods better than others. And while the ultimate goal for eating during the first trimester is to continue to eat an anti-inflammatory diet, we have found that people respond to the same foods in a variety of ways. In our experience, we have seen that when you follow a diet that is similar to your ancestors, it will have the least inflammatory results.

Look at the foods that your ancestry is linked to, and see if you tolerate those well. For instance, if your ancestors are from a part of the world where they grow plantains, you might be able to tolerate them better than bananas during the first trimester. If potatoes aren't grown where your family is from, then potatoes might be more inflammatory to your system compared to someone of Irish heritage.

If you don't know enough about your ancestry or if you are really unsure about where certain foods come from, you can check what your microbiome has more affinity toward digesting, and what has less likelihood of inflammation or negative effects. Viome's home stool-testing kit we discussed during preconception can identify your gut's microbiome and then create a personalized diet that is best suited for your individual needs.

First Trimester Avoidance Policy

Your doctor may tell you to avoid certain foods and substances because they contain toxins or can be contaminated with bacteria and parasites that can have adverse health effects on both mother and baby. These include

1. Alcohol
2. Caffeine
3. Cigarettes
4. Genetically Modified Foods (GMOs): Watch for new labeling! Some are now stickered with "bio-fortified."
5. High-mercury fish (tuna, shark, swordfish, king mackerel)
6. Organ meats
7. Processed foods
8. Raw eggs
9. Soft cheeses

10. Undercooked or raw fish and shellfish
11. Undercooked, raw, and processed meats
12. Unpasteurized milk, cheese, or fruit juices

The Difference Between Processed Foods and Ultra-Processed Foods

Even if you make all your food at home from scratch, some processed food is unavoidable. In fact, there are degrees of processed foods that are not only acceptable, they are advantageous. Minimal processing cleans fruits, vegetables, fish, poultry, and meats. It removes inedible parts like the outer skin of a coffee bean. Certain processing features include refrigerating, freezing, fermenting, pasteurizing, and vacuum packaging. Most cooking oils pressed from nuts, olives, or seeds are also minimally processed.

Ultra-processed foods are the ones we really want you to avoid because they almost always contain additives, artificial colors, preservatives, and lots of sugar, salt, and fat but very little nutrition. Ultra-processed foods, even organic or vegan options, often contain ingredients with unrecognizable names that you wouldn't find on a farm. They include artificial colors and flavors, preservatives, and ingredients, such as emulsifiers, meant to make the look or texture of the food more appealing. During the first trimester, and really, throughout your pregnancy, avoid

- Ready-made snacks, cookies, and cakes
- Bottled or canned soft drinks, sweetened teas, or juices
- Boxed cereals
- Luncheon meats
- Store-bought frozen prepared meals

Listen to Your Body: Food Sensitivities

If your obstetrician tells you to increase dairy consumption in the first trimester because it's high in calcium that's good for your baby, but you know that you're sensitive to dairy, eating more of it is not doing you or your baby any favors. First, discuss any food sensitivities you have with your doctor, and you can work together to find the best nutrient-rich food options for you. In this case, there are plenty of other healthy options that are high in calcium, like nut cheeses, goat and sheep cheeses, or dark, leafy greens like kale or collard greens, all of which are more easily tolerated and have just as much calcium as a glass of milk.

For instance, Anita's patient Debbie came in to the office covered in hives around her elbows and knees. Debbie shared that her primary care provider once told her to increase her calcium intake after she became pregnant, so she had started drinking two full glasses of milk a day. Anita explained that the hives are a typical reaction to food sensitivities and were likely related to the milk intake, and suggested that instead of milk, Debbie could eat leafy greens that were also high in calcium yet wouldn't affect her immune system. Once she stopped drinking the milk, her hives went away.

Why You're Not Drinking Alcohol

There's clear evidence that links consuming high levels of alcohol during pregnancy to negatively affecting a child's physical health. Studies now show that even low levels of alcohol during pregnancy are correlated to a child with mental health issues, including anxiety, depression, and behavioral problems.[20]

All alcohol is, by definition, a liver toxin, and it's a concentrated source of sugar, both of which we're trying to avoid in pregnancy. Any type of alcohol will also exacerbate other pregnancy symptoms. It will make getting a good night's sleep more difficult. And if you're already nauseous, it could upset your stomach and your microbiome. So there you have it: there's really no added benefit of even an occasional glass of wine.

Supplements to Consider

The best way to get the vitamins and minerals you'll need during pregnancy is through eating nutrient-rich foods like the ones we discussed. However, vitamin supplements are an easy and effective way to make sure that you are meeting your nutritional requirements. During the first trimester, we typically prescribe

- **A prenatal vitamin with iron.** Prenatal vitamins typically contain more folic acid than standard adult multivitamins. Folic acid is necessary to prevent your baby from developing serious abnormalities of the brain and spinal cord. Make sure the one you choose has iron, which is necessary to support the baby's growth and development and helps prevent you from developing anemia.
- **Methylated folate and vitamin B12.** When these two are combined, they can help to prevent spina bifida and other spinal and central nervous system birth defects in your baby. However, some women can't break down folic acid, and a methylated variety is easier to absorb so that the body can use it appropriately.
- **Magnesium.** Increasing magnesium during pregnancy can help prevent the uterus from contracting prematurely. Magnesium also helps build strong teeth and bones for you and your baby.
- **Vitamin D.** Vitamin D may benefit both you and your baby. For maternal health, it is thought to help regulate blood pressure and blood sugar balance. It is also associated with key growth issues, including birth weight, birth length, and head circumference.
- **Probiotics.** Probiotics are thought to help your digestive system work more efficiently. They most notably lessen the presence of bad bacteria so that you are sharing more beneficial bacteria to your baby.
- **Fish oil.** Fish oil provides two essential omega-3 fatty acids. EPA supports the heart, immune system, and inflammatory response for both you and your baby. DHA supports development of the baby's brain, eyes, and central nervous system.

WISDOM

During these first few months of pregnancy, reach out to that close friend, a sibling, a parent, or whomever you feel comfortable with, and ask for support. Even though the common tendency these days is to keep your pregnancy to yourself and your partner until after the first trimester, we think it's better to share your news with someone close to you, because then you can lean on them as much as you need. Support is very beneficial to your wellness and your baby's wellness, and reaching out to someone can help to ease your day-to-day worries.

If you don't have a partner, all the more reason to pull a close friend or relative into your experience. Let them get closer to you and they can help release your worries. They can also help you with the difficulties of daily life (preparing meals, chores, etc.) later when you are physically limited. Start that relationship now, not when you begin showing—you won't regret it.

Embrace Your Culture's Wisdom

Every culture has its own superstitions and customs surrounding pregnancy. When Patricia was pregnant, her mother shared that in the Greek culture they believe that a pregnant mother can focus on one physical trait she wants passed down to her baby. During her third pregnancy, Patricia imagined her baby with big, beautiful eyes. She began thinking about those eyes in the first trimester and kept that in her thoughts when she connected with her baby throughout the pregnancy. When she gave birth to her daughter, everyone was mesmerized by her big, beautiful eyes, which is still one of her most defining physical characteristics.

What does your family believe in? Ask your family and connect with those customs.

Music May Be the Key to a Happy Pregnancy

Listening to music is one of the most important practices to incorporate during the first trimester. Studies have shown that music improves one's ability to relax by lowering cortisol levels, which leads to a reduction of overall anxiety,[21] decreases depression, and puts you in a good mood.[22] It also is known to enhance the immune system[23] as well as improve sleep.[24] Specific studies on pregnant women found that music improves the ability to relax during pregnancy and can reduce the anxiety of its related stress or physical discomfort.[25]

We have also found that surrounding yourself with music allows you to connect with yourself and with your baby. One reason may be because it blocks out the negative noise of day-to-day living, like those jarring car horns that negatively affect your nervous system. When you listen to the music you love, it helps to make your day a little lighter. And it really doesn't matter what you listen to as long as you enjoy it. You might want to play music that reminds you of when you were dating your partner. Maybe it's just a new song that you absolutely love to hear. At night when you're reading a book or talking to your baby, you can switch up the beat and play soothing music that will heighten the experience.

If listening to music is something you love doing, you can incorporate it into the things that you need to do in your day. Whether that's making a meal, folding laundry, exercising, or commuting, we want you to switch off the news and stop listening to stressful things. In your first trimester, you don't want to hear the latest podcast covering some natural disaster. You don't want to listen to somebody yelling at you about politics. You don't want to be exposed to a stimulus that will make you fearful or put you in a stressed state.

You can listen to music playing out loud and filling the room, or in privacy. Remember to use air tube headphones that surround your entire ear instead of ear buds. Not only will you be avoiding the EMFs, the headphones that go inside your ears negatively stimulate the bones in the ear canal.

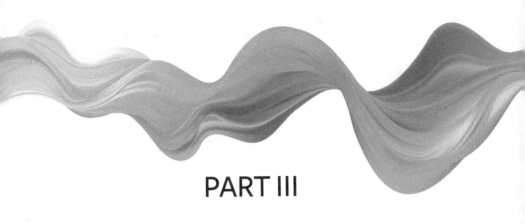

PART III

The Second Trimester: Three Months to Get Fit and Strong

The second trimester is an exciting time of pregnancy, as you will very likely begin to feel stronger, with less nausea and more energy. You'll be able to socialize, see friends, get out in nature, and work on your mental and physical health. In short, now is the perfect time to set your intentions, and your energy, in a direction that can positively influence the rest of your pregnancy.

As a wise woman, use the next few months to connect and stay with the joy of all the wonderful changes going on with your body and how they relate to your growing baby. You'll actually start to feel your baby's movements, so make sure to take time to pause and enjoy them.

Over the next three months, continue to build on the healthy habits that you have learned, which will ensure that you maintain a balanced state throughout the rest of your pregnancy. We know that *balance* equals *wellness,* and *wellness* equals *balance.* For the mother-to-be, wellness means feeling good physically and mentally every day, and maintaining good energy. One important goal is to continue to support a *quiescent,* or calm immune system. Whenever we have an inflammatory environment within, the body has to work hard to reduce that inflammation, and consequently, it doesn't function to the best of its ability. Instead, we want all our cellular processes and organs to work freely and optimally, and continuing to support it by following an anti-inflammatory lifestyle will help you reach this desired immune state. What's more, lowering inflammation also enhances the wellness of your growing baby by positively impacting the baby's epigenetics and setting the stage for optimal health throughout its life.

One traditional perspective you can keep in mind throughout this trimester is the ancient Hindu teachings of Ayurvedic medicine, which is entirely based on the principles of nature. In Hindi, Ayur means *The Life* and Veda means *The Knowledge,* and together it is known as the science of life. Its overall philosophy is aligned with ours in that it recognizes the definition of health as balance: a complete state of mental, physical, social, and spiritual well-being. When any one of these areas is out of balance, you cannot have wellness. Throughout this trimester, see how many Ayurvedic practices you can put in place. The effects of many of these tools are cumulative and are meant to ensure that you have a sense of peace and harmony within.

YOUR BODY:

RESTORATIVE BREATHING:

MOVEMENT:

NOURISHMENT:

WISDOM:

YOUR BODY

By the beginning of the second trimester your baby is about the size of a clenched fist. Its entire body is coated with downy body hair, called *lanugo*, which keeps it warm through the rest of your pregnancy until it gains enough body fat. As the weeks go by, your baby's body will be recognizable on ultrasound, and you'll be able to see hands, feet, and facial features. By the end of the sixth month, your baby will start to develop its senses: it can hear you talking, taste the foods you're eating via the placenta, and perceive light and darkness.

As your baby grows, your body is constantly going through its own little changes, even within a twenty-four-hour period. Your hormones cause the dilation of blood vessels, which then increases your breast size, your rib cage, and, later in the trimester, your pelvis. Your cardiovascular system is also affected. Your blood volume increases by as much as 50 percent; your heart rate also increases, and you may have fluid retention. These changes are responsible for episodes of palpitations, especially when you lie down at night, as well as lower leg swelling (you might notice sock marks at the end of the day), and frequent and large volume urination.

> ### Maintain Good Immunity by Practicing Social Distancing
>
> A wise woman really doesn't want to get an infection during pregnancy. You will be limited in the types of medications you can take because many will cross through the placenta and influence your baby's health. In fact, an infection you catch may negatively impact your baby's mental health later in life.
>
> Remember, your body is resilient and strong, especially because you are taking such good care of yourself. Yet the best course of action is always the safest: stay away from sick people. Practice social distancing and avoid handshakes and hugs with those who might be sick. If it makes you feel more secure, wear a disposable or washable mask when you're out in public.

Common Second Trimester Complaints

While you will generally be feeling healthy and vibrant in the second trimester, you may experience some of these common complaints. Discuss any of these issues with your obstetrician during your monthly visits:

Itchy Belly

As the belly grows the abdominal skin is stretching, which often leads to an itchy belly. This feeling may continue throughout the rest of your pregnancy. Avoid scratching, which can lead to damaging the exterior tissue. Instead, apply a thin layer of organic coconut oil (which is anti-inflammatory and cooling), sesame oil (which is antibacterial and warming), or a combination of the two (in equal parts) daily.

Unsteadiness

As you move through the second trimester, the uterus moves up and into the abdominal cavity, and the muscles that support it begin to get stretched and weaken. Most noticeably, you're going to feel your belly start to expand.

You might feel more "pregnant" as the day goes on: eating fills your bowels, and your belly will distend. The next morning you'll feel a little less pregnant. This constant shift makes it a bit difficult to maintain balance, good body mechanics, and good posture.

If this is your first pregnancy, your ligaments and connective tissue, called your *fascia*, will remain tight, particularly in your pelvis and abdomen. As your belly expands, this tight fascia acts like a barrier that creates a positive, passive tension that provides you with some core stability. Yet toward the end of the second trimester, as you're getting bigger, the fascia will start to loosen up, which is why you may feel unsteady on your feet. However, once you are deep into your third trimester, the abdominal fascia and pelvic ligaments adjust to being stretched, and will again support your growing belly due to the tensegrity that results. The concept of *tensegrity*, which stands for *tensional integrity*, occurs when there are adequate levels of both tension and compression, which causes an increase in stability within your musculature. Your intra-abdominal pressure will increase as the baby takes up more space, and at the same time, your ligaments and fascia will reach their maximal level of tension. The tensegrity that results will allow for optimal support even though it occurs in a completely passive way. So don't worry that the unsteadiness you're feeling now is only going to get worse; in fact, you're going to become more stable as the pregnancy continues, and the exercises in the program that support your deep musculature will add an extra layer of stability.

At the same time, your pelvis is slowly widening and shifting, and you may feel some discomfort. You may also feel unsteady on your feet and further lose the connection to your center of gravity as it shifts forward. Be very careful when you are going down stairs or walking off a curb. If you miss a step, you can actually create a greater shift in your pelvis. You may notice that you are bumping into walls or chairs, or that you have a greater tendency to lose your balance or drop things. Just be aware that your body has shifted quickly and will take a little time to adjust your inner sense of location and balance.

Your feet may also begin to swell and arches may drop, which decreases your ability to have a strong, grounded base of support for your pelvis. The exercises created for the second trimester will help address any discomfort, and develop the musculature you need to avoid it; you will be strengthening the muscles of the spine, the core, and the pelvic floor in order for your pelvis to be fully supported as it opens and prepares for delivery.

Back Pain

As the belly expands, pregnant women typically compensate by developing a more pronounced *lordosis*, or a curvature in the lower spine. This happens slowly and unconsciously as the spine is pulled forward toward the baby. This causes an accentuation of the curve of the low back, making it a slightly larger C. If your breasts become heavy, you might also develop a rounding of the shoulders, which pulls at the cervical core. Both of these postural changes can cause your head to drift forward, which inhibits your ability to engage the deep abdominal core. As your shoulders round forward, your head naturally inches into a forward posture, with your chin sticking forward. The more prominently your head moves forward, the more your core muscles shut down. You lose the automatic connection to your core and its activation is reduced. While some changes in the curves of the spine are okay since they are a response to your body's innate way to balance the growing belly, if they are not supported or become too pronounced, your head will significantly misalign (drifting forward excessively) and consequently, you will feel strain in either the spine or pelvis. Strengthening your core muscles and maintaining good posture when seated or standing will support the appropriate changes to your posture and keep you feeling great.

Upper or lower back pain might be caused by the pressure of your belly growing against the newly lax ligaments of the pelvis. Your deep, supportive muscles may become sluggish, especially if you have weakness in your back from a previous injury. When these muscles stop responding appropriately, they can shut off completely, making the superficial system (the superficial muscles that move your joints) take over, which leads to pain. The exercises created for the second trimester should help both avoid and relieve back pain. In fact, these exercises are more important than stretching. The truth is, stretching is not going to relieve tension or make the deep muscles develop or engage, but the exercises will. By really sticking with the exercises, you are activating the deep, supportive muscles to engage more, which leads to less gripping with your superficial muscles (where you may feel tight or strained), and you're actually going to feel better.

Lower Back Pain Relief

If you are ever feeling tension or pain in the lower back region, try the Step Forward Arm Lift exercise to activate a deep low back supportive muscle group to reduce or eliminate the pain.

START POSITION: Stand tall with arms by your sides.

SEQUENCE:

STEP 1. Inhale, take a step forward with your right leg, keeping your left foot on the ground, and allow your heel to lift. Most of your weight will shift to the front right leg. Simultaneously, lift your left arm straight up in front of you, overhead. Hold this position for the rest of your inhale.

STEP 2. Exhale, step the right leg back, and drop your arm to return to the start position.

STEP 3. Perform this movement 10 times while very slowly coordinating your breath, and then repeat 10 reps with the left leg stepping forward and the right arm lifting. You may repeat this sequence 2–5 times /day. If you are in a lot of discomfort, you may do a few reps on each side at the top of each hour until bedtime.

Pain That Points to Seeing a Professional

If you have a history of lower back pain that is not adequately addressed by the exercises in this chapter, you may want to seek the help of a physical therapist specializing in pregnancy/women's health for a more personalized approach.

Sciatic Pain and Nerve Sensitivity

Sciatic pain is caused by tension in the *sciatic nerve* and can present as buttock pain or a shooting pain that runs down the back of your leg. In some cases, as the baby grows, there may be asymmetric pressure put on your back or pelvis, which can cause sciatic pain. In other instances, when there is more laxity in the pelvis, the sciatic nerve's natural movement may be restricted, or the nerve may become *stretch sensitive*. As certain fascia become stretched, so does the connective tissue surrounding the nerve, which can make the nerve sensitive and reactive, leading to pain in the buttock or down the leg.

The best way to calm a sensitive nerve is to "floss" it. In a manner similar to the way you floss your teeth, you want to move your body so that the tissues surrounding the sciatic nerve move with a nice glide. Flossing can help you feel looser, decrease numbness/tingling in the legs, reduce muscle spasms, and keep fluids moving to decrease tension and swelling.

Nerve-Flossing Exercise

Perform this exercise any time you feel tightness in your lower back, buttocks, or back of the thigh(s). This flossing exercise will relax the tissues surrounding the nerve so that the nerve can move more freely. The movement is very small. Only move as much as you can and stop when you feel any type of stretching sensation.

Do not perform this exercise first thing in the morning or when you have been sitting for a long time; instead, you can do this after a shower or once you've walked around a bit, after the exercise program, or right before bed. If there is any increase in symptoms, stop doing this exercise. If your pain doesn't resolve within forty-eight hours, consult your physical therapist or medical doctor.

SEQUENCE:

STEP 1. Sit tall on the edge of a chair or stool. Inhale and slowly straighten your right knee while arching your back, sticking out your chest, and looking up to the ceiling. If you feel a stretch, back off and don't extend your knee all the way.

STEP 2. Exhale, lower your leg back down, and slouch, curving your spine into a C with your head dropped, looking down at your lap.

STEP 3. Repeat these motions in a smooth, continuous fashion at a slow pace; count 1-2-3 for step 1 and step 2. Perform 7 to 10 reps on the right, and then

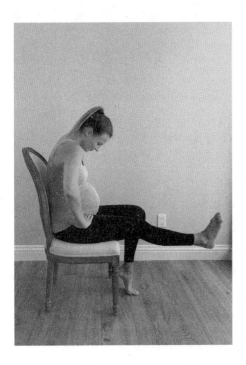
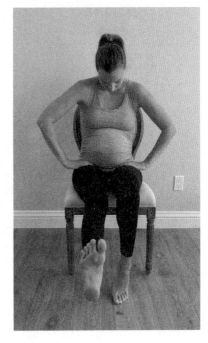

repeat 7 to 10 reps on the left. Stay within a range where you do not feel like you are doing much of anything. This will ensure you are not exciting the nerve or muscle fibers in a negative way.

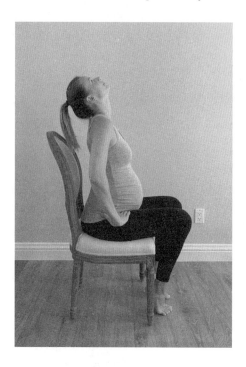 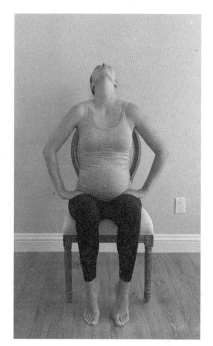

Diastasis Recti

As you enter into the later phase of the second trimester (around month six), you may start to see a gap between your right and left abdominal wall muscles as the *linea alba* thins out. This stretch happens for 100 percent of pregnant women and should resolve on its own after pregnancy. Maintaining a healthy abdominal wall postpartum is essential not only for maintaining posture but for urinary continence and pelvic organ support.

Having good *collagen*, the primary structural component of connective tissue, will help the linea alba thicken after delivery and generate the appropriate tension to restore the abdominal wall. However, having good collagen is genetic: if you have thin skin—which can look more transparent or bruises/

tears after minor injuries—you may produce less collagen. Some women have reported benefits from taking collagen supplements.

About 30 percent of women have a diastasis problem after pregnancy. In order to avoid this, you will be supporting that central seam beginning in this trimester through the exercise program. We also want you to avoid activities that create pressure through this area, which will stretch the linea alba further. This includes curl ups, sit-ups, or abdominal exercises where you lift your head off the floor when lying down on your back, or hover your legs parallel to the ground.

If this is a second pregnancy, or you are carrying multiples, have had previous abdominal surgery, or are already feeling that your belly is starting to feel heavy, follow the diastasis guidance for third trimester on page 232.

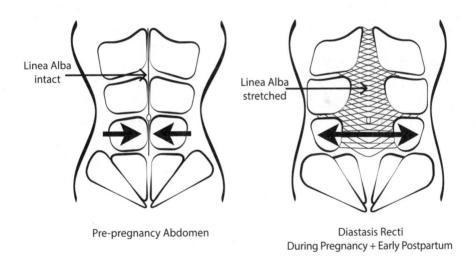

Pre-pregnancy Abdomen

Diastasis Recti
During Pregnancy + Early Postpartum

Varicose Veins

Varicose veins are the enlarged, swollen, and twisting veins that can appear on the legs and feet. They show through the skin with a blue or dark purple hue. These normally invisible veins become distended and potentially painful during pregnancy because of the increase in blood volume. This increase is responsible for a rise in fluid that needs to be distributed throughout the blood vessels, and in some cases, this will lead to varicose veins, which can be painful. Some pregnant women describe the pain as an aching or cramping in the legs. They may also cause burning, throbbing, tingling, or a general feeling of heaviness in the legs.

You are at an increased risk to develop varicose veins if you had them in a prior pregnancy or if you are carrying multiples. Standing and walking increase pressure on the veins, especially during pregnancy. They are also thought to occur when you maintain the same position for long periods of time, either standing or sitting. Make sure that you're moving around during the day, and take short breaks from any position every hour or so.

Pain from varicose veins is usually relieved by elevating the legs or by wearing support hose. You can also try the supplement diosmin, which is a natural plant extract found in citrus fruits and is safe to take in pregnancy. Diosmin helps to redistribute the blood flow from the superficial varicose veins to the deeper blood vessels that can handle the blood volume more easily.

Varicose veins will naturally recede within six weeks after delivery. However, in some cases they may persist and require treatment from a vascular surgeon or a dermatologist. However, none of these treatments are typically performed during pregnancy: your blood volume only continues to increase through the third trimester and will ruin any benefit of these treatments.

Hemorrhoids

Hemorrhoids are varicose veins that appear on the anus and rectal area. They may occur due to the changes in blood volume as well as the increased tendency toward constipation, fluid retention, and stress. Symptoms of hemorrhoids include

+ A raised area of skin near your anus
+ Bleeding after a bowel movement
+ Burning

- Itching
- Painful bowel movements
- Swelling

Being constipated, or straining when you go to the bathroom, can worsen the situation, so it is very important to soften your stool if you have hemorrhoids. The following are ways to ease the discomfort:

- Apply an over-the-counter remedy, such as witch hazel, directly to your anal area.
- Avoid sitting for long periods of time. Sitting puts pressure on the veins in your anus and rectum. Whenever possible, lie on your side or stand up. If you must sit, take frequent breaks or sit on a hemorrhoid pillow, also known as a ring cushion or doughnut.
- Consider natural ways to reduce constipation: supplement with vitamin C, magnesium, or a medium-chain triglyceride (MCT) oil like coconut oil. The supplement diosmin may also help.
- Drink plenty of fluids throughout the day.
- Eat more vegetable fiber.
- Soak in warm water.

Incontinence

While the need to go to the bathroom doesn't let up in the second trimester, the cause is different. By this point in your pregnancy, you may start feeling pressure on your digestive tract, including your bladder, because the baby is growing. Incontinence can happen anytime during pregnancy and depends on the position of the baby. If you're a petite woman or athletic, you may feel the effects a little bit earlier and a little more drastically. If you have a more average frame, you may feel fewer effects.

Increasing the support in your pelvic floor, lumbar spine, and abdomen will not erase the sensation of having to go to the bathroom, but it will help prevent incontinence. The fix is to continue doing the Kegels with Resting Squats (page 62) and proper diaphragm breathing throughout your pregnancy. Maintaining proper posture also helps because poor posture actually compresses the abdominal cavity, which then forces urinary frequency. Interestingly, incontinence is not caused by the lordosis issue; the way you carry your higher, thoracic core is more influential. If you are rounded forward from the top of your body, you are actually increasing pressure into the abdominal cavity, which then leads to pressure on the pelvic floor. By maintaining good posture, you can continue to lift the top half of your body and engage your diaphragm, relieving that pressure.

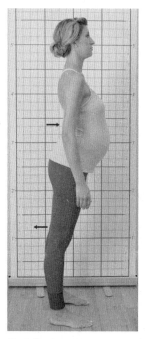
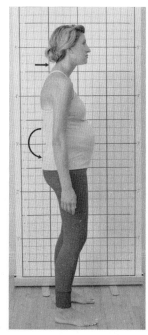
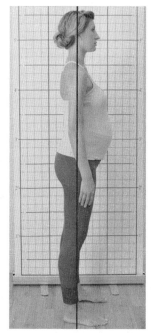

Poor Posture   *Poor Posture*   *Good Posture*

Gestational Diabetes

Gestational diabetes is a form of diabetes diagnosed during pregnancy through a simple urine test. Gestational diabetes causes high blood sugar that can affect your pregnancy and your baby's health. Having gestational diabetes puts you in a greater risk category for developing type II diabetes later in life. It also creates an increased risk of lifetime diabetes for your baby.

There are many ways to naturally keep your blood sugar regulated during pregnancy despite such a diagnosis. You can control and even reverse gestational diabetes by eating healthy foods, particularly lowering your intake of processed, sugary foods. Follow the same recommendations we've outlined to promote a more balanced sugar and insulin level: a gluten-free, anti-inflammatory diet that focuses on fiber-rich foods, plenty of fruits and vegetables, fewer grain-based foods, and healthy proteins and fats (see Nourishment section in preconception for a complete listing).

Lowering stress is now thought to be critical to improving blood sugar balance, and using the techniques mentioned in this book can help. In one 2018 study, blood sugar levels of pregnant women with "optimistic" life approaches toward coping with stress were lower than those who had a more negative outlook.[1] Reducing your toxin exposures, particularly to heavy metals found in fish as well as pesticides and chemical exposures in your food, filtering drinking water, improving air quality in the home, and minimizing chemicals found in beauty and makeup products are critical to reduce your chances of developing gestational diabetes.[2] Exercise not only reduces stress but limits the risk of gestational diabetes by improving insulin receptor sensitivity in the muscles. Lastly, adequate sleep impacts stress hormone levels as well as growth hormone production, both of which are important for blood sugar control.

Your doctor may recommend that you start insulin medication if you are diagnosed with gestational diabetes. The following supplements can be tried under a doctor's supervision before starting an insulin regimen:

- **Alpha-lipoic acid.** This antioxidant can enhance glucose uptake and inhibit sugar from coating proteins and enzymes (which increases free radical, oxidative damage). It can also help treat and prevent diabetic neuropathy, the nerve damage that often accompanies diabetes.
- **Calcium.** A 2017 study proved that higher dietary calcium intake was inversely associated with the risk of gestational diabetes.[3] The best way to increase your calcium levels is to eat calcium-rich foods like kale, broccoli, and almonds, but you can supplement as well.

- **Magnesium.** This mineral supplement helps to promote healthy insulin production. Magnesium glycinate is the best form to take, as it has less of a laxative effect than other forms of magnesium, such as magnesium oxide or magnesium citrate.
- **Vitamin D.** Research has shown that there is an association between vitamin D deficiency and gestational diabetes. Some studies suggest that vitamin D supplementation can reduce the risk of developing gestational diabetes.[4] We recommend Thorne liquid vitamin D that comes with vitamin K3.

Laura Reversed Gestational Diabetes

Laura came to see Anita when she was diagnosed with gestational diabetes during her second trimester. Her obstetrician had recommended that she start insulin medication, yet Laura was unsure if this suggestion was really right for her. Anita first recognized that Laura was stressed about her diagnosis and gave her a simple meditation practice to start at home that would help her lower her stress. She also outlined specific dietary guidelines that removed toxins from her diet, including removing inflammatory processed foods, and instead focusing on organic fruits, vegetables, and proteins that did not have harmful chemicals. She also recommended the supplements that help improve sugar-insulin balance and started her on a daily thirty-minute walk to increase her aerobic exercise. By following this protocol, Laura was able to control her sugar, and she did not need to go on medications for the remainder of her pregnancy.

Dizziness

Some women complain of dizziness or lightheadedness during the second trimester. This may be caused by reduced blood pressure, especially if you haven't had enough water to drink in the day, if you typically get low blood sugar or are hungry, or if you are standing for prolonged periods of time. Dizziness and feeling faint are also made worse if you allow yourself to get overheated or are in a crowded room.

When you feel dizzy, try to jog out your legs. Monitor your water so that you can stay hydrated. Add salt to your foods, or a dash to your water, both of which are healthier options than snacking on salty potato chips. Dress in layers to avoid getting overheated, and avoid crowds if possible.

You might also find that it's not as comfortable to be on your back, especially during exercise and when you are sleeping. By the eighteenth week of pregnancy, you may start to feel some pressure from the baby on your abdominal aorta, which is the largest artery of the body that runs the length of the abdomen. This pressure can reduce blood flow, which might make you feel lightheaded or nauseous. Switching to sleeping on your side instead of your back can help alleviate these feelings.

Congestion

Up to 30 percent of women experience *pregnancy rhinitis*, a fancy term for stuffy nose. This symptom is very common in the second trimester and is caused by hormonal changes. Unfortunately, many nasal decongestants will cross over to your baby via the placenta. Instead, we recommend using a saline nasal spray or neti pot whenever you feel stuffy. A humidifier, particularly at night, can help to keep your nasal mucous membranes moist. If you are very uncomfortable, discuss your symptoms with your doctor or an otolaryngologist, otherwise known as an ear-nose-throat specialist, to make sure you haven't developed nasal polyps that can obstruct your breathing. These polyps are a benign growth that is very common in pregnancy.

Vaginal Discharge

You may experience an increase in the amount of vaginal discharge. As the cervix and vaginal wall soften, the body produces excess discharge to help prevent infections; this discharge will become heavier toward the end of the third trimester. If you wish to use a cotton panty liner for comfort, please choose organic cotton and avoid tampons, douching agents, or other over-the-counter medications.

Normal vaginal discharge, termed *leukorrhea*, is thin, milky, white, and mild smelling. It should not have a strong odor or be accompanied by itching. Call your doctor if you develop any of the following signs, which could signal an infection:

◆ Burning pain

◆ Itching, redness, or swelling of the vulva

◆ Pain with urination

◆ Strong foul-smelling odor

◆ Yellow-, green-, or gray-colored discharge

Suddenly Forgetful?

A recent study found that pregnant women experience a slight loss of memory—and in many cases, the forgetfulness may continue *up to a year after* childbirth.[5] In the study, participating women reported that their ability to multitask declined, and they had difficulty retrieving new memories. Researchers believe that the abrupt hormonal changes pregnant women experience, combined with frequent sleep disturbance, may be the cause of the problem.

Balance Immunity with Reflexology

Gentle massage with organic oils—sesame, coconut oil, even olive oil—is an Ayurvedic tool that promotes overall well-being, stress relief, and pleasure. Studies show that during pregnancy, massage releases hormones into the body's circulation that both combat pain and discomfort and increase our capacity for love and bonding.[6,7] What's more, a relaxing massage from a massage therapist certified in pregnancy, prenatal, and postpartum massage, or even from your partner or a friend is equivalent to hours of deep, restorative sleep. We've found that self-massage during pregnancy is difficult to do correctly.

One preferred mode of massage during pregnancy is reflexology, an ancient practice that is both a science and an art. It is a method for activating the healing powers of the body in order to balance its systems. In this energy practice, the body is mapped into ten zones that run the length of the body from head to toe. By applying pressure to specific points on the feet and hands, we release energy blocks along these pathways, affecting the corresponding areas of the body within that zone. In many ways reflexology is just like acupuncture, where there are meridians and points on the body that correlate to organ systems and functions.

Reflexology is particularly useful for regulating the mind-body connection. The brain and body are connected through the nervous system, which is comprised of three parts: the *central nervous system* connects the brain to the spinal cord, the *peripheral nervous system* connects muscles and skin to the brain and spinal cord, and finally, the *autonomic nervous system* regulates bodily functions such as digestion and heartbeat. The autonomic nervous system is further divided: *the sympathetic nervous* system controls hormonal output and the "fight or flight" response, and the *parasympathetic nervous system* is responsible for the body's ability to "rest and digest" as well as heal. Reflexology stimulates the parasympathetic nervous system that keeps us calm.

Wellness is achieved when we can respond to life in a parasympathetic mode, even when we are working, eating, and being social. This is particularly important during pregnancy because you want to maintain a stress-free disposition so that you are restful, calm, and happy. When the reflex points of the feet and hands are worked on, the parasympathetic nervous system is activated and restores the body to a state of calm. Reflexology is also thought to activate the release of endorphins, leading to a sense of calm, joy, and optimism. Many of the pregnant women we see report feeling less stressed afterward.

Reflexology is also a great way to connect with your partner because you can take turns working on each other as a form of foot massage. It's such a beautiful way to bond and to be able to do something for your partner, bringing you both into the present moment. You can literally feel that person's energy. What's more, there's power in a loving touch: it releases the feel-good hormone oxytocin, which naturally lowers stress.

A reflexology massage doesn't have to last very long—typically less than thirty minutes. Both you and your partner should be comfortable, either lying in bed or sitting on a chair. If the person receiving the massage is lying down, use pillows to support the upper chest and under the knees. Keep the lines of communication open so that you and your partner can provide feedback on what feels good or when there is too much pressure. A great resource is Laura Norman's book, *Feet First: A Guide to Foot Reflexology*. There are many reflexology socks you can buy online to instruct you as well.

When you are providing reflexology massage to your partner, think about their body and their health and what your body is going through.

Your partner can massage the area that corresponds to the diaphragm, spine, chest, and lungs. If you feel any sort of discomfort, stop immediately. Avoid the areas corresponding to the uterus, bladder, kidney, and thyroid. Discontinue any foot or leg massaging in the third trimester because it could bring on labor.

New Ways to Relieve Stress Now That You're Feeling Strong

Now that you're physically feeling better, some of your mental stress may naturally dissipate. However, new worries can creep in, especially if you have become backlogged because you didn't feel so great during the first trimester. Alleviating stress is critically important in the second trimester because when you reduce stress, it reduces the baby's stress. In fact, when the baby is bombarded with your stress-producing cortisol via the placenta, it can lead to neurodevelopmental disorders for the baby. Practicing stress relief techniques can reverse and prevent this.

Ayurvedic medicine teaches that the mind controls the body, and so during pregnancy, women should be protected from negative emotions such as jealousy and anger and should not be exposed to upsetting news on television or from other sources. Negative emotions not only affect the physical body by creating stress, they are thought to influence the baby and how the baby will ultimately respond to your emotions. A pregnant woman should therefore only have pleasing thoughts and be exposed to the emotions of love and attachment. Her mind should be peaceful, and she should focus on joy, which is exactly our recommendation for this trimester.

Dance Your Way to Joy

If you're looking for exercise that is definitely going to bring you joy and keep your mood up, look no further than dancing. Did you know that dance has more health benefits than meditation? The reason is that its effect is amplified because in one activity you are getting three endorphin stimulators known to reduce stress: movement, music, and socialization.[8] What's more, dancing also promotes mindfulness. When you're dancing, you have to focus on the music and your movements, so you're not thinking about your to-do list or something else that stresses you out.

You can try any type of dancing that interests you, as long as you're not doing a lot of jumping or hopping. You can dance around your living room or participate in a formal dance class that's either virtual or in person. You can also dance alone or with a partner. The same research study shows that dancing with someone else lights up areas of the brain that stimulate a sense of oneness and connection. And when you're pregnant, you're automatically dancing with your baby!

We also think that dancing is a great way to bond with your partner. When Patricia was pregnant, she and her husband took Latin dance classes. She believes that it was wonderful for her marriage to try an activity that was new to each of them, wasn't stressful, and was really a lot of fun.

Dance Cultures and Customs

In certain parts of the world as far apart as Israel and Taiwan, whole towns gather at the local piazza or square to participate in group dancing. Someone may be playing live music or blasting the loudspeakers. There's typically a leader, and people gather just to dance because they know that dancing creates moments of joy.

Street and social dancing is popular in Latin America, where on Sundays, the parks and plazas across Mexico City host groups of amateur Latin dancers who gather to practice and socialize. In Buenos Aires, locals gather regularly in plazas and squares to dance the tango. In Brazil, a dance craze known as *passinho* (a mix of breakdance and funk, combined with Brazilian traditional dance moves), is done in the streets throughout the *favelas* of Rio de Janeiro.[42] In China, *guang-chang wu,* or "plaza dancing" has exploded in popularity. Women meet in the early mornings and evenings to perform synchronized dance routines.

Calm the Mind with Meditation

During meditation, one is at peace and harmony. A regular meditation practice can be very helpful to reduce the chatter in your brain and promote higher level development, which can come in handy during the second trimester when we tend to be more forgetful. What's more, studies have shown that mothers who meditate rarely have babies with heart disease.

Different types of meditation are linked to different benefits. For example, researchers have found that a mindfulness practice cultivates discipline, greater attention, and emotional regulation.[10] Taking a few quiet moments and paying attention to your breath or watching the flame of a lit candle as you practice your diaphragm breathing will pull your attention into the present and away from your worries, which then calms the mind.

Transcendental Meditation or Vedic Meditation techniques both use scientifically backed ways to provide calmness in the mind. They are thought to promote calmness, restful alertness, and a heightened sense of self-awareness.[11] We have found that these programs are quite effective for those of us who can't stop ruminating on thoughts or to-do lists. To try these, take just a few minutes every day to be in complete stillness, focusing on a one-word mantra. If you like, go back to the meditation in Preconception (see page 87), which you can use throughout your pregnancy.

There are many books and apps for meditation that are easy to use. One of our favorites is a collection of meditations from Agapi Stassinopoulos's book, *Wake Up to the Joy of You*. There is an app called InsightTimer, which connects people who are meditating at the same time around the world. There are also meditation tools that can provide biofeedback in real time. One of them is called Muse, which is an electronic headband that you wear during meditation. It interprets your brain activity to keep you on track to get the most benefits out of meditation. When your mind is calm and settled, you hear peaceful weather. When your focus drifts, you'll hear stormy weather that cues you to bring your attention back to your meditation practice.

RESTORATIVE BREATHING

Good diaphragmatic breath holds the key to reducing stress and achieving relaxation. Yet as you progress through your second trimester, you may find your breathing is becoming more difficult. Once your belly starts to grow, you naturally lose access to your diaphragm. Your breathing can become more labored, you might feel like you have to take a deep breath all of a sudden, or you're yawning more often.

We want to correct breathing issues quickly because they can cause real symptoms, including

- Anxiety or low mood
- Dullness to your senses
- Fatigue or low energy
- Feeling light-headed or dizzy
- Forgetfulness or brain fog
- Nausea that comes in waves

Breathing with Inverted Postures

Practicing appropriate diaphragm breathing can shift you back into a positive place. The cupping technique that we reviewed in the first trimester will also help if you feel any sort of distress or any of the symptoms listed.

If you're comfortable lying on your back, the partially inverted position using a few pillows under your hips or legs can help (see the inverted breathing technique on page 47). However, you may no longer be comfortable lying on your back, especially later in the second trimester. Instead, try going into an inverted position like Downward Dog yoga position or bending forward while seated. These positions take the pressure off the diaphragm so that it can expand a little bit more than when you are upright. The more expansion through the diaphragm, the easier it will be to get a more efficient breath. Breathing will never be truly easy or efficient until after pregnancy, but practicing the following inversions in the second and third trimesters will definitely help.

Consider Pranayama

Pranayama is a category of yogic breathing exercises. One we like to recommend that is part of the Ayurvedic tradition is called *alternate nostril breathing*. It is exactly what it sounds like. All you need to do is close up one nostril with your thumb and breathe through the other and then repeat on the other side. This exercise balances and equalizes the sympathic and parasympathetic nervous system, which helps to restore balance to the mind and to the body.

Try any of these inverted positions for 3 to 5 minutes, consecutively and mindfully, whenever you are having difficulty breathing:

+ **Downward Dog.** Gently place your hands and knees on the floor or a yoga mat. Extend both elbows and knees to a comfortable range without locking them and assume an inverted V position. Keep your hands under your shoulders. Your inner elbows should face each other. Your heels will be lifted depending on how flexible your calves and legs are, and your knees should remain slightly bent. Relax your head and neck:

imagine that your head is a cherry hanging from a stem. Focus your breath coming in through the nose: imagine that it is moving down a tube that bypasses your chest and spreads to each side of your ribs. Let the sides and back of your lower ribs expand outward with your inhale and come back together on your exhale. Be careful not to take very deep breaths, which is counterintuitive. Simply stay quiet with your breath and don't let your shoulders or neck move or tense up. Less is always more: think of this movement as starting small in your ribs, and then you will be more successful as the muscles and connective tissue lengthen and release.

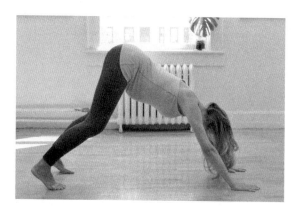

If Downward Dog is not comfortable, use the same breathing technique with any of the following positions. Quietly and gently breathe into the back and sides of the lower ribs:

- An all-fours position on the floor on your hands and knees: make a fist if your wrists hurt.

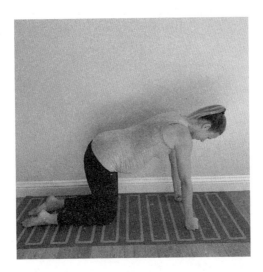

- Half-standing: Place your elbows on a countertop, allowing your belly to hang.
- Lying on your side.
- Seated bending forward: while sitting on the edge of a chair, bend your body forward over your thighs. You may cross your arms over your head and hang them down.

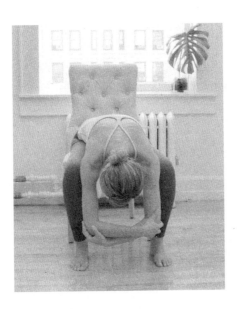

MOVEMENT

Remember, the number one way to relieve stress, reduce depression, and boost self-esteem is through exercise, especially when you are doing an activity you really enjoy. Exercise floods your whole system with endorphins like oxytocin, the feel-good hormones that combat anxiety. What's more, you don't have to exercise for long: a 2001 study found that participants who exercised for just ten to twenty minutes every day have improvements in their overall mood, with no additional improvement for longer periods.[12] This is one reason why the exercise routine for the second trimester can be broken up throughout the day, whenever you need that hit of endorphins!

Exercise and physical activity is recommended for pregnant women under Ayurveda, and conversely, so is sleep. Do activities that are aligned with the rhythm of the universe: exercise during the day, and sleep at night. In fact, 10:00 p.m. is the recommended bedtime after a full day of activity—it's the time when the mind starts to slow down.

The Second Trimester Exercise Routine

Thirty-Plus Minutes of Aerobic Activity

During the second trimester we recommend continuing thirty-plus minutes of regular walking a day, preferably in nature. You can now increase your intensity and elevate your heart rate. Doctors used to recommend that pregnant women keep their heart rate during exercise below 140 BPM (beats per minute), but we believe this thinking is not only outdated, it doesn't have much scientific validation. Instead, listen to your body and base your comfortable level of exertion on how you used to exercise prior to pregnancy. To find your range, monitor your heart rate, noting when you feel good and when you feel too taxed. We do not want you to exercise to exhaustion.

Think of your rate of exertion as a scale from 1 to 10, where a rate of 1 is hardly working and 10 is a maximum intensity workout. We want you to stay within the 6 to 7 range for the duration of the aerobic activity.

The biggest change to your resting heart rate usually happens during the second trimester. It can become as much as 10 bpm higher than your pre-pregnancy resting heart rate because of the increased circulating blood volume. This means that you may have a harder time doing the same level of exercise that you did prior to pregnancy. Don't beat yourself up if you can't sustain the same level of intensity; you'll be able to return to your old levels of exertion soon after the baby arrives.

We also want you to shorten your stride when you walk. As your pelvic ligaments begin to stretch, the wider the stride you take, the more you pull on those same ligaments. You will be in less pain if you walk with a slightly shorter stride. Lastly, continue to remain properly hydrated and wear layered clothing so that you don't overheat during aerobic exercise.

When to Modify Your Routine

There are a few situations in which you should not increase your level of exertion during the second trimester. These include carrying multiple babies, experiencing preterm labor, or if you have been diagnosed with gestational diabetes, vascular disease, hypertension, vaginal bleeding, incompetent cervix, sickle cell anemia, or renal disease.

When you are exercising, stop right away if you are feeling dizzy or nauseous, and let your doctor know that you are having difficulty. Avoid supine exercise (lying on your back) and standing still for more than 15 minutes at a time after the first trimester.

Thirty Minutes of Eccentric Strengthening and Lengthening

The second trimester is where Patricia's ballet training really comes into play. You will focus on exercises that elongate the spine and neck while toning the arms and legs. Elongation produces positive support for all the joints and activates a spiraling support that maintains optimal length and prevents spinal compression and back pain, reduces the gravitational load, and effectively activates the three cores of the body. You will also work on specific muscle strengthening and lower leg stretching as well as new exercises for the lumbar, pelvis, glutes, shoulder blades, and core that feature eccentric contractions, which are the most difficult contractions for muscles to do.

These exercises promote good posture, reduce nerve compression and varicose veins, and reduce the risk of developing a diastasis. We will also shift the focus to strengthen and ground your body in the legs—you'll need strong legs to support you now and in the next stage of your pregnancy. As we strengthen the joints and pelvic floor muscles, not only is it going to help you now, but it will help make labor and delivery easier. Afterward, these same muscles can help reduce back pain or your chances of incontinence after you have the baby.

The upper body exercises will target the muscles that enhance strength necessary for handling the baby later on. Proprioceptive, balance exercises become important now to restore grounding in the whole body and keep you confident during activities of daily living.

You'll see that a few of the exercises below are traditional yoga poses. They will help you lengthen areas of the body that usually shorten with pregnancy, like the spine and the diaphragm, providing you with more space for your internal organs and your baby. They can also increase your endurance in the supportive muscle groups, which will help you feel more limber and will help ground you while still challenging your balance and core control.

In the second trimester, you will drop any of the previous exercises where you are on your back unless you are still comfortable to do so. Continue with Kegels with Resting Squats, Foot Doming, and the Ballet Arms Series and add the following new routine.

Exercise Equipment You'll Need

- A mat or towel
- Basketball
- Firm chair
- Physio ball, a large beach ball, or two thick pillows
- Tennis or small ball

Exercise: Pelvic Self-Correction: Push-Pull Series

EQUIPMENT: A bed or a mat/towel on the floor.

PURPOSE: To correct the alignment of your sacroiliac joints for relief of pain, clicking, or soreness in the back of the pelvis or the lower back.

START POSITION: Lie on your back or on your side and pull one knee directly over your hip. Keep your hands clasped under the back of the thigh. If you can't reach, use a towel.

SEQUENCE:

Gently push your thigh away from your chest and resist this motion with your hands. Hold this position, pushing for 5 seconds. Then hug the knee a couple inches closer to your chest. Repeat the 5-second isometric resistance. Bring it a little closer and repeat. You will perform a total of 5 (5-second push/

pulls) sets, incrementally bringing your knee closer in each time, but angle the final 2 sets toward the shoulder. Do this before you take your first steps out of bed, before and after you exercise, and before bed at night.

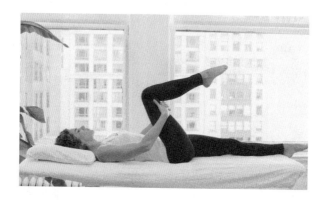

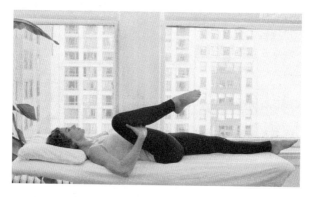

Exercise: Ball Release for Feet

EQUIPMENT: A chair and a tennis ball.

PURPOSE: To release and lengthen the fascia and small muscle groups under the feet. This exercise will also reduce some swelling and make you feel more grounded in the feet.

START POSITION: Sit in your chair with your feet on the floor. Place the ball under the toes of your right foot.

SEQUENCE:

STEP 1. Roll the ball under the foot starting at the toes, moving to the middle of the foot, and ending at your heel. Keep firm pressure on the ball to release the tissues on the bottom of the foot. Do 5 times backward and forward.

STEP 2. If you feel tight anywhere under the foot, stay at that spot and lean your elbows on top of your thigh to increase pressure on the ball. Take 3 breaths and then release. Repeat this at each tight spot as needed.

STEP 3. Roll the foot back and forth on the ball 10 times, then switch feet and repeat.

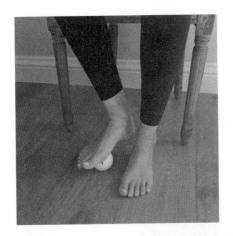
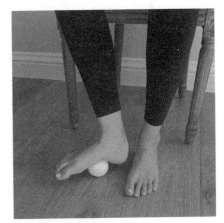
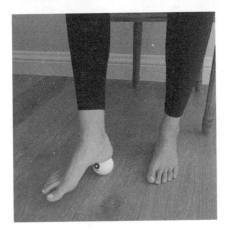

Exercise: Pliés and Wall Slide

EQUIPMENT: A Physioball and/or a sturdy chair.

PURPOSE: To strengthen the hips, legs, and pelvic joints.

START POSITION: Stand with arms by your sides and lean your back on a large ball against a wall. You can also hold a chair *or* put your back up against a wall without a ball. Place feet shoulder width apart with toes slightly pointed out.

SEQUENCE:

STEP 1. Inhale, bend your knees, and track the center of your knees out over your second toes as you lower your body about 45 degrees. Exhale and press through your heels while keeping toes on the floor to accentuate the lower glutes (buttocks) and pelvic floor firing on the way up. Repeat 10 reps for 2 sets.

STEP 2. Return to the start position. This time place your feet hip width apart and toes pointing straight ahead. Inhale, bend your knees, and track the center of your knees out over your second toes in comfortable range. Get close to a 90-degrees knee bend if you can tolerate that. Hold for 10 to 20 seconds or so, until you feel some fatigue. On an exhale, press through your heels (while keeping toes on the floor) and straighten your knees back to standing. This will help accentuate the lower glutes firing on the way back up. Repeat 2 more sets, going to fatigue each time (which will take less time with each set).

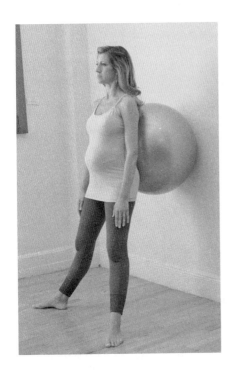

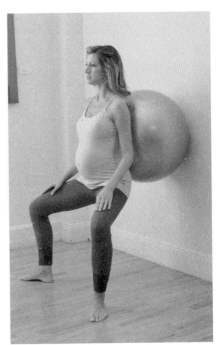

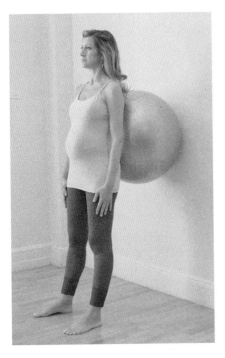

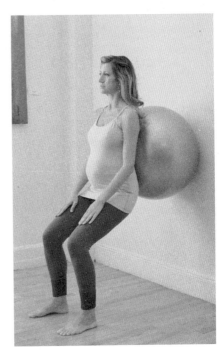

Exercise: Upper Body and Spine Release

EQUIPMENT: A chair.

PURPOSE: To reduce tension, lengthen, and relax the upper body, neck, and spine. This inverted position will also open the diaphragm to improve breathing.

START POSITION: Sit or stand (with soft knees) bent forward with arms crossed above your head and hands holding your elbows.

SEQUENCE:

STEP 1. Let the head, spine, and arms (crossed) hang freely as you hold this position for 3 breaths, relaxing further into the release each time.

STEP 2. Hang toward the right and use your diaphragmatic breathing for 3 breaths, expanding the sides and back of the lower ribs. Relax the head and neck as well.

STEP 3. Change sides and hang to the left in the same manner.

STEP 4. Repeat this sequence 2 to 3 times for as long as you are comfortable. If you feel lightheaded, stop. Each time, try to relax deeper and allow for a larger diaphragmatic breath into the back and sides of your lower ribs. Many pregnant women love being in this position, especially as their belly gets larger. Feel free to repeat the sequence a couple times per day if it feels good.

Sit...

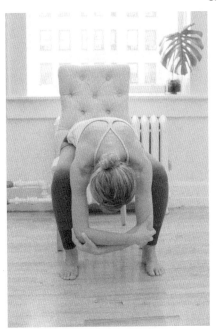 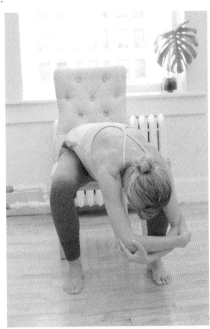

...or stand

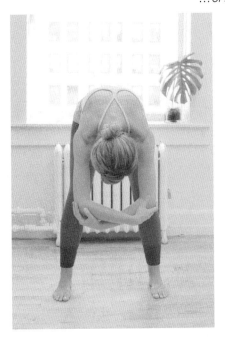 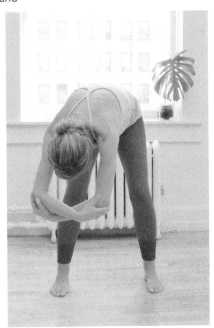

Exercise: High Lunge to Warrior II

EQUIPMENT: A yoga mat or towel.

PURPOSE: To open the chest and lengthen legs, hips, and the side of the body, while strengthening the legs [All Cores].

START POSITION: Stand tall in the center of a yoga mat or towel with your arms at your sides.

SEQUENCE:

STEP 1. Inhale, take a lunge forward with the right leg, and raise both arms up to the ceiling in-line with your ears. Palms should face each other, and the back heel is lifted. Activate the legs by pressing all toes down into the floor and the front heel into the floor. Your legs will feel as though they are coming in toward each other even though they don't move. Reach tall with both arms through the crown of your head up to the ceiling. Hold this position for 3 to 5 breaths.

STEP 2. Gently turn the left thigh so that your foot is toed out at a 45-degree angle, with the left foot staying in-line with the front right foot. Your back left knee should stay straight. Lower your arms down to your shoulders and stretch them out to the sides; your right arm is now in front of you, and the left arm is outstretched over your back leg. Make sure to keep the front right knee bent so that the knee is over your foot at a 90-degree angle in-line with the second toe. Both palms should face down to the floor. Keep your gaze out over your front hand in-line with the second finger. Feel your front thigh and hip rotating outward and your back hip and thigh rotating inward, even though they shouldn't move. Grow tall through the center of your body. Your core will naturally activate. Maintain this pose for 3 breaths.

STEP 3. Repeat the High Lunge to Warrior II sequence 3 times and then switch to the other side for 3 sets.

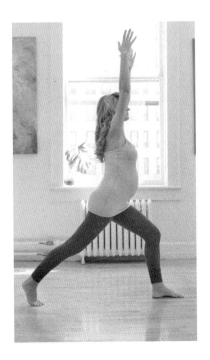
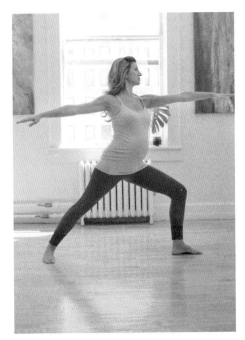

Exercise: Trikosana/ Modified Triangle Pose

EQUIPMENT: A mat or towel on floor.

PURPOSE: To lengthen trunk, inner thighs, and hamstrings, improve breathing, and stabilize spine. This pose can also improve digestion [All Cores].

START POSITION: Stand tall in final Warrior II position (see previous exercise).

SEQUENCE:

STEP 1. Slowly straighten both knees. Reach and hold your left shin with your left hand. Extend your right arm to the sky with palm facing forward. Look up toward the right arm or, if your neck feels strained when you look up, modify the pose and look straight ahead. Feel the lengthening in left inner thigh and hamstring. Keep both arms and your trunk elongated. If holding your shin is too intense, hold a spot higher, closer to your thigh so you do not overstretch. Breathe into the right side of the body for 3 to 5 breaths.

STEP 2. Slowly release the pose, and shake out both legs. Switch to the other side from Warrior II going into this Triangle Pose. Repeat a 3- to 5-breath hold into the left side of the body. You can do 2 to 3 sets on each side.

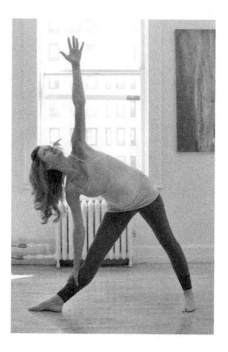

Exercise: Sun Salutation into Downward Dog Marching

EQUIPMENT: A mat or towel on the floor.

PURPOSE: To open the chest, lengthen leg muscles, and strengthen the core and hips [All Cores].

START POSITION: Stand tall in the center of your yoga mat with your feet close together and your arms by your sides.

SEQUENCE:

STEP 1. Inhale and reach arms up and over your head. You may gaze upward to follow your hands above your head. Exhale and release your arms back down by your sides. Each time you repeat the Sun Salutation sequence, reach higher up to the ceiling with energy flowing out your fingertips. Only raise your arms as high as you feel comfortable. You can remain looking straight ahead if looking up is difficult.

STEP 2. On your exhale, bend forward toward the floor, placing both hands on the floor, and soften your knees as you bring one leg back at a time into the Downward Dog position. Keep your elbows neutral (not locked) and knees soft to avoid extreme stretching, but if keeping your knees relatively straight feels fine, then do so. Your heels will lift off the floor. Relax your head like it is a cherry on a stem. Feel like someone is lifting your hips to the ceiling as you hold for 3 breaths.

STEP 3. Bend one knee and then the other, essentially pumping your heels up and down, alternating one heel coming closer to the ground as the opposite knee bends. Do this movement 10 times, alternating knee bends. Then walk one leg forward toward hands, followed by the other and roll body up gently, keeping both knees bent.

STEP 4. Repeat this sequence 1 to 3 times.

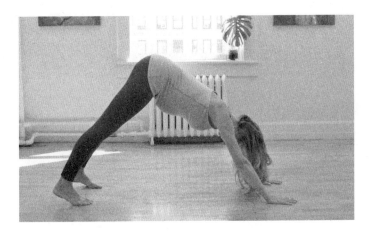

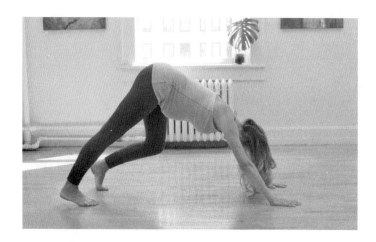

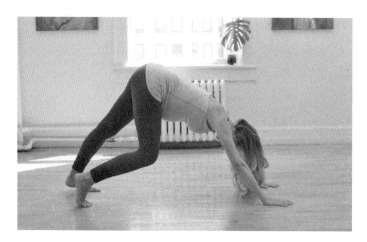

Exercise: Sidebending Whole Spine Release

EQUIPMENT: A yoga mat or towel on the floor or a chair.

PURPOSE: To reduce tension and lengthen upper body, neck. and spine [Thoracic Core].

START POSITION: Sit on the floor with legs crossed or in a chair with feet on the floor. Arms should be out at your sides.

SEQUENCE:

STEP 1. Inhale and reach left arm up to the ceiling while pressing the left sits bone into the floor or a chair in opposition. Feel expansive in the left side of your body as you lengthen and reach.

STEP 2. Exhale and slowly bend over to the right side, maintaining that lengthening/reaching feeling. Right arm rests on the floor (or on the chair seat) to the side of you with palm up. Make sure to stay long on both sides of your trunk. Hold position and keep the lengthening/reaching feeling going for 3 breaths. If this is difficult, modify by changing the right hand position so that your fingertips or flat hand is on the floor beside you. Use the right hand to push your body away from the floor, even though you are bending to the right.

STEP 3. Repeat on the other side. Then repeat a complete set 3 times. If you are feeling stiff on a particular day, you may repeat this exercise 2 to 3 times per day.

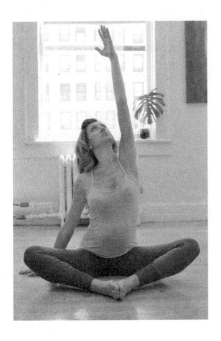 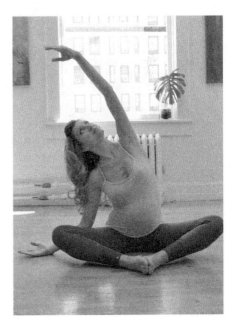

Exercise: Arabesque Ball Squeeze

EQUIPMENT: A physioball and sturdy chair.

PURPOSE: To strengthen the legs and hips while activating your abdominals [Lumbar Core].

START POSITION: Stand tall, with both hands holding the back of a sturdy chair in front of you. Place the physioball behind your left ankle.

SEQUENCE:

STEP 1. Inhale and place your right ankle/leg onto the physioball behind you. You may need to roll the ball away from you so that your right ankle and foot are on top of the ball. Place your leg in a slightly turned-out position (hips rotated/toes pointed out). If it doesn't feel good to lift your leg onto the ball, slide your leg behind you on the floor, actively pointing your toes behind you with your leg turned out.

STEP 2. Lengthen your body from the crown of your head; stretching the sides of your body, feel your whole body elongating, which will draw your central abdominal core inward. Exhale and, press your rotated leg into the ball gently as you continue to grow tall through your center. Keep your standing leg strong with all your weight on the foot on the floor. You may keep the standing leg slightly toed out as well. Hold the gentle pressure into the ball with your right leg for 10 seconds as you continue to breathe, expanding the lower ribs apart.

You will feel your core and both inner thighs working. Keep your mind connected to your outer hip muscles that help support the turned-out position of the leg on the ball. You should not feel pressure in your lower back; if you do, it is a sign that your leg is lifted too high.

STEP 3. Perform 10 reps. Repeat on the other side.

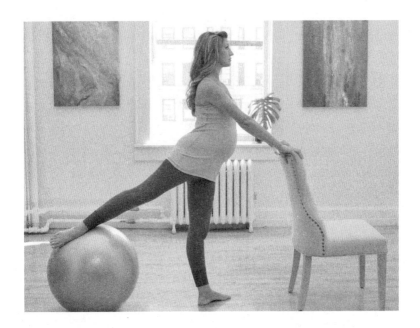

Exercise: Inner Thigh Squeeze with Ball

EQUIPMENT: A basketball or physioball (choose a ball size that feels more comfortable; a smaller ball is easier than a larger ball) and a sturdy chair.

PURPOSE: To strengthen the legs and hips while integrating your abdominals. This exercise also lengthens your trunk and works on creating more space for breathing [All Cores].

START POSITION: Place the ball next to you and the sturdy chair. Stand tall, with the left hand holding the back of the chair next to you. Your right arm is lengthened over your head, palm facing in. Both hips and legs are slightly toed out.

SEQUENCE:

STEP 1. Roll the ball so that it is in front of you between both legs, with your right leg turned out to a 45-degree angle. Keep the ball in place with your right leg at the front and your left ankle/shin at the back of the ball.

STEP 2. Inhale and lengthen through the crown of your head with your chin tucked down. The sides of your body should be long. Reach the right arm to the ceiling. Your abdominal muscles will naturally contract; don't force them to. Exhale and gently squeeze the right leg into the ball toward the standing leg with your heel flexed (toes up). Keep the left leg still and actively supporting you. Hold the gentle pressure into the ball for 5 seconds as you continue to breathe, expanding the ribs apart, then release. You will feel both sides of your gluteals working as well as the inner thigh and quads of the right leg.

STEP 3. Perform 15 reps. Repeat to the other side. If you feel any gripping or muscle activity in the front of the hip, use a smaller ball and hold the squeeze for only 3 seconds for 10 to 15 reps. Visualize the inner thigh, glutes, and core doing the work.

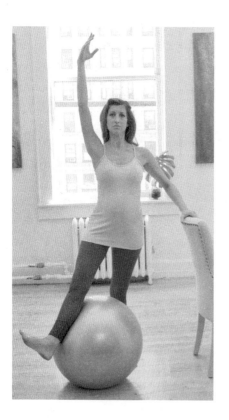 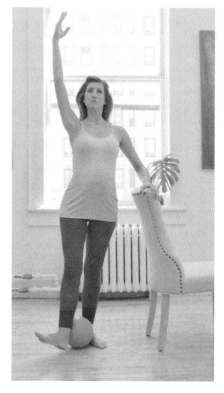

Exercise: All Fours Leg Lift and Attitude Bent Knee Lift

EQUIPMENT: A yoga mat or towel.

PURPOSE: To improve hip strength, core support, and spinal control [All Cores].

START POSITION: Get down on the mat on your hands and knees. Position hands on the floor under your shoulders and the inner elbows facing each other. Remember to keep elbows relatively straight but not locked into hyperextension.

SEQUENCE:

STEP 1. Keep chin tucked into chest so that ears are in-line with your shoulders. Look toward the floor in front of you on a spot between your hands. Keep head and whole spine in a straight line. Slowly extend right leg back with toes pointed. Only lift leg as high as comfortable but not higher than hip level. Hold this position, maintaining the elongation through your whole body with the leg reaching long away from you. Hold for 2 diaphragm breaths, then lower the right leg back to starting position.

STEP 2. Repeat with the left leg. Control the transition so your pelvis stays level the whole time, like you are balancing a tray on your sacrum/back of the pelvis. Repeat this sequence alternating legs 5 times. If your wrists/hands are uncomfortable, take a break or switch to resting your fists on the floor.

STEP 3. Take a break and shake out your hands. Then get back on all fours. Lift your right leg and this time flex the foot and bend the knee. Keep the knee lifted higher than the foot. The knee can be in-line or higher than the hip, if tolerated. Hold this position while maintaining a lengthening feeling throughout your spine and neck. Shoulder blades should feel active, separated apart as you ground through your palms with your chin tucked into your chest. Your gaze should still be on the floor between your hands. Hold this position for 3 diaphragm breaths. Only stay in the position as long as you can maintain your body in a straight line, with your spine in a neutral position.

STEP 5. Repeat 5 times as tolerated on each side, being mindful to slowly transition between sides with control.

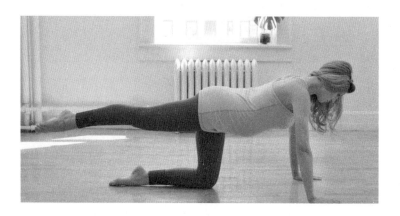

If this exercise is uncomfortable, try a standing variation. Hold onto the back of a sturdy chair with your left arm and hold your right arm out to the side. Stand tall and lifted through the crown of your head. Gently extend your right leg behind you with a pointed foot on the floor. Bend your knee and lift the whole leg with the knee remaining bent and toes pointed. Feel the deep outer right glutes working at the side of the hip. Hold this for 3 diaphragm breaths and return the foot back down to the floor. Repeat 5 times and then switch legs.

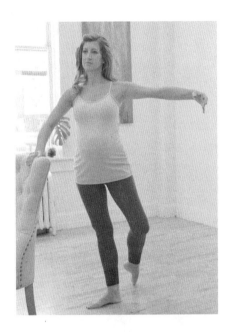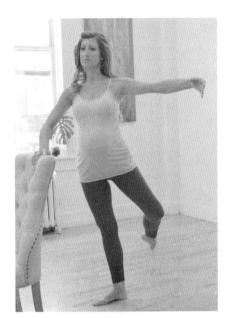

Exercise: Bowler

EQUIPMENT: A sturdy chair.

PURPOSE: To improve hip strength, core support, and lumbar control [Lumbar Core].

START POSITION: Stand and hold onto the back of a sturdy chair with one or both hands.

SEQUENCE:

STEP 1. Inhale and lean into the left hip with your right leg behind you, keeping the right knee bent and foot relaxed. This position should remind you of bowling, when you are getting ready to release the ball.

STEP 2. On your exhale, press through the left heel and engage your deep outer hip muscles to bring your pelvis level again. Make sure to not use the right hip, back, or leg to help; the work should solely be in the left gluteal area.

STEP 3. Repeat until fatigued, approximately 10 to 20 reps. Then perform the same with the right leg.

If you feel like you can isolate your deep outer hip muscle better with the Airplane exercise from the preconception routine (see page 63), you may swap that one back in instead of this Bowler progression.

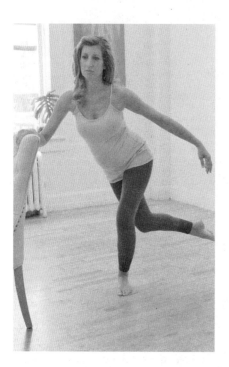
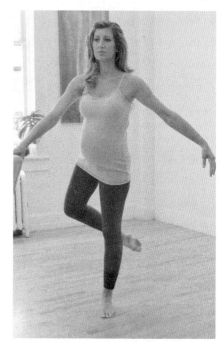

Exercise: One-Legged Heel Raises

EQUIPMENT: A sturdy chair.

PURPOSE: To strengthen and gain control in the stabilizing muscles of the feet and ankles. This exercise will strengthen the calves to support good standing posture and improve balance.

START POSITION: Stand tall with shoulders lifted up and back; elongate your neck as if a string was pulling you up through the crown of your head. Hold on to a sturdy chair for help with your balance.

SEQUENCE:

STEP 1. Transfer your weight onto your right leg and bend your left leg; point your left toes.

STEP 2. Keeping right knee straight, slowly lift your right heel. Keep your arch in-line with the center of the right foot with your ankle in a neutral position. If you find that your arch or foot rolls outward or that you are wobbling, don't come up as high.

STEP 3. Lower your right heel with control and without releasing the leg into a stretch. Controlling the heel down is the key part of this exercise. Maintain good posture and breathe diaphragmatically and consistently.

STEP 4. Alternate to your left foot. Repeat each foot for 10 slow reps, 1 to 2 sets.

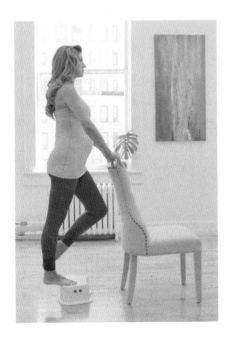 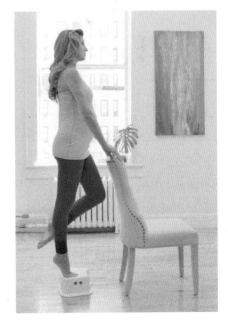

Exercise: Tree Pose/Passe Modification

PURPOSE: To improve balance; helps strengthen and gain control in the stabilizing muscles of the hips, legs, feet, and ankles [All Cores].

START POSITION: Stand tall near a wall with arms by your sides and both feet slightly toed out.

SEQUENCE:

STEP 1. Inhale, lift both arms out to the sides and overhead as you transfer your weight onto your right leg. Exhale and put your left heel on top of your right ankle. Left toes stay on the ground. Feel lifted through the spine, keeping your chin relaxed down and your eyes looking straight ahead. You should feel a counterforce grounding your left foot into the ground. Hold this position for 5 diaphragm breaths.

STEP 2. Repeat on the other side. If this exercise is difficult, hold onto a wall in front of you for support. You may also hold this position for less time if you begin to wobble.

STEP 3. *Modification:* Perform this once you have mastered the exercise: lift your whole left foot and rest it on your leg either over the right ankle or a little higher up toward the shin or knee. The higher you place your left foot, the more challenging the exercise will be. Maintain a tall, elongated posture; your standing leg should be active and grounded on the floor as you work on this balance position for 3 to 5 diaphragmatic breaths. Repeat on the other side and perform 2 to 3 sets as tolerated.

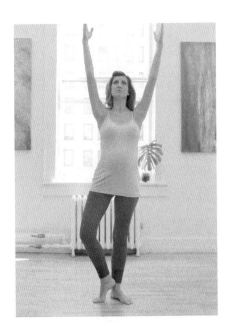 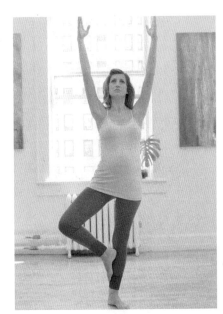

Exercise: Tendus and Pliés

EQUIPMENT: A sturdy chair.

PURPOSE: To strengthen the hips, cores, legs, and feet [Thoracic and Lumbar Cores].

START POSITION: Stand tall with your left hand on a sturdy chair and your right arm out to the side with the elbow slightly lifted. Keep heels together and toes slightly apart. If this doesn't feel comfortable, keep feet relatively close together with toes slightly apart.

SEQUENCE:

STEP 1. Grow tall from the crown of your head, chin relaxed down, lengthen the sides of your body, and feel your whole body elongating, which will draw your central core inward. Inhale, transfer your weight onto your left leg, and extend your right leg out to the side while pointing your right toes.

STEP 2. Exhale, slowly bring your right leg back to the starting position, allowing your right heel to meet the left heel. Keep your right foot in contact with the floor the whole time. Slide the toes along the floor until both heels meet in the center, and center your body weight on both feet.

STEP 3. Inhale and perform a plié: a small knee bend with knees tracking over the center of your turned-out feet. Exhale and rise back up to standing. By putting a little extra pressure through both heels as you straighten your knees, you can accentuate the activation of both lower glute muscles.

STEP 4. Repeat 10 slow reps of this sequence, and then perform the same with the left leg. Repeat 1 to 2 sets as tolerated.

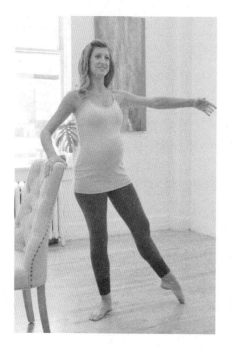 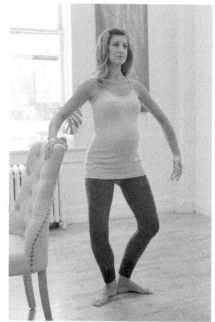

The Wise Woman's Pregnancy Stretching Program

Continue with all the stretches from first trimester except for Happy Baby, to avoid being on your back.

NOURISHMENT

You can expect your appetite to return at the beginning of the second trimester, and there's good reason: your baby is counting on you to properly grow and develop. The quantity and quality of nutrients that reach the baby via the placenta are strongly influenced by your nutritional intake as well as your overall health.

This increase in nutrition is perfectly timed to a returning tolerance for different foods. Now that you are less likely to be nauseous, you can expand your meal plans to a variety of different tastes. By doing so you are also expanding your baby's palate. During the second trimester, your baby will start to develop their own sense of taste, so it's a good idea to vary your diet so that the baby can be exposed to a diversity of options. While this doesn't influence development now, familiarity with a range of tastes will help them be more open to a variety of foods as they get older, which then will give them the diversity of nutrients necessary for a life of optimal growth and development.

We strongly recommend a diet that helps avoid gestational diabetes and keeps you from gaining too much weight. We now know that a baby with a high birth weight is often a consequence of gestational diabetes and poor maternal nutrition. These same babies are at a higher risk for a lifetime of illness, including obesity, heart disease, and diabetes.[13] To make things more complicated, we find that many women are hungrier and have more of a desire to eat carbs in the second trimester. The key to success for amplifying your diet is to plan ahead. Instead of focusing on starchy, processed foods, continue to follow the nutritional guidelines from first trimester. In short, choose polyphenol-rich fruits and vegetables and healthy gluten-free grains like quinoa, which is a grain-like food that has a higher amount of protein. And since you can tolerate a wider variety of foods now, try to eat all kinds of colored fruits and vegetables to get your carb fix.

The fruits and vegetables that have the most health benefits are saturated with color throughout. For example, a cucumber that is green on the outside but white inside isn't as nutrient-dense as spinach, kale, or asparagus. Each color has distinct positive effects that support your health and your pregnancy:

- *Red*: watermelon, pomegranate, beets, raspberries
- *Orange and yellow*: carrots, papaya, pumpkin, peaches, sweet potato
- *Green*: spinach, kale, avocado, kiwi, broccoli, asparagus
- *Blue*: blueberries, black beans, dark grapes
- *Purple*: plums, purple kale, blackberries

You will also need to eat plenty of protein, in addition to healthy fats, to keep you feeling full and satisfied. The optimal environment for building healthy cell membranes for both the mother and the baby require healthy fats from plant sources, like olive oil, and they should be included in every meal/snack. Our favorite is Kosterina Organic Extra Virgin Olive Oil because it is harvested early to maximize polyphenol content. Polyphenols are antioxidant plant-based micronutrients that are a rich source of potential health benefits. They are thought to combat inflammation and its related diseases.[14] To be deemed extra virgin, an olive oil needs to have 55 mg of polyphenols; Kosterina has 430 mg, which is far more nutritious.

The Power of Olive Oil

Olive oil is a staple in the Mediterranean diet that you have been following since preconception. Some believe that history's greatest thinkers, philosophers, and warriors came from the Mediterranean regions, and their success is due in part to a diet rich with the brain- and body-boosting benefits of olive oil.

Have a Pantry Makeover

Just because you are hungrier doesn't mean that you can eat whatever you want. The following are foods or ingredients that should be avoided because they aren't beneficial to you or your baby. Become a food detective and read labels carefully.

- Artificial sweeteners, found in condiment packets and in sugar-free packaged foods
- BHA/BHT, preservatives found in candy and processed meats
- Carrageenan, found in ice cream and dairy-free milk substitutes
- Cottonseed oil, corn oil
- Foods with artificial coloring, including energy drinks, pickles
- High fructose corn syrup
- Hydrogenated oils, found in some nut butters and baked goods
- Potassium bromate, found in some store-bought baked goods
- Products with MSG (or "flavor enhancer (621)"), included in salad dressings, mayonnaise, ketchup, barbecue sauce, and soy sauce or low sodium flavoring products, seasoning blends, and bouillon
- Texturized soy/soy protein isolate, found in energy bars, cereal, bread, veggie burgers, wraps, tortillas, and smoothies

Consider Ayurvedic Eating

Ayurveda also addresses maintaining balance with food. In these teachings there are six tastes: sweet, salty, sour, bitter, astringent, and pungent. Problems arise when we ignore some of these tastes and focus only on one or two. Beginning in this trimester, try to have some of each of these tastes in each meal:

- *Sweet:* Fruits, grains, rice
- *Salty:* Natural salt, sea vegetables like seaweed
- *Sour:* Oranges, tomatoes, yogurt, fermented foods
- *Bitter:* Spinach, kale, dandelion greens, herbs
- *Astringent:* Legumes, raw fruit, vegetables
- *Pungent (spicy):* Chili peppers, garlic, ginger, spices (Be creative in your food preparation adding spices that you like as long as they don't give you an adverse reaction like acid reflux.)

There are also traditional thoughts about certain aspects of eating that can be followed:

- Before each meal, wash your hands so that you may touch your food. Be present, relaxed, calm, and grateful when you eat.
- Avoid eating dairy and citrus fruit together.
- Avoid eating dairy and fish together.
- Avoid heated honey. The chemical composition of honey changes when heated and is not thought to be healthy. If you want to put honey in tea, let the tea cool down a bit first.
- Each meal should be an opportunity to engage with your senses. Enjoy the taste and smell of your food. Prepare dishes that are pleasing to the eyes and have different textures.
- Cook with spices to help strengthen the digestive system and to reflect the six tastes.

- Drink warm water instead of cold water: warm water is mildly laxative and aids in digestion. Starting your day with warm water and a squeeze of lemon if you like can help get the elimination process started.

- No fried foods, especially if you are feeling nausea. If you are sautéing meats or vegetables, add a little water to the pan to protect the food from frying. Or, stick with boiling, baking, and steaming.

- Prepare your food with love and care, maintaining a balanced emotional state. Let go of anger and jealousy as you cook.

- When we eat, we should fill our stomach half with food, a quarter with water, and a quarter should be left empty.

- Finish eating at least two hours before bedtime.

- During the day, eat as often as you feel is necessary based on requirements of your body. Do not fast, do not go hungry, and do not overeat.

Ice Water in Other Cultures

In Patricia's Spartan culture, ice-cold beverages are not helpful when you want to have a balanced and strong body. One historical story is that warriors would give ice to their opponents to weaken them before battle.

WISDOM

Even in pregnancy, wellness comes when every aspect of life is in balance. Paying attention to your body and mind is the first step. Once you are in tune with the changes happening to your body, you will be able to relax into them and develop an intuition that you can trust. This is when wise women really come into their power.

As you've learned, Ayurvedic medicine teaches that feeding your spirit is just as important as taking care of your body and mind. Beyond exercising and eating well, you can nurture your spirit. This helps you develop a deeper understanding of who you are and the kind of mother you want to be. Spiritual insight can come from solitary exploration such as a private meditation practice, a mindfulness activity, spending time in nature, pursuing a craft or hobby, praying in your home, or reading a book that moves you. Or you may find that being social and surrounding yourself with friends and family adds to your sense of spirituality. In the company of others, you may be able to fully let go, be joyful, and have fun. Whatever provides balance is the way to go!

Your Partner and Your Pregnancy

The second trimester is an important time for tending to relationships, especially with your partner. Enhancing the emotional bond between the two of you can help you reduce stress and therefore positively impact the baby's development. In one 2014 study, researchers found that pregnant women who believed that they had strong emotional support from their partners during the second trimester had lower emotional distress postpartum, and their infants were generally less distressed.[15] This is why it is so important to use this time to get your relationship in order.

The love that you give to your partner will come back to you. So if you're not feeling supported, focus your conversations on what you need rather than what stroller or what car seat you're going to get. Your partner can't help you if they don't know there is a problem. Talking about the things that are bothering you or symptoms you're feeling are ways to let them into your inner life. Don't just try to be a strong person and close them out.

Paying attention to your partner will help them feel like they are truly a part of the pregnancy because, in many ways, your partner may feel like the understudy. During the first trimester it's understandable that your partner was supporting you. Now that you have your energy back and are feeling better, it's time to check in and see what your partner needs. Sex, physical touch, and spending time together doing activities that bring you both joy will deepen your bond.

Every person has both a feminine side and a masculine side. The balance between those two energies creates your internal harmony, and we need to have that same balance within your relationship. If one of you is more masculine or more feminine, you need to purposefully balance each other out in order to bring out the best qualities in your relationship. If you can achieve that balance in your relationship in the second trimester, it will build cumulatively throughout your pregnancy and ultimately make you both better parents and better able to handle the challenges of having an infant, toddler, and young adult(s).

If you are without a partner, either suddenly or since the beginning of your pregnancy, you can create these same relationships within your larger tribe of family members, friends, coworkers, neighbors, or even your doctor. Whoever is providing you with support now, let them know that you're grateful and that you would like to lean on them throughout your pregnancy. It's important for you to formalize this relationship, even if you are feeling fine now. And just like you would support your partner, you can offer support to this special person as well.

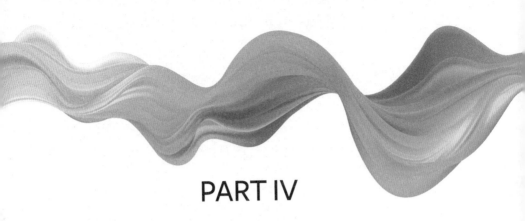

PART IV

The Third Trimester: Three Months to Get Ready to Deliver

The third trimester often brings a surge of energy and excitement. You'll be experiencing both your baby's movements and seeing your own body change in new and wondrous ways. You might even be starting to think about what your new life as a mother will be like.

As you're heading toward the pregnancy finish line, there's so much that will change over the next few months. As a wise woman, you know that you need to prepare for all of it. Now is the time to get your home in order, so that once you give birth, you will have forty days to simply rest, recover, and bond with your baby. It's like when you're on a plane and the flight crew reminds you to put your own mask on before you attend to your loved ones: you need to have everything in place to support this new baby well before arrival.

So put your attention on you, and continue to maintain and enhance your own wellness. Every day that you are managing stress, eating right, and exercising is like giving yourself and your baby an extra bonus of good health. In this section we will teach you how to modify the way you go about your day so that you can glide through the next few months pain free. You'll continue with your diaphragmatic breathing, and learn how to adapt it to labor. You'll amplify the fitness program, focusing on new exercises that prime you for delivery and postpartum. You'll learn why it's critical to cook nutritious foods in advance and freeze them so that they're ready for you after childbirth.

So enjoy these next few months because this really isn't the end of the race, it's the beginning of a whole new you.

YOUR BODY:

RESTORATIVE BREATHING:

MOVEMENT:

NOURISHMENT:

WISDOM:

Please make sure to read the next section—Labor and Delivery—during this trimester!

YOUR BODY

By the seventh month of pregnancy your baby can weigh as much as four pounds, and by the end of the trimester, it can gain another five. The placenta is becoming heavier as well, so it's no surprise that you may have already gained eight to ten pounds.

Your baby is developing a strong sensory system and will begin to notice the difference between light and darkness, respond to sound, and recognize both taste and smell, particularly your unique smell. These sensory experiences formed in utero will last a lifetime.

Yet all this development can take a toll on you. Your body is changing to accommodate the baby's growth in both size and weight, and the first victim is often your posture. At the same time, the placenta is excreting the hormone *relaxin*, causing a slackening in your musculoskeletal connections that's necessary for both supporting your baby and preparing for the birth. Your ligaments—the short bands of flexible tissue that connect your bones/joints or support an organ to keep it in position—will be softening, affecting the stability of your neck, rib cage, pelvic girdle, and the thoracic (upper) and lumbar (lower) spine. This new laxity is one of the reasons why you are more likely to misstep, feel off balance, or possibly adopt a compensatory, and totally avoidable, waddle.

Toward the middle or end of your third trimester, the tensegrity we discussed in the second trimester will occur. Your abdomen will begin to naturally feel supported—you may feel like something else is all of a sudden holding the belly up—as the internal pressure increases and the ligaments and fascia get to their maximal tension levels. This is good because we don't want you overgripping in any core muscles due to the stretching that is occurring in the linea alba.

By the third trimester all women will have stretching of the *linea alba*, the central seam of the abdomen, whether they notice it or not. This stretching is the *diastasis recti* that we mentioned in the second trimester section. We've treated many women who believe that a diastasis is an actual tearing of the abdominal seam, and if they have it, they won't be able to ever get a toned core back. This is a misconception. First, the abdominal seam doesn't actually tear into two halves: it stretches and widens so that the two sides of the rectus abdominis muscles are farther apart. For the vast majority of women, these muscles naturally regain their original form postpartum. When these tissues remain supple, buoyant, toned, and adaptable through exercise and proper breathing, they will more easily recover and return to their pre-pregnancy state. As you've learned, the fix is not about pushing or strengthening the abdominals more; it is about protecting and supporting your body as your abdomen expands, and coordinating the deep abdominal system to bring the tissues together to produce positive, supportive tension.

Easy Modifications for Daily Life

Prevention is the name of the game in the third trimester: we don't want to create any unnecessary strain or tension across the vulnerable abdominal seam through everyday movements or exercises that require curling. A sit-up motion increases pressure and may exacerbate a diastasis, making it more difficult to regain functional tension postpartum.

The following modifications not only prevent diastasis as well as other injuries, they better prepare the body to recover after delivery. The less strain you put on your body during this time, the less you have to deal with afterward.

For instance, if you lift something or pull/push a heavy package improperly, you will put pressure in places you shouldn't, leading to strain that can impede your overall recovery. Worse, in some cases, the discomfort from a strain may continue after delivery.

Continue with these modifications throughout your third trimester and postpartum. If you plan to breastfeed, your ligaments will not return to their previous supportive tension capacity until ten months after you stop breast-feeding. So being careful about how much stress or strain you put on your joints is a wise idea. These small adjustments can help anyone prevent injury and strain, so you can utilize the tools indefinitely.

Approaching Steps and Curbs

If your foot hits the ground suddenly, it jars the pelvis, which can actually make it rise and misalign. It can take a while to get it back into a neutral position, and in the interim you can experience pain. What's more, if you usually have a long stride when walking, it will make you more susceptible to misalignment, so learning to take smaller steps is just as important as watching where you are going.

Some women feel more stable later in pregnancy when they are walking in flatter shoes. This is because the lumbar lordosis curve accentuates as the belly grows, which shifts your center of gravity. When you wear heels, this curve becomes further accentuated, which puts too much pressure on your lower back. Supportive shoes, like sneakers, offer the most support and actively neutralize these curves. Stay away from ballet flats or sandals that have zero support. If you feel more supported with a slight pitch, limit your footwear choices to no more than an inch and a quarter of a heel, as long it has proper arch support. If your shoes don't have good arches, add an insole; we like the ones from Superfeet and Spenco.

If you've experienced a fall or a misstep, you can help your body reverse the misalignment through exercises that target the supportive muscles of the pelvis and hips. For instance, Andrea, one of Patricia's clients, came in during her third trimester. She was complaining that she couldn't walk without limping and waddling. Andrea thought the limp would just resolve on its own, yet two weeks later, it was still there. Patricia quickly noticed that her pelvic joint was misaligned and, because of this, her normal supportive muscle groups couldn't fire/engage. Patricia let Andrea know that she could correct her alignment herself. She showed her how to engage and fire up the stabilizing muscles in the pelvis/hips. After just a few minutes, Andrea was stunned that she could walk without a limp comfortably. She felt empowered and grateful. Then, Patricia taught her how to do other corrective and stabilization exercises for the pelvis to help combat future misalignments, whether they come on suddenly or gradually.

Bending Down/Squatting

Whether you are bending down to sit in a chair or load a dishwasher, washing machine, or dryer, or lift a basket of laundry, you need to do these activities with awareness. The key is to employ a flat back, make sure that your feet are level, and widen your stance. Then bend with a neutral spine, hips hinging back, and go into a flat back squat. Even when you're washing your face at the bathroom sink, bend with a nice straight, flat back squat. If you need to squat all the way down to the floor, lift your heels. Your hips should be facing in the same direction, straight ahead, pointed toward the object you are interacting with: you never want to twist where your hips are pointing in one direction and the rest of your body in another. This twist can excessively load your spine and cause discomfort.

Do not lift or push heavy objects, even if you feel like Wonder Woman. These movements may seem innocuous, but they put compression through the body, and because your tissues are in such a lengthened position, you're not going to be able to do them in a properly supported way like you used to before you were pregnant. Don't test the waters with cumbersome packages or moving furniture. You'll thank us later.

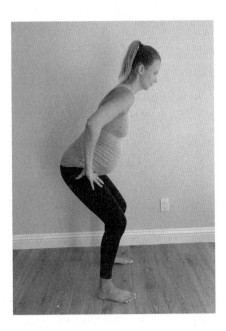

Cooking/Standing/Sitting for Long Periods of Time

If you have to stand for a long period of time—let's say over the sink while you wash dishes, or while you are preparing and cooking a meal—open a lower drawer and put one foot on top, using the drawer like a step stool. If you don't have a lower drawer, use a step stool or a three-inch-thick book, placed on the floor in front you. You can alternate lifting your legs if you are standing for more than twenty minutes; taking a small break is also a good idea. This small movement will reduce some of the pressure on your lower back.

When you sit down for an extended period of time, your body is being compressed by gravity, and your key supportive muscles will start to fatigue. It's good practice to take a short break by standing up and shaking your legs, which will bring circulation back into your body and refresh your deeper muscles. One trick is to take phone calls standing up and stick to sitting for computer work.

Then reset your posture as you go back to your seat, using a flat back squat to properly descend into a supportive chair. This movement allows you to automatically land on your sitz bones—the *ischial tuberosities* pelvic bones that you sit on—for an improved seated posture.

The best position to sit in is with your feet on the floor (never cross your legs) or on a step/box under your desk/table, holding your body tall and your core muscles engaged. Your lumbar lordosis should be supported by a thick sweatshirt or pillows—ideally a bedroom/standard pillow placed vertically so it runs from your tailbone to your shoulder blades. Your ears should be in-line with your shoulders and your chin relaxed down. If your chair has the ability to lean back, use this feature from time to time when you need to take a break and reduce loading on your spine.

Getting Dressed

To avoid falls when you're putting on pants, leggings, or pantyhose, watch that you're not testing your balance. Hold onto something or sit as you pull them up. Be careful that you're not pulling your leg through your clothes too forcefully or abruptly. This movement can cause muscular tension, a strain on your connective tissue, or misalign your pelvis at the *pubic symphysis*, your pubic bone, which is the front central attachment of both pelvic bones. Since the pelvis is naturally widening, the pubic bone at the front is stretching apart and can be vulnerable to strain.

Getting In and Out of a Car

The best way to get in and out of a car toward the end of pregnancy is going to be totally different than the way that you were doing it before. Vans and most SUVs are a little bit easier than regular cars, but the motion will be the same. First, open the car door as far as you can. Place yourself at the side of the car, standing with your back to the car. Your calves or the back of the thighs will be up against the side of the car. Keep your hips and shoulders square as you perform a flat back squat to lower your body into the car seat. Then, swing your legs and your shoulders around in one motion so that you are facing forward. As always, remember to put on your seatbelt.

To get out of the car, repeat the motion in reverse. Shut off the engine, then swing your whole body to face the side of the car, get your feet on the floor, and stand up with the same flat back squat mechanics. If you are unable to get out of the car without using your upper body, use your hands to push off the bottom of the seat or the side frame of the car.

If you're carrying multiples or if this is your second or third pregnancy, and you are feeling looser through your pelvis or less coordinated, you may need additional help. Hold onto someone's hands/arms/shoulders or lean on them in front of you as you descend and ascend from the seat of the car in the same way as previously described.

Additional Support to the Rescue!

If you feel weak through your core, have discomfort in your back, or if you're starting to see a cone-like bulge through the center of your abdomen, you may have an increased diastasis and can benefit from using a pregnancy belly band or pelvic belt. These belts provide external support by taking some of the pressure off the back and pelvis, lifting the belly almost like a corset lifts the breasts. With this help, the overstretched muscles don't have to struggle to support the belly at a time when they have become overstretched. The Baby Belly Pelvic Support belt by Diane Lee is our favorite.

If you are still having difficulty or pain with functional tasks, even with the support belt, you may need the assistance of a physical therapist who specializes in prenatal and postpartum health. This professional can create an individualized strategy that will bring the tissues of the abdomen together for improved support.

Sleep More Comfortably

During sleep, your body automatically, and very naturally, shifts positions. Under normal circumstances you probably sleep through this shifting, but during pregnancy, when there is just more of you to move, even the smallest shift can disrupt your sleep. You may have to fully wake up to roll over. Even getting into a comfy position to start the night off with can be challenging.

The goal for sleeping is to remain in the most neutral position possible so that the spine, joints, and muscles can rest and recover from the day's worth of walking and moving with more weight and possibly swelling. Body pillows provide great support to all your new curves so that you experience less pulling. You can adjust them to support your hips, knees, or your belly, or any combination of these three pressure points. Some are marketed specifically as pregnancy pillows. If you are able to sleep on your back or lie in a reclined position with a wedge or pillows behind you, putting pillows under your feet to elevate them can reduce leg swelling.

You also need a good pillow that supports the curve of your neck. Good pillows will allow for malleable support but not flatten over time. One of our favorites is The Clean Pillow from Kate Klein; it is both hypoallergenic and washable for the times when you might be sweating. It is a down pillow with an inner spandex core that prevents the down from flattening. Because of this construction, it provides more neck support to keep the cervical spine neutral.

Often women in second or third trimesters will feel nerve pain or numbness in the arm(s) when they sleep. Proper support from this type of pillow will help mitigate this pain. For instance, Rachel came to see Patricia during her third trimester because she wasn't sleeping well and couldn't take the constant fatigue and pain any longer. She had nerve pain in both her arms due to swelling/water retention. Her doctor had diagnosed her pain as gestational carpal tunnel syndrome and told her to just "deal with it" during the last stage of pregnancy.

First, Patricia explained that we never have to learn to live with pain. She then recommended The Clean Pillow. She also taught her how to use the pillow to optimally support the crook of her neck, which would reduce the pressure to the nerve; the trick is to only place the head on the pillow so that the firm ends are supporting the nook of the neck. With these tweaks, Rachel was able to finally sleep without nerve pain and could wake up feeling refreshed so that she could finish preparing for the baby's arrival.

Lastly, remember to practice good sleep hygiene as discussed in preconception. It is very important to prioritize sleep and "hoard" sleep/naps as it is almost guaranteed that you will have disrupted sleep once the baby is born.

The Best Way to Get Out of Bed

When you wake up, no matter what position you were sleeping in, roll onto your side at the edge of the bed, facing away from the bed. If you are on your back, bend the knee farthest from the edge of the bed and keep that foot on the bed. Push through the foot to roll your whole body as one unit onto your side. Then as the photos on the next page show, reach across your body with your top arm near the edge of the bed, and push into the bed with that hand and your bottom elbow as you press up to sit.

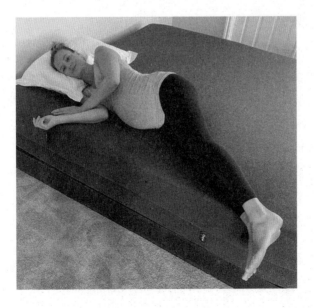

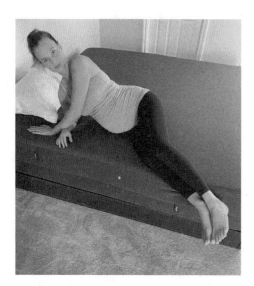 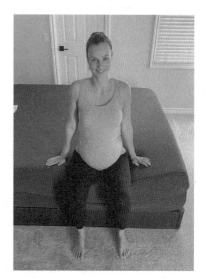

Common Third Trimester Complaints

Acid Reflux

You may experience acid reflux and other digestive complaints in the third trimester that are caused by the increased size of the baby and your uterus and how they are compressing your digestive organs around it. In addition, progesterone, the dominant hormone of pregnancy, tends to reduce the effectiveness of the esophageal sphincter, the muscle that opens and closes to allow food to travel from the esophagus to the stomach. This can also result in reflux. Progesterone also causes a slowdown in your intestinal motility, which can cause constipation and reflux.

Consider the remedies listed in the First Trimester section that may have provided relief for you, or try any of the following new ones:

- Drink coconut water, which may help neutralize acidity.
- Don't drink *during* meals; have the bulk of your daily hydration between meals.
- Elevate the head of your bed six to nine inches to keep stomach acids from reentering the esophagus while sleeping.

- Fennel seeds can soothe indigestion and reduce acid and inflammation. Crush a teaspoon and add to hot water or chew on them after a meal. Don't use this remedy too frequently, as it may lead to cramping. We recommend once a day after your largest meal.
- Peppermint tea may help settle your stomach.
- Wait two to three hours after eating before lying down.

Incontinence

Third trimester incontinence is not only triggered by pressure on the bladder; it also can result from losing access to the diaphragm caused by poor posture. When the diaphragm is active, it acts like a conductor for your core, allowing all the core muscles to engage together, including the pelvic floor. However, it's quite common to lose this capacity in this trimester, so we have to work harder at maintaining proper posture in order to recruit the muscles of the pelvic floor. When you exercise proper posture during the day, you are

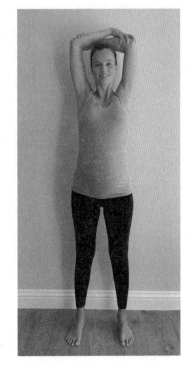

getting more engagement of the diaphragm and more tone and buoyancy in the pelvic floor, which will prevent incontinence. The diaphragm breathing, along with the Kegels, Deep Squat, and PNF Diagonal exercises, will also strengthen these connections, which will help with incontinence now and for labor/delivery, and postpartum.

If you are feeling acute pressure on the bladder, urgency, or incontinence, you can also try lengthening your thoracic core, which will help reduce some of that pressure. Crossing your arms overhead can lengthen the sides of your body (the thorax) and may give you some extra ability to engage your pelvic floor for reinforcing continence.

Group B Streptococcus (GBS) Infections

Many pregnant women develop Group B Streptococcus (GBS), a bacteria that colonizes in the vagina and could cause an infection to the baby during delivery. If you have had frequent urinary tract infections during pregnancy, ask your doctor to test for this bacteria. The goal is to avoid taking antibiotics during the third trimester and during labor, which would knock, out not just the Group B Strep ("GBS"), but the mother's entire microbiome, including all the beneficial bacterial we have been cultivating.

Instead, talk to your doctor about these remedies, and if you can, try them each before starting a course of antibiotics:

- Probiotics that contain *Lactobacillus rhamnosus GR-1* and *Lactobacillus fermentum RC-14* can reduce the presence of pathogenic bacteria and yeast and have been shown to eliminate overgrown GBS. You can take them orally and vaginally, and the best course of treatment is to combine these two methods. Insert the capsules at night as far as your finger can push them up, enough so that they don't fall out. Insert gently so that you do not scratch the vagina. Metagenics UltraFlora® Women's or Jarrow Femdophilus® 5 Billion are good brands to consider. *Saccharomyces boulardii* is another strain of probiotics that has been shown to reduce the presence of GBS and can also be taken orally and vaginally. *Lactoferrin* can also decrease GBS levels. Brands we recommend include Life Extension Apolactoferrin and Jarrow Lactoferrin.
- Insert allicin, a concentrated nutrient from garlic. Insert one gel cap or one half fresh garlic clove (must be cut or pierced for allicin to release) every night for four weeks, then once every three days for the rest of pregnancy. The allicin brand we like is Design's for Health Allicin.

Back and Nerve Pain

By this point you may feel pressure on the hip joints, and when your legs swell because of increased fluid retention, they put further pressure on the feet, ankles, and veins. By this time, the spine is at its maximal lordosis curve, which can create compression and back pain. What's more, the nerves closest to your spine or under the pelvis/at pelvic floor may be pressed as the baby grows and shifts position. The nerve flossing you learned in the second trimester (page 174) is very helpful to improve the mobility and fluidity of the neural tissues, minimizing and preventing back pain and nerve pain. Performing the Pelvic Self-Correction exercise (page 197) and any of the exercises that engage the "lumbar core" will help mitigate back or nerve pain in the legs. Massaging the muscles around the area of pain may loosen restriction. The diaphragmatic breathing and pelvic floor exercises you have been doing should also help to prevent sudden nerve pain in the pelvic floor region. Buoyancy, flexibility, and coordination of the pelvic floor with your breath is integral and will help immensely.

During the third trimester, your breasts become heavier in preparation for breastfeeding, and this additional weight affects the thoracic core, forcing a rounding of the midback known as a *kyphosis*. This motion stretches the cardiac ligament, which tugs on the neck, making your head move forward. The shoulders will then round forward along with the head, which further reduces the activation of all three core areas. The exercises you will learn in the Movement section are going to work the shoulder blades and the neck muscles to keep the neck more supported and elongated so that there's less compression of the nerves. When the neck is more aligned, the nerves that go out to the wrist and arms are less compressed and less affected by any increase in fluid around your wrist, as well as other small compartments along the length of the arm.

If you lightly strain a muscle at your spine or extremities, you can try to relieve some of the pain with ice for the first twenty-four to forty-eight hours. If you are still in pain after the third day, switch to heat in the form of a warm shower or a moist heating pad. Do not use a heating pad directly over the abdomen, but you can apply it by your hips. Depending on where the strain is, a supportive belly or pelvic belt can be helpful as well. If you feel like you significantly strained a joint or muscle, and it doesn't resolve in three to five days or the pain intensifies over time, reach out to your physical therapist, ob-gyn, or a prenatal/postpartum chiropractor.

Round Ligament Pain

The round ligament connects the front of your uterus to your groin. You may experience pain in this region—from underneath the belly to the groin—when there is a sudden increase in intra-abdominal pressure, like when you sneeze or cough. You may also get a burst of pain when you move to get up from sitting.

To avoid this pain, move slowly between positions, making your transitions smoother. A mild heating pad or warm shower can help, but be mindful not to use heat longer than fifteen to twenty minutes at a time. When coughing or sneezing, brace yourself by softly bending over toward your belly. This will bring slack to the tissues and decrease the pain.

Achiness in the Legs

Feelings of heaviness and achiness in the lower legs, particularly after a long day standing up, is primarily related to increased fluid retention. Excess water weight tends to pool in the hands, feet, and legs. This is magnified in the third trimester because of the growing uterus and compression on pelvic blood vessels responsible for shunting blood away from the lower extremities.

The following suggestions will reduce swelling. These practices need to be followed daily, as excess fluid retention will continue each day throughout the rest of your pregnancy.

- Compression socks, or maternity pantyhose or leggings, provide an added boost toward getting your circulation system to be more efficient. They reduce the amount of swelling that can pool in your lower legs by compressing the veins and lymphatic vessels that then support the flow of blood and fluid back to the heart. Rejuva is a brand of socks and leggings that come in fun patterns and look like trendy socks instead of grannie hose.

- ◆ Recline on your sofa or bed with a wedge or pillows to elevate your legs above the level of your heart for at least thirty minutes and up to two hours. At a minimum, elevate your legs one to two feet from the floor in the afternoon or after work.
- ◆ In the elevated position described above, "pump" the fluid out by flexing and pointing your feet twenty times when you first enter your elevated position and twenty times again before getting out of the position.
- ◆ Magnesium sulfate, or Epsom salt, foot soaks are helpful to draw out excess fluid.

Leg Cramps

During pregnancy, it's quite common to have lower than usual levels of the electrolytes potassium and magnesium. These minerals are important for regulating muscle contractions and reactivity, and without them, you can develop painful leg or foot cramps known as a *Charley horse*.

You can easily increase potassium with the following foods if you have at least one every day. Many of the same foods are also high in magnesium (see asterisk):

- ◆ Beans and legumes, including lima beans, pinto beans, kidney beans, soybeans, lentils*
- ◆ Beef
- ◆ Broccoli (cooked)
- ◆ Brown and wild rice
- ◆ Cucumbers
- ◆ Dried fruits, including prunes, raisins, dates
- ◆ Eggplant
- ◆ Fish, including halibut, cod, trout, rockfish*
- ◆ Fresh fruits, including bananas, oranges, cantaloupe, honeydew, apricots, grapefruit

- Leafy greens (cooked)*
- Mushrooms
- Nuts*
- Peas
- Potatoes
- Poultry
- Pumpkin
- Sweet potatoes
- Zucchini

You can also take a daily, bio-available magnesium supplement: look for a magnesium glycinate, malate, or citramate formulation. Topical magnesium oils can be applied to areas where you get cramping; we like Ancient Minerals magnesium lotion or Aimee Raupp Beauty's Mag-Ease Oil.

Braxton Hicks Contractions

Braxton Hicks contractions can begin as early as the second trimester but are most commonly experienced in the third. The muscles of the uterus tighten for 30–60 seconds and sometimes as long as 2 minutes.

Braxton Hicks are also called "practice contractions" because they prepare you for the real event and allow the opportunity to practice the breathing exercises. Although it isn't clear why these non-labor contractions occur, they may play a part in toning the uterine muscle and increasing blood flow to the placenta. They might also have some impact on softening of the cervix. Don't worry if you don't feel them; your uterus is ready for what's ahead, regardless.

A Braxton Hicks contraction can be described as

- Irregular in intensity
- Infrequent
- More uncomfortable than painful
- Not increasing in intensity or frequency and often disappearing within two hours

Braxton Hicks contractions can occur when you or your baby is very active, if someone touches your belly, when your bladder is full, if you're dehydrated, or even after sex. You may need to bring down your pace on your walks, give yourself a little more time to commute, or reduce the resistance or speed of any exercise.

The Recipe for a Productive Bed Rest

There are many different reasons why your doctor may require that you be put on bed rest. In fact, according to WebMD, almost one out of five pregnant women is placed on restricted activity or bed rest at some point during her pregnancy.[1] Even with our best intentions, and following the best advice for consistent exercise and a high quality diet, issues arise that can affect your health or the health of the baby. The goal of bed rest is that by taking it easy, you should be lowering the risk of preterm birth or pregnancy complications.

If this happens to you, listen to your doctor. Even though you may be asked to stay in bed, the rest of the program still holds. Following the guidelines in this book can help you make the best out of your situation. However, you must make the following modifications:

Modify diaphragmatic breathing:

If you've been put on bed rest, you can either rest in a reclined position or on your side. Review the breathing exercises and find the cues that work best for you and continue using them in these positions. For example, if you lie on your left side, think of expanding your lower rib cage upward, widening the ribs apart. If you are in a reclined position with a wedge or pillows supporting your back and head, visualize your ribs expanding apart as you breathe into the back and sides of your lower ribs. If you are still comfortable lying on your back, add extra pillows under your pelvis/buttocks to raise that area up. This will put you in a mildly inverted position and can help you access a better diaphragm breath.

Modify your exercise routine:

Even though you will no longer be able to do a thirty-plus minute daily walk that we recommend, we want you to continue the strengthening exercises in order to keep your muscles toned. These modifications will continue to support your health and get you ready for delivery. What's more, there's a real consequence of prolonged bed rest related to atrophy and deconditioning, which can be very problematic when you deliver the baby.

The following modifications can be made to exercises you already know. However, discontinue the program if you have any pain, bleeding, or other symptoms, and contact your doctor.

For Reclined Positions

Instead of standing or sitting upright in a chair, you can do the following exercises lying on your side *or* somewhat reclined with pillows supporting your back and head, as long as you're comfortable and feel that you can breathe properly while in these positions. Do the same amount of reps as you would standing or seated. Feel free to do less or more depending on your comfort with these modifications:

- The Ballet Arm Series (page 126)
- Kegels (See page 62)
- Standing Rotator Cuff with Resistance Band (page 133)
- Transversus Abdominis Activation with Marching (page 405)
- Sun Salutation (page 138)
- Sidebending with Twists (Arms Overhead) (page 271)
- PNF Diagonals (page 269)
- Glute Bridges (page 64)

Bicep Curls with Resistance Band. Bend both knees with feet on your bed while you are reclined on your back. Tie the resistance band in a loop around your thighs and hold the band (or loop both forearms into it) to do your bicep curls. You can also do one at a time in a similar fashion when lying on your side—place the looped resistance band under your thigh and pull the forearm to bend the elbow. Perform 2 sets of 10 reps with a focus on controlling the arms on the way down.

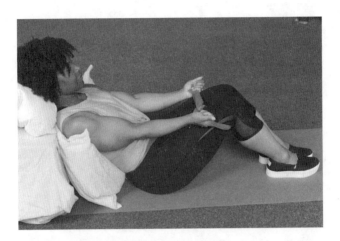

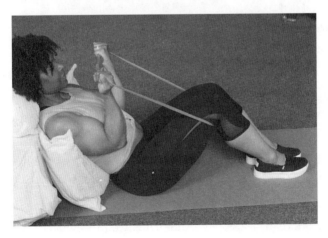

+ **Triceps Extensions.** Hold the resistance band with one hand behind your back down by your waist and with the other hand at the top by your upper back. Pull the band with your top hand going from an elbow-bent position to an elbow-straight position. Perform 2 sets of 10 reps with each arm.

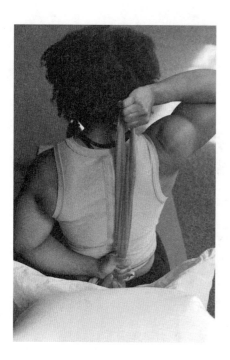
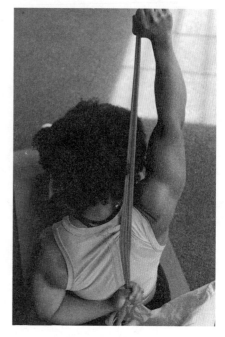

- **Lower Glute and Inner Thigh Isometric.** Lie on your back. Bend both knees with your feet on the bed, keeping feet and knees together. Place a small folded towel between knees. Press your feet into the bed with a little extra pressure into the heels to activate your lower glutes as you squeeze the knees together into the towel. Hold this squeeze for 10 seconds, and repeat 10 times.

- **Heel to Buttocks Isometric.** Lie on your back. Keep knees bent with feet and knees together. Squeeze the glutes at the lower gluteal region just as you did in Glute Bridges. Imagine pulling your feet closer to your buttocks to activate your hamstring. No motion should occur, just a muscle activation. Hold for 10 seconds, and repeat for 10 reps, 1–2 sets as tolerated.

- **Quad Squeezes (front of thigh).** Flex your quadriceps muscle at the front of your thigh with your knee straight in any position you are in. This will straighten your knee more. Hold the contraction for 10 seconds for 10 reps.

- Ankle Circles. Lie on your back. Place one leg on a bunch of pillows so that the knee is straight and the ankle is above the level of your heart. Perform ankle circles (20 clockwise, 20 counterclockwise) and ankle pumps (flexing and pointing feet 20 times). Repeat 1 to 2 sets. Do on both sides, one side at a time.

Modifications for Reclined Releases and Stretches:

- **The Preconception Exercise Routine** (see page 55)
- **Stiffness Relief Ball Rolling.** Use a tennis, pinky, or softer/squishy balls to release any muscles while you're lying on your back. Put the ball under your hamstring and roll the hamstring around, moving the ball from side to side along the length of your thigh. Place the ball under any trigger point/tight areas at the buttock. Or use the ball under your calf while on your back, rolling it to release any pressure points.

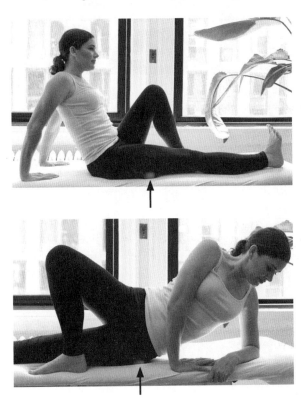

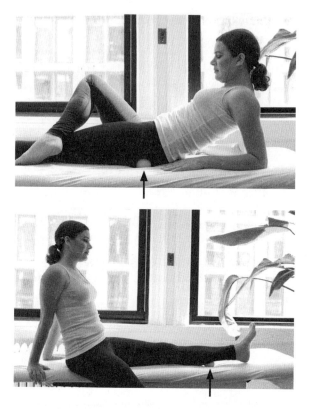

- **Pec Stretch.** Lie down on the side of the bed and open up one arm at a time into a 90-90 position with your arms (like cactus arms). Allow gravity to pull it back, opening up the chest. The arm may swing below the level of your bed for a deeper stretch. Repeat on both sides.

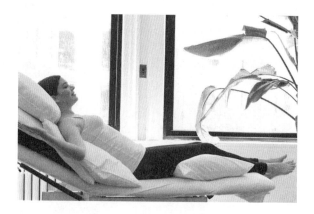

◆ **Hamstring Stretch.** Use a towel to bring one leg up toward your chest with a straight knee, keeping the opposite knee bent. Only bring the leg up to where you begin to feel a stretch. Push the leg away slightly into the towel and resist by holding the belt firmly so there is no movement. Maintain this pushing action for 5 seconds, pause, and then pull the leg in a little closer (it will be easier with more freedom of movement as you do this each time). Repeat this sequence 3 times. Hold the final stretch in the newly gained range of motion for 20 to 30 seconds. If the pushing and pulling is too difficult, simply perform a static stretch (go into the beginning of stretching range) and hold for 20 to 30 seconds.

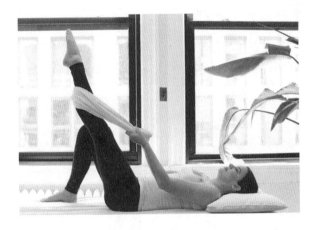

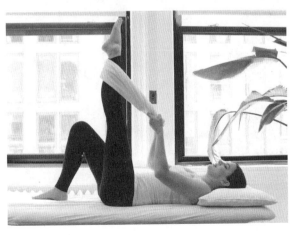

- **Calf Stretch.** Back off on the previous stretch by moving the leg a little farther away from you. Move the towel to your foot and pull the foot down toward you, with the knee staying straight to feel a stretch in your calf. Push up against the towel, pointing your toes, and resist by holding the towel firmly. Pause and then pull toes down toward you for a deeper stretch. Repeat sequence 3 times. Hold the final stretch for 20 to 30 seconds. If the pushing and pulling is too difficult, simply perform a static stretch (go into the beginning of stretching range) and hold for 20 to 30 seconds.

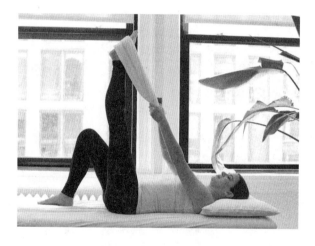

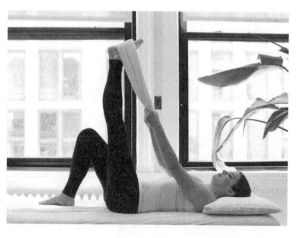

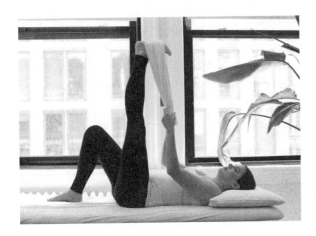

Seated Modifications

If you're allowed to sit up, try any of the seated exercises from the previous chapters, or modify the following by sitting on a chair or the edge of your bed:

- Seated Heel Raises (page 273)
- Stiffness Relief Ball Rolling with the foot (page 251)
- Pec Stretch (page 252): You can open your chest and strengthen your arms and shoulder blades by holding this 90/90 position as you diaphragm breathe. Hold for 10 to 20 seconds, for 10 reps.
- Ballet Arm Series (page 126)
- Sidebending with Twists (Arms Overhead) (page 271)
- PNF Diagonals (page 269)
- Seated Spine Roll with Ball (page 284)
- Bicep Curls with Resistance Band (page 248): Put the resistance band under your feet and bend your elbows while seated instead of standing.
- Triceps Extensions (page 249)

Exercises on All Fours:

If your doctor allows you to be in an all-fours position, you can do those exercises as described in each trimester. There are many great strengthening and stabilization exercises in the third trimester on all fours. They will be helpful for reducing spinal and pelvic pressure that builds up during bed rest while keeping your stabilizing muscles of all the cores engaged.

Practice Good Posture Even During Bed Rest

Be mindful when you are getting up those few times in the day to walk with good posture. Continue to practice growing tall through the crown of your head and holding a lengthened position. Whenever you are going to squat at the toilet, remember to have a flat back, hinge from the hips, and really use your legs. On the way up, use your lower glute muscles around the sitz bones with the flat back squat.

Dial Back Your Stress Response

We've already discussed how the way you handle stress can affect the growth and development of your baby. In the third trimester we want to be sure to not pass on any negative effects of acute stress. While we can't control the rest of the world—your boss harping on you—we can control how we choose to respond. Some people let stress fester: if something annoyed them for two minutes, they feel stressed for the rest of the day. Another person may have the same uncomfortable, stressful experience and brush it off within two minutes of it happening. You want to be that second person when you are pregnant. The reason: the negative effects of stress are entirely dependent on their frequency, duration, and intensity. Ideally we want to mitigate all three.

Having happy experiences helps create a positive mental state that gets stronger each time we cultivate and focus on the happiness and positivity in our lives. It is a loop that gets stronger through repetition. So while we can't avoid every stressful encounter, we can learn how to adjust our response to not have negative effects linger. If we focus on negativity, stress, worry, hurt, self-loathing, anger, jealousy, danger, etc., we are shaping our brains to react more readily and strongly to these types of feelings. However, if we can quickly shift our focus to positivity, kindness, happiness, gratitude, calmness, etc., our brains will wire in a way that makes them more reactive to these positive feelings. The truth is, your brain is more resilient than your baby's. It will not be affected by the negative effects of stress (cortisol response, inflammation, etc.) if we can release ourselves of the acute stress quickly.

As a wise woman, whenever a stressful situation occurs, be mindful of it. Observe how you are feeling; don't just rush and react to get that thing done for which you just got yelled at. You will actually be more productive and complete the task more successfully if you pause for a moment and take a diaphragm breath, think of a happy scene or doing something that brings you joy. Repeat your mantra to yourself, shower your baby with love, smile to remind your insides that you are calm and happy, channel love to your boss because they may not have realized what they did and how their actions affected you, and rise above the whole situation.

Above all, remember that you are safe, you are wise, and you are beautiful. In the grand scheme of things, everything will get done, and it will get done well. There is no bear chasing you; this is just an acutely stressful moment that needs to pass. You may need 3 to 5 minutes to fully reset. But those few minutes could make a world of a difference for your internal chemistry and your baby's overall health.

RESTORATIVE BREATHING

Most pregnant women will have difficulty breathing during their third trimester, and it will be especially noticeable if you haven't had this problem so far. By this point you can no longer fully access your diaphragm because the baby is taking up that space, so you can't possibly expand and contract your lungs in an efficient way. This situation causes *hypocapnia,* a condition where you do not have enough carbon dioxide in your lungs to keep the internal pressure at an ideal level. You may feel like you can't catch your breath or that you have to suck more air in on your next inhale. In reality, you're stuck in a negative feedback loop where you are actually breathing harder than normal and blowing off too much carbon dioxide. This carbon dioxide deficit then triggers you to take a deeper breath in, and you suck in more air than you need, so you end up blowing off more again.

You may experience different symptoms that are letting you know that you aren't breathing as well as you can. Memory loss or brain fog, nausea, or fatigue might be attributed to having too much on your plate, yet the cause may be related to breathing. As we learned, this lack of carbon dioxide reserves in the lungs causes a cascade of effects on your internal chemistry. The negative feedback loop leads your red blood cells to hold on to oxygen instead of distributing it out to both the body and brain.

Improving how you breathe during this trimester will not only help you feel better, but it will also help you get your body back after pregnancy. Your diaphragm can act as that wonderful conductor of your core, involuntarily activating your core with everything you do in your day functionally. It will also keep you in a parasympathetic state that prevents cortisol from taking over, which can stall your metabolism, making you more likely to hold onto the weight you've gained.

Try any of the following suggestions when you feel like you need to access better breathing. It is good to get into a habit of performing this mindful breathing for at least three to five minutes, five times per day or at the top of each hour. You can also incorporate the breathing cues into your meditations or prayers:

- Extend your exhale. Slow down your exhalations and let yourself get to the very end of your exhale. Pause, and you will feel the reflex kick in to take the next inhale.
- Continue with the inverted postures that you learned in second trimester; they will help to decompress the spine and get you back into a position where you can improve your breathing. If you can't completely get into an inverted posture, you can hang off the edge of a chair or put your forearms on a countertop or table. Let the belly just relax forward and hang.
- At any time or in any position, you can use cupped hands, a paper bag, or mask around your nose and mouth to get a little boost in your internal chemistry. You will be taking in some of the previously blown off carbon dioxide. After a few breaths in this manner, you actually start to increase the carbon dioxide reserves in your lungs, which leads to a more peaceful, settling response that stops the negative, vicious cycle.
- When seated, or standing, cross your arms at the top of your head and breathe mindfully, in and out, softly and quietly through your nose. This position will take pressure from the shoulder girdles and arms off the thorax to open more space for the diaphragm and lower ribs to expand.

- Focus on breathing gently and quietly in and out through your nose, which will naturally produce nitric oxide, which can improve overall blood circulation.

- When you think of something joyful or happy, your breathing immediately shifts to amplify that experience, which automatically puts you into a better state with your breathing. Try diaphragmatic breathing while imagining a pleasing scene to calm your mind and put yourself in a more relaxed state.

Practice Breathing for Labor and Delivery

Because you've learned how to breathe to the best of your capacity throughout your pregnancy, and you have been coordinating your breathing throughout the exercise programs, you will naturally be more efficient during labor because your body is primed to utilize your breath in coordination with your muscles. This will provide for a smoother delivery.

During labor, your breath affects your pelvic floor and can help it widen and open smoothly when it is time for delivery. The following observations can help you connect your breathing with your pelvic floor:

- Sit on your hands while seated on a physio ball or a cushioned chair. Feel how your pelvic floor relaxes and feels like a balloon descending down into your hand as you inhale. Your sitz bones may feel like they widen and relax.

- Observe what happens as you exhale. You should feel a mild drawing in or mild tension. The sitz bones will gently come closer together.

- Be mindful that the pelvic floor muscles are shaped like a diamond. Since many of us sit for long periods of time, the back half of the diamond—the posterior pelvic floor—will be tighter. We will want to open that area with a few mindful inhales.

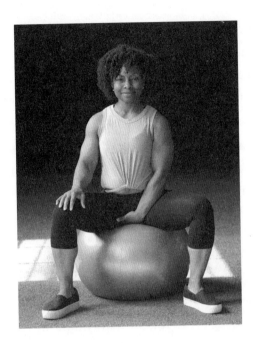

Labor Breathing Exercises

Now that you have an idea of how your pelvic floor moves while breathing, you are ready to train your breath for delivery. Practice this technique once to get a sense of the experience, but save the larger effort for practicing the week before your due date.

The body's innate and natural response to pain is to pull up and clench the pelvic floor. However, during labor, we need to release into the pain. Just as athletes visualize their hardest shot or moving swiftly across the court or track to be successful at game time, we want you to use visualization with these exercises. In our clinical practices this method has improved women's success in labor and delivery.

- ♦ Relax the pelvic floor on an inhale, and as you exhale, continue the relaxation of the pelvic floor. This will feel different than what we just observed. In labor and with pushing, we want to optimize the contraction's ability to slowly push the baby down and out. The pelvic floor must be relaxed with both the inhale and the exhale to allow for this. Practice this pelvic floor relaxation for a few breaths.

- On an exhale, as your ribs come down and in, allow the upper abs to gently contract, pressing the lower ribs together. Release as you inhale to restore length and space again to your ribs and tummy. When you are ready for pushing, you will be able to push the baby downward by activating these same muscles. Try this a couple of times just to get the hang of it. Please note that your lower tummy (lower abdominal area) should stay relaxed.
- During the final stage of labor, you may be told to not push by your ob-gyn/doula/midwife/nurse. It is important to prepare for this by softening your breath like you are blowing out birthday candles. Practice blowing gently on a tissue to become familiar with this effort.
- Sometimes women can tolerate pain better when they are panting. Practice gentle panting, short inhales and exhales, while relaxing the pelvic floor at the same time.
- Sometimes women can tolerate pain better when they are making sounds. Using low sounds like a long, low *G* or *O* or even an *Om* as you exhale can prove to be relaxing.
- Throughout labor, visualize the baby descending down and out, especially with each contraction.

MOVEMENT

*A wise woman knows how to listen to her body. During this last tri-*mester, do the exercises as long as you feel up to them and they feel good. Each day will feel different depending on what you've done the day before or the baby's movements or position: you may be a little more fatigued, or sore, or uncomfortable. Don't feel like you have to push through. If you can't get into certain positions, use the modifications. Ideally we want you to do the exercise program exactly the way it's laid out, but if you need to break up the program, feel free to do so. You can insert a ten-minute walk or a stretch or two in between exercises. Make sure that you are taking sips of water throughout. Change your clothes if you're getting warm.

Most important, stay positive. Allow yourself to take it day by day and adjust the program as you need.

Fitness Activities to Put on the Back Burner

Now that you're in your third trimester, we do not want you jumping or bouncing at all. These physical activities either have a high risk of injury or falling or carry a risk of losing your balance:

* Bicycling (a stationary bike is fine)   * Contact sports

- Diving
- Gymnastics
- Horseback riding
- Ice skating
- Scuba diving
- Mountain climbing or exercising in higher elevations than normal
- Skiing
- Volleyball
- Water skiing

Don't worry. You'll be able to get back to your favorite activities after about three months following childbirth.

The Third Trimester Exercise Routine

Thirty-Plus Minutes of Aerobics

One pregnancy fact is that the further along you are in pregnancy, the less oxygen you have available for aerobic exercise. Modify the intensity of your daily walk according to how you feel. Your daily walk may need to be broken into segments to prevent unnecessary fatigue. It is important to warm up before your workout, perform your workout with good form, and then cool down and stretch.

Even though we don't want you to constantly monitor your heart rate, recent research has shown that women in their third trimester can work out within 60 to 80 percent of their age-predicted maximum maternal heart rate.[2] You can modify intensity based on your perceived exertion rating: rate your exertion as a 6 or 7 on a 1 to 10 scale; this means you should be able to talk as you exercise. High-intensity or prolonged exercise in excess of 45 minutes can lead to low blood sugar, so make sure that you eat before exercise, or limit the intensity or length of the exercise to minimize this risk.

Continue to take walks outside in nature. Christiane Northrup, MD, author of *Women's Bodies, Women's Wisdom,* believes as we do that walking directly on the earth for at least 20 minutes a day grounds you and can reduce inflammation by 20 percent.

Thirty-Plus Minutes of Eccentric Strengthening

Continue with the following exercises from the previous chapters: Foot Doming (page 70), Step Forward Arm Lift for Lower Back Pain Relief (page 173), and, if still comfortable, the Pelvic Rotation on Hands and Knees (page 129; or seated hip rotation). You should continue with the Kegels with Resting Squats but use a yoga block or book under your pelvis in the squat if you feel like you need that assistance to hold the position. Begin your daily routine with the Standing Pelvic Self-Correction to make sure the pelvis is in improved alignment each time you begin. This exercise routine relies heavily on resistance bands. Refer to page 124 to make sure that you are using them correctly.

At this point we are modifying some of the exercises so that you can continue to engage your deep supportive muscle groups. This will help you prevent misalignment and discomfort. We have tweaked the exercises to amplify proper tone and buoyancy in the pelvic floor for successful labor/delivery. Many women sit a lot in their day, especially those who work or commute long hours. Because of this there is a tendency to have a tighter posterior area of the pelvic floor. The deep squats that you will be doing in this trimester will help to lengthen the posterior pelvic floor.

The following exercises continue to focus on maintaining proper posture and strengthening the midback and neck to compensate for increased belly girth, breast volume, and stress on the spine. Centering/grounding exercises for the core and feet are added, along with proprioceptive/balance exercises for the increased challenge of belly girth. Stretching the calves is very important in this trimester as well. There are exercises that focus on strengthening the arms, legs, and lower gluteal muscles to prepare the body for the various positions for labor and to compensate for not being able to use your outer abdominal muscles for bending down or controlling your core when you are going up and down stairs due to increased belly girth. We're also getting your upper body ready for life after delivery, specifically for baby holding and breastfeeding.

What's a Valsalva?

Valsalva is the push that you do while holding your breath, like when you are trying to pass a bowel movement. In the third trimester, we want to avoid creating a Valsalva because it changes your blood pressure, and you can unintentionally increase your intra-abdominal pressure, which can lead to hemorrhoids or organ prolapse (the dropping of the rectum or bladder down the vaginal canal). Keep your breathing continuous as you exercise and avoid bearing down.

Equipment Needed

- Physio ball
- Resistance band
- Step stool
- Sturdy chair
- Tennis ball
- Yoga block or hardcover book at least 3 inches thick
- Yoga mat or towel

Exercise: Pelvic Self-Correction: Push-Pull Series: Standing (Modified)

EQUIPMENT: A sturdy chair or a wall; towel (optional).

PURPOSE: To correct the alignment of your sacroiliac joints for relief of pain, clicking, or soreness in the back of the pelvis or the lower back region. Do this before and after you exercise, anytime you feel discomfort in the pelvis or lower back, and before bed at night.

START POSITION: Stand tall and hold the back of a sturdy chair with your left hand. Grab hold of your right leg under your thigh with your right hand or forearm. Position the knee outward toward your shoulder at roughly 90 degrees of hip flexion. If you can't reach under your thigh, use a towel to pull your leg up.

SEQUENCE:

STEP 1. Using the glutes and back of your thigh muscles, gently push your thigh away from your chest and resist this motion with your hands. This is called isometric resistance. Hold this push for 5 seconds.

STEP 2. Hug your knee a couple inches closer, moving your leg toward your shoulder. Repeat 5-second isometric resistance. Hug it in a little closer and repeat. You will perform a total of 5 (5-second push/pulls) incrementally bringing your knee closer toward the shoulder each time.

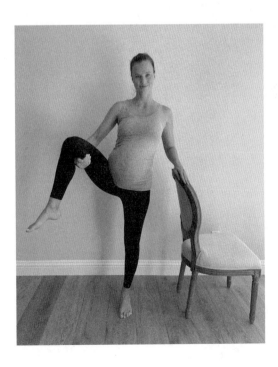

Exercise: Cactus Arm Squat

PURPOSE: To strengthen the legs, glutes, and stabilizing muscles of the shoulder and shoulder blades. This is a neutral spine squat that can be used (without the arm movement) when you are doing activities of daily living (like loading the dishwasher, doing laundry, and bending to pick up something light) and soon, when handling baby [All Cores].

START POSITION: Stand tall with feet shoulder width apart, or a width that feels comfortable. Grow tall from the crown of the head and stay grounded in your feet with both feet pointing straight ahead.

SEQUENCE:

STEP 1. Lift your arms 90 degrees out to the side and then bend at the elbow 90 degrees, hands pointing toward the ceiling.

STEP 2. Inhale and bend your knees to go into a neutral flat back squat. Your ears should be in-line with your shoulders, your chin in, and you should still "grow tall" from the crown of your head. Your body will bow forward, and the front of your hips should crease/fold as your buttocks lifts behind you. Your head should stay in-line with the spine as you look out at the floor. Keep the arms wide, chest open, and shoulders rotating back so that your wrists are close to or in-line with your elbows as much as possible.

STEP 2. Exhale and continue to diaphragmatically breathe as you hold this position for 5 to 10 seconds. Focus on staying grounded in the legs and keeping your arms/shoulders working to maintain an open chest with shoulders rotating behind.

STEP 3. On an exhale, press through the heels to activate the lower glutes (muscles by the sitz bones of the pelvis) as you rise up to standing with arms relaxed down. Repeat this 5 to 10 times.

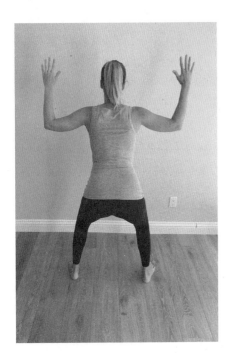
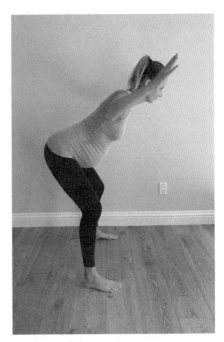

Exercise: Peripheral Neuromuscular Facilitation (PNF) Diagonals

EQUIPMENT: Resistance band.

PURPOSE: To strengthen the shoulder blades and arms while integrating your core and posterior muscles of the spine. This is an exercise that works the diagonal muscle patterns of the body that we need to perform functional tasks well. We have certain patterns of movement that calm our nervous system; these diagonals patterns both calm and strengthen our body [Thoracic and Lumbar Cores].

START POSITION: Stand tall with your feet hip width apart. Shoulder blades are slightly lifted, floating up and slightly back toward the back of your ears.

SEQUENCE:

STEP 1. Put one end of a resistance band under your right foot and hold the other end with your left hand, which is placed in front of your left hip with thumb down, as if you are pulling a sword out of your left front pants pocket.

STEP 2. Inhale, pull the band across your body, and turn your hand outward, like you are drawing a sword, lifting the arm overhead. Your eyes can follow your hand, looking up at your arm if that is comfortable. You can position your arm farther away from the head if the one o'clock position is uncomfortable. If you have pain in your arm, do not extend the elbow to its end range; instead, keep it soft. Make sure to keep the body feeling tall and keep the shoulder blades lifted.

STEP 3. Exhale and return to the start position, lowering the arm slowly and with control. Repeat this 10 times, then perform with the right arm. Complete 2 sets (20 reps total) on each side. Each time, the movement begins with the hand turning downward first.

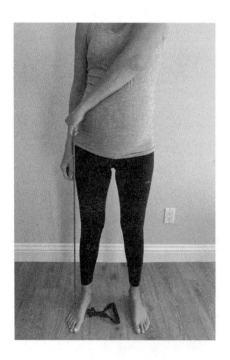
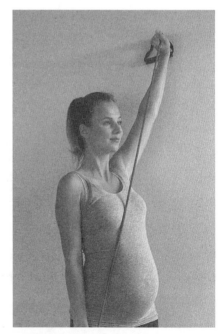

Exercise: Sidebending with Twists (Arms Overhead)

PURPOSE: To elongate the trunk, making space for improved diaphragm activity and to stabilize the thorax, shoulders, and shoulder blades to support better posture [Thoracic Core].

EQUIPMENT: A resistance band; chair (optional).

START POSITION: Stand tall *or* sit tall on the edge of a firm chair and bring arms overhead in a V while holding a medium resistance band with tension in both hands.

SEQUENCE:

STEP 1. Grow tall from the crown of your head with chin relaxed down as you look straight ahead. Inhale and gently bend to the right side, keeping your arms in a V overhead. Keep your left foot (or your left sit bone if you are sitting) firmly planted. Make sure you stay lifted in both sides of the body even though you are bending to the right. Exhale and take another inhale in this position.

STEP 2. Exhale again and return to the start position. Repeat on the left side. Alternate and do 5 times on each side.

STEP 3. Return to your tall, lifted, standing or seated posture with arms in the V position overhead. Inhale and rotate the whole body toward the right. Allow your head, body, and hips to rotate gently in comfortable range. Your right foot will roll outward and your left foot inward as you perform this gentle twist. Stay in this position, actively lengthening the sides of your body with your exhale and another inhale. Exhale and return to center.

STEP 4. Inhale, and repeat the movement to the left. Perform 5 times, alternating each time. Take a break to relax the arms from the overhead position at any time as needed.

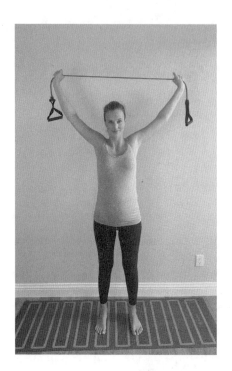

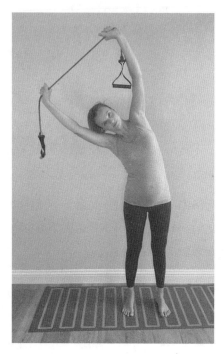

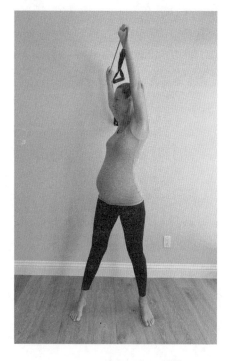

Exercise: Seated Heel Raises

EQUIPMENT: A sturdy chair, tennis ball.

PURPOSE: To strengthen and gain control in the stabilizing muscles of the feet and ankles, including the deep muscles of the calves. The exercise will strengthen the calves to support good standing posture and blood circulation and to improve balance.

START POSITION: Sit tall on the edge of a chair. Keep feet pointing straight ahead and place a tennis ball between your heels.

SEQUENCE:

STEP 1. Inhale and raise your heels to come up to your tippy-toes. Keep the ball between your heels/ankles.

STEP 2. Exhale and slowly lower the heels with control. The ball will keep your arches and ankles in-line with the center of your feet (into a neutral position). You may experience a bit of jaggedness to the movement as your heels lower: Your calf may not lower smoothly, like it is having little hiccups. That is normal; just keep the movement slow and as controlled as possible.

STEP 3. Controlling the heels down to the floor is the key part of this exercise. Maintain good posture and breathe diaphragmatically throughout the exercise. Repeat 10 slow reps, for 1 to 2 sets.

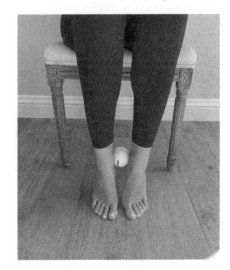

Exercise: Hip Sink and Lift

EQUIPMENT: A sturdy chair, a step stool or step, yoga block or thick book.

PURPOSE: To strengthen the gluteus medius muscle and gain control of the pelvis amid a changing center of mass and ligament laxity. If you have difficulty activating the deep outer hip muscle when you do this exercise, return to the Pelvic Rotation on Hands and Knees (or seated pelvic rotation modification) [Lumbar Core].

START POSITION: Stand with your left foot parallel to the step with the bannister in front of you or on a step stool with a chair at your side. Stand tall with shoulders lifted up and back and neck elongated, as if a string was pulling you up through the crown of your head. Your right leg should be dangling by your side toward the floor, which will make your right pelvis drop below the level of the left that you are supporting yourself with. Hold onto a sturdy chair or the bannister to help with your balance. Keep feet pointing straight ahead the whole time.

SEQUENCE:

STEP 1. Exhale and press through the left foot. Use the muscles in the deep outer left hip to bring the pelvis to a leveled position. Avoid using any back muscles or muscles on the right side of the body. Hold this position for 5 seconds.

STEP 2. Inhale and slowly, with control, allow for the pelvis to tip again where right pelvis/hip drops down (left hip is higher) and right leg dangles to that lower position again.

STEP 3. Perform 10 slow reps and then repeat with the right leg supporting you. Repeat for 1 to 2 sets.

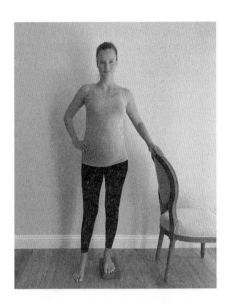 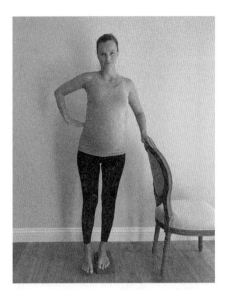

Exercise: Bicep Curls

EQUIPMENT: A resistance band; a sturdy chair (optional).

PURPOSE: To strengthen the biceps and integrate postural muscles. This exercise will help prepare you for lifting and carrying the baby (and all the equipment!) after delivery [Thoracic Core].

START POSITION: Stand tall with your feet hip or shoulder width apart with the right foot placed slightly in front of the left. Keep toes pointing straight ahead. Grow tall from the crown of your head, chin relaxed down, with eyes looking straight ahead. This exercise can also be done seated if you prefer.

SEQUENCE:

STEP 1. Place the middle of the resistance band under your right foot and hold both ends with both hands. Make sure your spine stays neutral (maintain proper curves of the spine), both hips are still, and keep shoulders and shoulder blades lifted and still.

STEP 2. Exhale and bend both elbows up slowly with palms up. You should be able to get through the whole range of motion of bending your elbow and feel moderate resistance toward the second half of the range of motion. If you can barely bend your elbow due to the resistance tension, you need more slack in the resistance band or to drop to an easier resistance level. Hold this position as you continue to exhale and take an inhale.

STEP 3. On your exhale, lower your arms down to your side, extending the elbows, super slowly with palms continuing to face up. Take double the amount of time to lower the arms (extend the elbows) than to raise them. This focuses on the eccentric (lengthening) contraction. Repeat this movement, with this specific timing, for 10 repetitions. Shake out your arms.

STEP 4. Perform 10 repetitions with the left arm. Complete 1 to 2 sets total on each side. Take a break on either side if you can't maintain neutral posture or if you begin to fatigue.

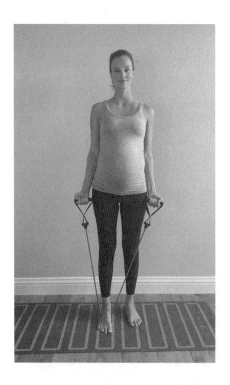
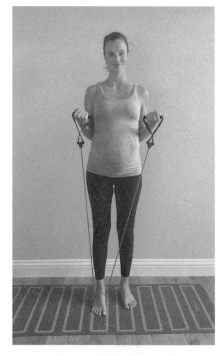

Exercise: Standing Leg Slide

EQUIPMENT: A sturdy chair, a towel.

PURPOSE: To strengthen and lengthen the inner thighs while also strengthening the gluteus medius muscle. This exercise will help you gain pelvic and hip control [Lumbar Core].

START POSITION: Stand tall on a smooth floor (no rug or carpet) holding a chair or the wall with your left hand. Place a small towel under your right foot.

SEQUENCE:

STEP 1. Inhale and slide the right foot out at your side, using the towel to allow for a smooth gliding movement. Your body may bow forward a small amount with the spine staying neutral and controlled. Only go as far out to the side as you feel you can control; do not go out into a large stretch.

STEP 2. Exhale and slowly, with control, slide the leg back to the start position. Focus on pressing the right straight leg down into the towel and smoothly gliding it back in.

STEP 3. Perform 10 slow reps and then repeat with the right leg supporting you. Do 1 to 2 sets.

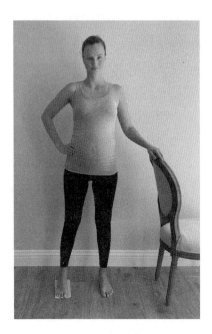 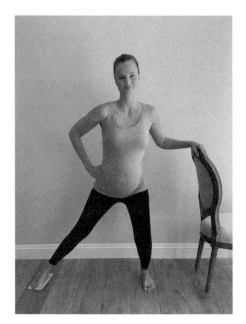

Exercise: Side Stepping with Resistance

EQUIPMENT: A resistance band.

PURPOSE: To strengthen the legs and hips, particularly the *gluteus medius* muscle and promote centeredness amid a changing center of gravity [Lumbar Core].

START POSITION: This exercise travels with steps to the right and left so do this in a hallway or wide/long room. Stand tall, grow tall from the crown of the head, with feet hip width apart. Feet should point straight ahead with knees bent, tracking over the second toes. Place a resistance band around the middle of the thighs, above the knees. Hold the band with mild tension in the start position.

SEQUENCE:

STEP 1. Inhale and step to your right with your right foot. Make the step as wide as you can control. Your spine should stay straight, and your body should simply transition to the right as one unit. The final photo shows improper form.

STEP 2. Exhale and transfer your weight onto the right leg, allowing for the knee to bend just like the left. Stay stable in the pelvis and spine and focus on grounding your weight in your legs.

STEP 3. On your next inhale, step the left foot toward the right, maintaining hip width distance or come in a little closer. Continue to step toward the right 10 times slowly and with control. Feel the focus of the work in the left deep outer hip muscles. The lumbar (abdominal) core should be activated naturally as you keep stillness and stability in the trunk and pelvis.

STEP 4. Switch sides and step toward the left. Place your focus on the right outer hip. Perform 3 to 5 sets, working both legs.

Step 1

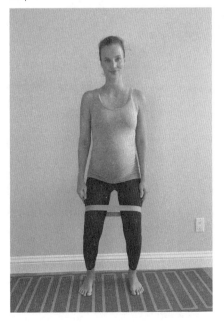

Step 2

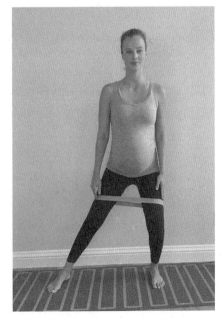

Step 3

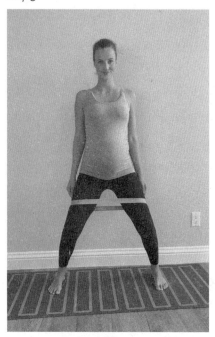

Improper Form

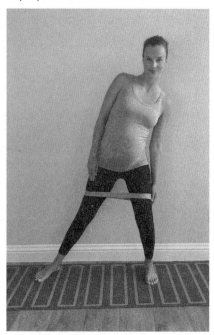

Exercise: All Fours Arm Lift to the Side

EQUIPMENT: A yoga mat or towel.

PURPOSE: To strengthen the stabilizing muscles of the spine, neck, shoulder, arms, and shoulder blades. These muscles are very important to maintain proper head posture and combat rounded shoulders [All Cores].

START POSITION: Get onto hands and knees (all fours position) on a mat or towel on the floor. Position your hands (or fists) under your shoulders and your whole spine in neutral with the head in-line with the spine, chin tucked in slightly.

SEQUENCE:

STEP 1. Press shoulder blades apart gently. Inhale and raise your right arm out to the side to 90 degrees, keeping the elbow straight. Your thumb should point up to the ceiling throughout the exercise. Focus on the right shoulder blade coming closer to your left one as you lift your arm. Do not hitch the shoulder up to your ear. Make sure the spine stays neutral (maintain proper curves of the spine), both hips are still, and that the left shoulder and shoulder blade are supporting you. Exhale and lower the arm down to the floor at your side with control.

STEP 2. Repeat this movement at a slow tempo for 10 repetitions. Shake out your wrists/hands and then perform 10 reps with the left arm. Shake out your wrists again. Perform 1 to 2 sets total on each side. Take a break if you can't maintain neutral posture or if you begin to fatigue on either side.

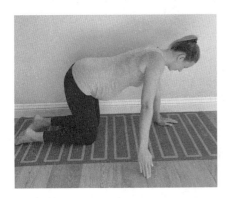 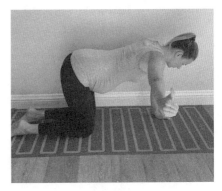

Exercise: All Fours Crawling

EQUIPMENT: A yoga mat or carpet/rug on the floor.

PURPOSE: To strengthen the stabilizing muscles of the spine, neck, pelvis, shoulder, arms, and shoulder blades. This exercise works on coordinating your spinal muscles to reduce spinal tension, improve alignment, and amplify control and strength. This exercise travels with steps to the right and left so do this in a hallway or wide/long room. It is a great exercise to do before you go out for your walk [All Cores].

START POSITION: Get onto hands and knees (all fours position) on a mat or carpet/rug on the floor. You can be on your fists if being on your hands is uncomfortable for your wrists. Position your hands (or fists) under your shoulders and your whole spine in neutral with the head in-line with the spine, chin tucked in slightly. Look down between your hands, keeping the head in-line with the spine.

SEQUENCE:

STEP 1. Press shoulder blades apart gently. Maintain consistent diaphragmatic breathing throughout this exercise.

STEP 2. Bring your right hand forward and your left leg forward followed by your left hand forward and your right leg forward in a reciprocal fashion. Stay slow and rhythmical with spine in neutral curves. You will need to work to keep your lower back curve in neutral, without letting it *sag* into extension.

STEP 3. Repeat this movement while diaphragmatic breathing for 3 to 5 minutes, for 1 to 2 times/day.

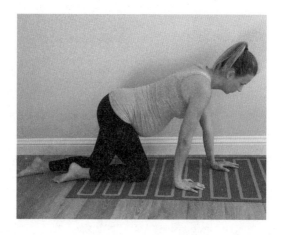

Exercise: All Fours Triceps Extension

EQUIPMENT: A mat (or carpet) on the floor; resistance band is optional.

PURPOSE: To strengthen the triceps muscle while activating the stabilizing muscles of the spine, neck, shoulder, and shoulder blades. This exercise helps to strengthen the back of the arms and shoulders, which will help when lifting and carrying your baby [All Cores].

START POSITION: Get onto hands and knees (all fours position) on a mat or towel on the floor. Position your hands (or fists) under your shoulders and your whole spine in neutral with the head in-line with the spine, chin tucked in slightly.

SEQUENCE:

STEP 1. Press both shoulder blades apart gently. Support yourself on your left arm, keeping shoulder blades apart and active. Inhale, and bend the right elbow at your side. Do *not* hitch the shoulder up to your ear. Make sure the spine stays neutral (maintain proper curves of the spine), both hips are still, and that the left shoulder and shoulder blade are supporting you.

STEP 2. Exhale and extend the elbow straight at your side. Feel the triceps activating. If this is too easy, place a resistance band under your knee and hold the other end with your hand as you extend the elbow.

STEP 3. After extending the elbow, focus on controlling the elbow back to the bent position at your side. Repeat this movement at a steady tempo for 10 repetitions. Shake out your wrists/hands and then perform with the left arm. Shake out your wrists again. Perform another set on each side. Take a break if you can't maintain neutral posture or if you begin to fatigue on either side.

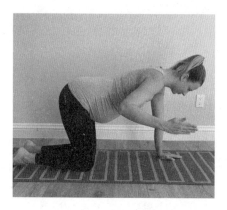
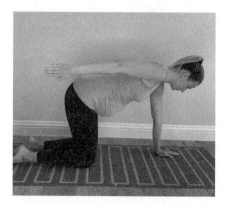

Exercise: Seated Spine Roll with Ball

EQUIPMENT: A sturdy chair and physio ball.

PURPOSE: To mobilize the spine segmentally and open the chest. This exercise will create more space in the body amid the growing belly, helping you feel more "free" in your breath as a result.

START POSITION: Sit tall at the edge of a chair with legs/feet apart so that the physio ball is on the floor in front of you. Place both hands comfortably on the physio ball.

SEQUENCE:

STEP 1. Start from the crown of your head and grow tall, lifting the sides of the body as you tuck your chin toward your chest. Continue to round the spine one vertebra at a time as you lower your body into a C curve. Keep your hands on the ball.

STEP 2. Continue to deepen the rounding of the spine and allow the head to drop farther as you move forward, rolling the ball in front of you with arms extended on the ball.

STEP 3. Allow your spine to extend starting from your tail, open the pelvis and hips, and allow the belly and chest to drop forward toward the floor. The chest will feel open. Focus on the chest opening and midback pressing downward (your lower spine is already in a heightened curve in the third trimester and doesn't need that much extension). This will feel great in your midback, especially if you have been feeling the increased weight in your breasts accompanied by rounded shoulders.

STEP 4. Gently and slowly curl from the tail and lower back, allowing the rest of the spine to curl until you get back to sitting on your sitz bones. Your head is the last to roll up with eyes looking straight ahead.

STEP 5. Perform 5 rolls forward and back as tolerated. Start with small movements that you can control, and as you get more steady and confident, you can increase the range of motion. Stay out of extremes of these motions since you have more flexibility in this trimester, and you don't want to spend time in the outer/end ranges of available movements to prevent pain. Keep the movement fluid and breathe through the diaphragm throughout.

Step 1

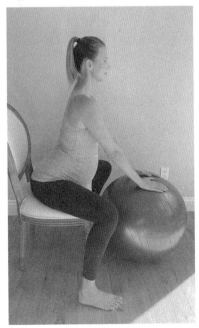

Step 2

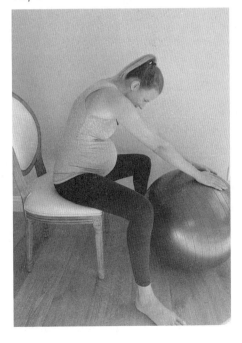

Step 3

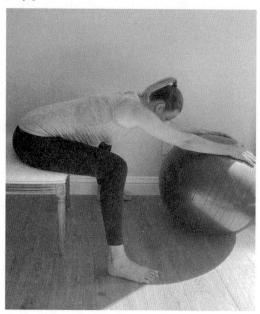

Step 4

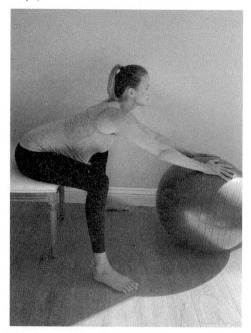

Step 5

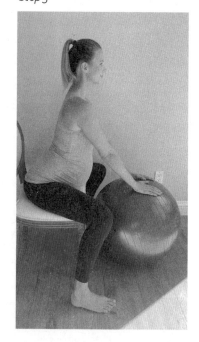

Exercise: Scapular Protraction and External Rotation on Wall

EQUIPMENT: A resistance band.

PURPOSE: To strengthen the stabilizing muscles of the shoulder, shoulder blades, and neck. This exercise targets the serratus anterior and rotator cuff, which are very important muscles to support the shoulder blades and thorax in proper alignment. When these muscles are strong, we can do more with our upper body with less strain and allow for the efficient cervical and thoracic spine curves to be supported/maintained [Cervical and Thoracic Cores].

START POSITION: Stand tall approximately 3 feet from a wall. Place your forearms on the wall. Keep palms facing each other so that the outer border of the forearms is in contact with the wall. Keep your whole spine in neutral with the head in-line with the spine, chin tucked in slightly.

SEQUENCE:

STEP 1. Exhale and press your forearms into the wall as you separate the shoulder blades apart. Your body will shift backward as you separate your shoulder blades, but do not lose contact with the wall. Keep chin in toward chest, and keep shoulder blades working to pull apart. Hold this as you continue to breathe for 10 seconds.

STEP 2. Slowly release the blades so that the body moves forward again and your shoulder blades relax back toward each other. This is the "rest" phase of the exercise. Repeat the sequence for 8 to 10 more reps.

STEP 3. Loop a resistance band around your forearms and return to the same start position. Repeat step 1 and press the blades apart by pushing on both forearms.

STEP 4. Keeping this feeling, separate the forearms/hands apart, stretching the resistance band. The movement of external rotation at the shoulder is very small, but you will feel the work in the back of the shoulders. Make sure the spine stays neutral (maintain proper curves of the spine).

STEP 5. Hold this position as you continue to breathe into the back and sides of the lower ribs, for 5 seconds. Relax the arms back in and relax the shoulder blades. Repeat 5 to 10 reps as tolerated.

Step 1

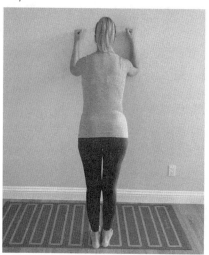

Step 2

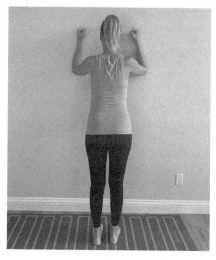

Step 3

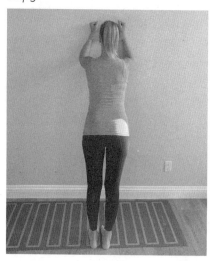

Step 4

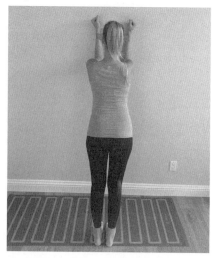

Exercise: Sun Salutation into Downward Dog Marching

EQUIPMENT: A yoga mat or towel.

PURPOSE: To open the chest, lengthen leg muscles, and strengthen the cores and hips [All Cores].

START POSITION: Stand tall with feet close together and your arms by your sides.

SEQUENCE:

STEP 1. Inhale and reach arms up and over your head. You may gaze upward to follow your hands above your head, or look straight ahead if looking up is difficult.

STEP 2. Exhale and release arms back down by your sides, flexing wrists so that your fingers are pointing up. Each time you repeat the Sun Salutation movement, reach higher up to the ceiling with energy flowing out of your fingertips. If this movement is restricted, only go as high as you feel comfortable.

STEP 3. On your next inhale, bend forward toward the floor, and place both hands on the floor, softening your knees as you bring one leg back at a time into the downward dog position. Keep your elbows neutral (not locked) and knees soft to avoid extreme stretching, but if keeping your knees relatively straight feels fine, then do so. Your heels will lift off the floor in this inverted V position. Relax your head like it is a cherry on a stem. Feel like someone is lifting your hips to the ceiling as you hold for 3 breaths.

STEP 4. Bend one knee and then the other, essentially pumping your heels up and down—alternating one heel coming closer to the ground as the opposite knee bends. Do this 10 times, alternating knee bends. Then walk one leg forward toward hands, followed by the other, and roll your body up gently while keeping both knees bent. Repeat this sequence 1 to 3 times.

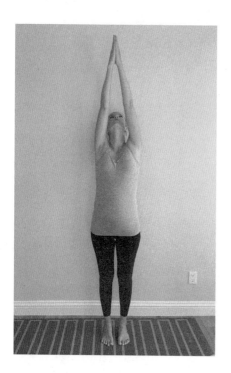

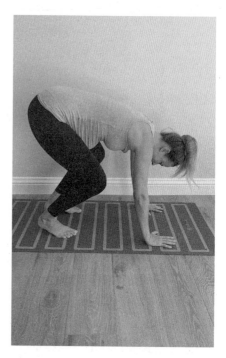

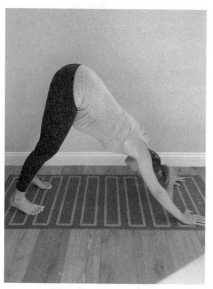

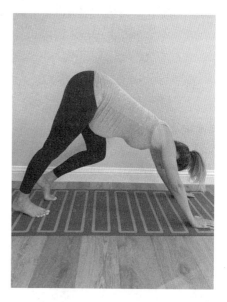

Exercise: Bird Dog

EQUIPMENT: A yoga mat or towel.

PURPOSE: To improve hip strength, core support, and full spinal control [All Cores].

START POSITION: Get down to the floor (on a mat) slowly again but this time onto hands and knees, all fours position. Position hands on the floor under your shoulders with the inner elbows facing each other. Knees should be under (in-line with) hips. Keep elbows relatively straight but not locked into hyperextension.

SEQUENCE:

STEP 1. Keep chin tucked into chest so that your ears are in-line with your shoulders as you press your shoulder blades apart. Keep your head and whole spine in a straight line like you are balancing a broomstick on your back.

STEP 2. Exhale and slowly extend your right leg back with toes pointed as you also lift your left arm up and forward. Lift these opposite limbs in a range that feels comfortable so that you can still maintain steady spine and pelvic control. Hold for one diaphragm breath and then switch sides.

STEP 3. Alternate for 10 repetitions on each side. Each time, focus on keeping the spine and pelvis still and reaching your leg and arm long, as if your hand and foot are being pulled in opposite directions.

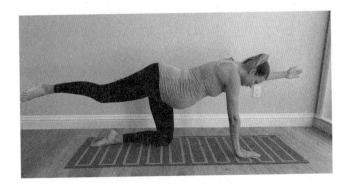

Exercise: Warrior II to Modified Side Angle Pose

PURPOSE: To open the chest, lengthen legs, hips, and the sides of the body, while strengthening the legs. The modified side angle pose can also improve breathing, stabilize the spine, and improve digestion as well [All Cores].

START POSITION: Stand tall, and grow tall from the crown of your head, with your arms at your sides.

SEQUENCE:

STEP 1. Inhale and take a step forward with the left leg so that the knee is roughly bent 90 degrees and tracking over the second toe. Gently turn (right) thigh out so that the foot is toed out at a 45 degree angle, with the foot staying in-line with the front (left) foot and back (right) knee staying straight. Stretch your right arm out in front of you as your left is stretched over your back leg. Both palms should be facedown to the floor.

STEP 2. Keep your gaze out over your front hand in-line with second finger. Feel a wrapping "out" feeling in your front thigh and a wrapping "in" in your back hip and thigh, even though they shouldn't move. Your legs will feel as if they are coming in toward each other; grow tall through the center of your body. Your core will activate. Maintain this *activation feeling* in this pose for 3 breaths.

STEP 3. Slowly bend your left elbow and place your left forearm on the left thigh. Extend the right arm out above your head, in-line with your body over your ear (or up to the ceiling if that is more comfortable). Feel lengthening in the left inner thigh and hip rotators. Keep energy in both arms and your trunk/spine long.

STEP 4. Breathe into the right side of the body for 3 to 5 breaths. Slowly come back up and shake out both legs and arms for a break. Switch to the other side and complete all steps of the sequence. You can do this sequence for 1 to 3 sets on each side.

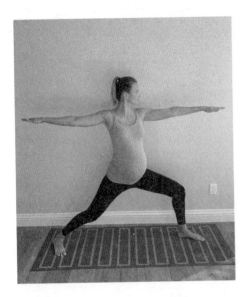 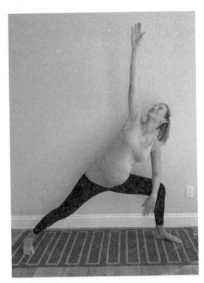

Wise Woman's Pregnancy Stretching Program

Continue with all the stretches from first and second trimester except for Happy Baby, to avoid being on your back. When you are performing Child's Pose, keep your knees wider to make room for your belly. Remember, you are looser in this trimester, so be mindful transitioning in and out of the stretches, and do not go into any extreme end ranges of movements.

NOURISHMENT

Continue to eat a variety of nutrient-rich foods as we have outlined previously. Important nutrients like healthy fats, lean proteins, fruits, vegetables (both in season and organic whenever possible), and gluten-free grains fuel not only the baby's physical growth but the formation of his or her *synapses*, the connections within the brain that provide the basis for learning. If you are not eating enough because you are worried about weight gain, you might be lacking enough calories, as well as nutrients, and vital brain development can be impaired.[3] However, if you aren't careful, excessive weight gain in the third trimester can have a powerful influence on your baby's lifelong health, as well as your own. Refer back to the chart on page 108 that shows what we consider to be the "Goldilocks zone" for optimal weight gain during pregnancy—not too little and not too much.

By the third trimester, your baby has developed its own sense of smell along with a sense of taste, as they are exposed to all the foods you are eating via the amniotic fluid. The least picky eaters will be exposed to a wide variety of foods in utero: A 2014 study published in the *American Journal of Clinical Nutrition* showed that six-month-old infants were more likely to eat carrot-flavored cereal and less likely to express distaste when their mothers regularly drank carrot juice during the last trimester of pregnancy. What's more, the study also showed that the foods a baby is exposed to in utero may be their preferred foods throughout his/her life.[4]

We also recommend that you continue to eat slowly and enjoy smaller meals more frequently. Perhaps more important, you need to drink more water than ever before, even if you feel swollen or bloated. While it might sound counterintuitive, being well hydrated helps to decrease swelling and inflammation because it helps to flush out the lymph system. Drinking lots of water, especially toward the end of the day, is necessary to hydrate the soft tissues, connective tissues, and muscles to reduce cramps and to optimize your stabilizing muscles so that you feel good when moving. Lastly, we want you to be well hydrated leading up to labor and delivery. Labor will be a challenging experience, and if you're not well hydrated, it can be all the more uncomfortable.

Make sure you drink half your body weight in ounces every day. So as your body weight increases, you want to increase your water intake. For instance, if you used to weigh 100 pounds and now you're 125 pounds, you need to up your water intake from 50 to 62 ounces. Whenever possible, it's best to drink room temperature water without ice; feel free to drink herbal teas and coconut water (which is especially good for controlling acid reflux). If you must have a caffeinated beverage, limit it to one a day, and keep it under 12 ounces. Eating lots of vegetables is another great way to keep you hydrated.

Take Meal Prep to a Whole New Level

The third trimester is a perfect time to start preparing for life immediately after birth when you come back home. One thing you can take care of now is to prepare and freeze meals. During the first few weeks you need to rest, recuperate, and bond with your baby; we don't want you to be cooking and cleaning. Now is a good time to put on your chef's hat and get some very nutritious foods cooked so that you can enjoy them later. Foods that freeze best are soups, stews, bone broths, and casseroles. You can cook them now and freeze them in two- or three-portion containers. Then, whenever you want to eat them, you can simply reheat one of those portions. You'll feel much better having a wonderful nutritious meal instead of grabbing something convenient but not that healthy. Remember also to cook with love and set your intentions on your health and baby's health as you are cooking.

Soups, stews, and casseroles are also perfect because during the first forty days after birth, we want you to be eating warm, nutritious foods. Soups and stews in particular are very easily digestible, which makes them perfect for a healing body that may also be breastfeeding. If you eat lots of cold foods during this time, like salads or cold yogurt, it will cool the body down, which is counteracting what your cells are doing and may delay healing. What's more, we want your body to start contracting back into the shape you had before. This contraction may affect your digestive tract, and you do not want to tax the digestive system with cooling raw foods that require more work to break down the nutrients. By eating warm foods that have already been cooked, they will be softer, easier to eat, and easier to digest.

Start Supporting Breastfeeding

If you are planning on breastfeeding, the diet we've been describing is the most beneficial for creating nutrient-rich breast milk: a balance of healthy fats, healthy proteins, and a multitude of vegetables is best for the quality of your breast milk. Again, staying well hydrated is important: if you're eating well yet not drinking enough, your milk production will go down.

WISDOM

Some wise women are often self-reliant, trying to take everything on themselves. We like to do things our way. However, the first forty days following childbirth is not the time for this attitude. In order for you to rest, recuperate, and bond with your baby, you will need to get your people in place and form a supportive community now, where you are at the center of attention, but not the center of the action. You will need someone to clean your home, do the laundry, and help out with grocery shopping, errands, or various tasks. The more others can do for you, the better off you will be, the faster you will recover, and the stronger and wiser you will be because of it. With these people in place, when the baby arrives, your household can continue to run like a well-oiled machine without you.

Historically in Patricia's Spartan culture and in other Mediterranean communities, following childbirth, all the other women in the tribe or town would gather to support and assist the new mom who was only supposed to rest, eat, and take care of the baby. For the past twenty years, we each have been instructing women to follow this ancient wisdom and create a support network. This idea was scientifically confirmed in 2018 when the American College of Obstetricians and Gynecologists issued new recommendations for postpartum care, including the suggestion that women develop a postpartum care plan during pregnancy.[5] And don't forget what we learned in preconception from our friend and colleague Dr. Elissa Epel: the number one strategy that helps a woman feel good during her pregnancy and create the healthiest baby is feeling supported. So while we certainly don't promote eating lots of fast food, you could sit around and eat lots of junk and have better outcomes if you're supported than a pregnant woman who has been eating the best things possible but is unsupported.

Even if your closest friends or family live miles away, you can still create a network of supporters. Look through your contacts, including your various networks, and see who you can enlist. Don't put the burden entirely on your partner or the one special friend you identified in the second trimester. Research postpartum delivery services local to your area, many of which are run by nutritionists. Or find an organic restaurant that delivers great soups, bone broths, and stews. Try them out now in the third trimester to see which ones you like best.

Think about how you want your first forty days postpartum to go and try to get everything taken care of so that you don't have to do it later. Then talk through with your team exactly what you need. Lay out your plan in a very organized way and have conversations with those people in terms of when you may need them and exactly for what.

Questions to ask your team:

* *For your partner*: Does your company offer paternity leave? Do you want to take it right away or after a few weeks?
* *For the grandparents:* How available are you able to be, and how do you want to help? Or you may direct them based on their availability: you choose the time frame and the exact chores/help you will need from each of them. Think of what they do best and put them in that role for a specified time frame or certain days of the week. For example, your mother may be able to come over Mondays and Wednesdays and be responsible for sterilizing bottles, cooking a meal or two, and doing the laundry.

- *For your friends:* Can someone set up a meal train? Put specifications of what type of diet you are eating, include details about any food allergies/sensitivities and mention your preference to soups, stews, bone broths, and warming foods. Heng Ou's book, *The First 40 Days*, has wonderful recipes for new mothers.

- *Professional help:* Can someone be on call to support you as you begin breastfeeding? Ask your ob-gyn or birthing professional for their best lactation consultant's contact information. Interview them now and discuss your breastfeeding plans and hear how they can help. If you are having a hospital birth, you may receive a lactation consultant visit before you leave the hospital.

- Ask your doula if they offer postpartum services: often doulas come for a couple of visits postpartum and have postpartum packages you can sign up for (see registry tips below). They can help with a wide range of services for your home: helping with breastfeeding, helping set up baby changing areas in an ergonomic way, teaching you to swaddle baby, and guiding you with body mechanics for you and baby in a hands-on way in your space.

Packing for Birthing

- ❏ Adult wipes (for gentle use after a bowel movement)
- ❏ Bath and face towel
- ❏ Bed sheet for labor
- ❏ Birth ball and/or peanut ball (see Creating a Birth Plan section)
- ❏ Birth plan
- ❏ Breastfeeding bra
- ❏ Car seat and car seat cover (if necessary for the season)
- ❏ Diaper bag (stocked)
- ❏ Extra-long charging cord (for mobile phone)
- ❏ Essential oils
- ❏ Filtered water (stainless steel water bottle) and/or coconut water; apple juice for flavor if preferred
- ❏ Granny/high-waist support panties or belly wrap
- ❏ Hairbrush and hairclips/hairbands/headband
- ❏ Healthy snacks (for after birth)
- ❏ Hoodie and/or sunglasses (to be able to shut out the environment if you need)
- ❏ Italian ice or granita (bring in Ziploc to store in freezer at facility)
- ❏ Music and music device; portable speaker for labor/delivery room
- ❏ Nightgown or pajamas
- ❏ Nipple cream
- ❏ Nipple pads
- ❏ Organic lip ointment cream (Aimie Raupp Beauty or Korres brand are great)
- ❏ Organic unsweetened electrolyte packet (like BioPure's Matrix Electrolyte Powder) or organic electrolyte drink
- ❏ Outfit for baby to go home
- ❏ Outfit for mom to go home—comfortable fabric for pants or skirt, nursing shirt
- ❏ Pediatrician's information
- ❏ Pillow
- ❏ Receiving blanket
- ❏ Robe
- ❏ Scarf/pashmina (to protect against drafts)
- ❏ Slipper socks
- ❏ Snacks for partner
- ❏ This book
- ❏ Tissues
- ❏ Toiletries
- ❏ Wired headphones and earbuds/airtubes

The Ancient Wisdom of Home Organization

The next thing you need to figure out is the baby's room, and while you are at it, now is a great time to clean up your environment and organize your home. We look to the wisdom of feng shui and Ayurveda to offer advice, as these practices are thought to amplify our health.

According to Andie (Nancy) SantoPietro, physical space is not benign. It's a living entity that we constantly interact with, and like any relationship, the quality of that interaction can range from energetically stressful to calming. If the energy of your home—both the people who live in it and the actual space—is stressed, you are going to feel continually overwhelmed.

In feng shui, for instance, one way to create a calmer environment is to make sure each room within the home is clean, organized, and uncluttered. The colors you choose, as well as your furniture placement, can either support or distract from the vibe you are trying to create. While there may be colors that you like, it doesn't necessarily mean that the energy that they offset balances you, your home, or family members.

Andie also recommends that you create a special place for breastfeeding with the calming tenets of feng shui in mind. For the baby's room, she advises placing the crib headboard against a solid wall. The headboard should be made of solid wood without openings in order to block discordant energies from flowing toward the baby's head. The more solid the surrounding you can provide the baby with, the stronger energetically the baby is going to be. Most important, the baby's head should not be facing toward the direction of the bedroom door, and the crib itself should not cross the entranceway or be directly in the line of sight from the door.

Ayurvedic teachings that encompass the science of architecture are referred to as *vastu*. Vastu practitioners believe that the northeast section of the home is the spiritual center and should remain clear of clutter for optimal energy flow. Use a compass to identify this section. However, the ideas of optimal crib placement are different than in feng shui: vastu practitioners believe that the baby's head should be in the south and the feet should be toward the north when sleeping in the crib. Vastu teachings also focus on color therapy and advise keeping dark colors away from the baby's room, like black, dark brown, or dark gray.

Creating a Birth Plan

A birth plan is a written document about your birth preferences that you can show your doctor and bring to the delivery. According to Denise Spatafora, author of *Better Birth*, a birth plan is both a document and an exercise. The point is to make sure that everything related to the birth is discussed ahead of time and that all of your questions are answered. Creating this document allows you to uncover your thoughts and feelings about birth, some of which could require some emotionally deep decision-making. However, this kind of preparation will preempt unnecessary surprises, breakdowns, anxiety, or even medical interventions during birth.

When you arrive at the hospital or birthing center, you will be asked a lot of questions, so it's very important to have all of your desires laid out because when you're having contractions, you may not want to be focusing on these questions. When you can hand over a printed birth plan, it's very clear as to what your wishes and preferences are for how the birth should go.

As you are crafting your birth plan, discuss your options with your health-care provider and decide what's right for you. Read through the next section to see exactly what your options are. Listen to your innate wisdom to see what feels helpful. The birth plan can include:

- Your thoughts surrounding an epidural.
- What type of birth you are aiming to have.
- Specific people who will be allowed in the delivery room.
- The type of music you would like to hear (or none at all).

- Additional birth tools you will want available: a physio ball (which you may bring yourself) or a peanut ball, a birth bar.
- Additional medications you agree to have, like Pitocin.
- Specific birthing postures you want to try, such as a squatted birth.

A birth plan is not a guarantee that everything will go exactly the way you envision it. However, by putting your intentions down on paper and discussing them with your medical professionals and your team, you are increasing the odds that you will have fewer surprises and more control over the birth experience.

Showering Your Baby with Love

The preparation and planning can be all-encompassing, so don't lose sight of the fact that the third trimester is also the perfect time to follow your instincts and really connect with your baby. We deeply believe that when you shower your baby in love and surround yourself with love, you can break the trap of getting caught up in the to-do list of the third trimester. While we must plan or we will have issues later, let's do it with a smile. Let's remember that all the planning is for this beautiful baby that will be coming into the world soon, so let's do everything with that intention and carry that love.

We also believe that your baby can feel your love when you speak to her, sing her a lullaby, or even read a book aloud. You can put your hands on your belly and tell the baby that you're really looking forward to seeing her. You can even insert your due date in your missives, so the baby knows exactly when she is expected! This connection of communication can be quite calming for both you and your baby, as it releases oxytocin and keeps you in a parasympathetic state, naturally lowering inflammation. If you are on bed rest, there's even more reason to communicate that the baby should be resting, for baby not to come early, as those intentions can go very far.

Music for You and Your Baby

You can play music you enjoy and music that is calming for you and baby. Put wired headphones on your belly for baby to hear. With a headphone connector, you can listen with your headphones at the same time.

Apart from simply listening to music, active singing and playing a musical instrument during pregnancy has shown to have a positive effect on the quality of mother-to-infant bonding. If you can combine soothing words, singing, or gentle touch to your own abdomen, your unique scent will be married to these pleasant experiences to form memories the baby will have for a lifetime.

In one 2017 study, pregnant women in their third trimester were taught to sing lullabies to their babies. The women who did this experienced significantly less stress than those in the control group. What's more, fetal heart monitoring showed that when the mothers were singing, the baby's heart rate decreased,[6] a sign of a calm and relaxed baby!

You're Ready, So Read On!

It's time to start thinking about delivery. In the next section, we'll go over all of your options and begin to prepare you in every way. Don't wait until you're in your ninth month to read the next section because the baby may come early, and you don't want to be going into labor unprepared. If you are tuned in to your body, as we've been training you this whole time to do, and keeping that open line of communication with baby, you will succeed. Even if you haven't done everything we've covered in this book, your openness to our thoughts and your positive attitude will help you have a smooth labor and delivery. So don't worry, read on!

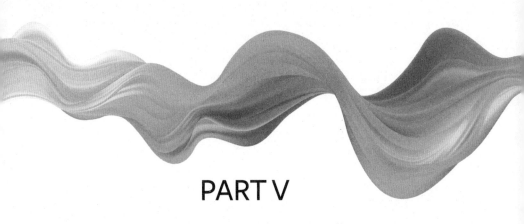

PART V

Labor and Delivery

To have faith is to trust yourself to the water.
When you swim you don't grab hold of the water,
because if you do you will sink and drown.
Instead you relax, and float.

—Alan Watts

All the ways that you have been taking care of yourself have prepared you so that you are ready to deliver. The process is elegant and efficient; you will be amazed to see exactly what your body can do. At the same time, there are aspects that you can control. Birthing is not an automatic response, and while the innate wisdom of the body should naturally take over, sometimes we get in its way. Or, the baby may need your help. The more you know ahead of time, the more likely you will be able to have the birth you've been dreaming of. So have faith, relax into the process, and make sure you fully understand the information in this chapter well ahead of your delivery date.

And, of course, know that we are here with you!

YOUR BODY:

MOVEMENT:

WISDOM:

YOUR BODY

The cervix, *which is the muscle of the lowest part of the uterus, is* normally very narrow, long, and hard. This helps to support the baby, the amniotic fluid, and the placenta throughout your pregnancy. By the end of the third trimester the cervix changes in preparation for the birth: it will shorten, thin out, and soften, which is referred to as *effacement*. As the cervix begins to thin and widen, the thick cervical mucus that has been accumulating in the cervical canal is released through the vagina. Passing your mucus plug is not necessarily a sign of labor: this can happen on the day you go into labor or as early as days or weeks before. It simply means the cervix has started to soften or slightly dilate. If there is no associated labor or bleeding, there is no need to be concerned about seeing the cervical mucus plug.

Once the cervix begins to soften, the baby can drop down low into your pelvis: this process is called *lightening*. The uterus changes from being pear-shaped to that of a watermelon and begins tipping forward, especially in the two weeks closest to birth. For most first time mothers, the uterus is curved on their left side and straighter on the right. If you are in your second or third pregnancy, it will be a bit more stretched and doesn't have this distinct shape.

As the baby comes down headfirst, it should be slightly angled to the left, facing the right side or your right hip. This position is following the natural curve of the uterus into the pelvis. The pelvis is wider side to side and narrower from sacrum to pubis; the baby's head is wider at the back of the head to the front and narrower ear to ear. The exercises and stretches you have been doing all along have helped to bring length and buoyancy in the pelvic muscles to ensure that the pelvis widens enough to make room for your baby's exit.

The Stages of Labor

There are three formal stages of labor. The first stage encompasses the time it takes for the cervix to dilate up to 10 centimeters. All the pushing occurs during the second stage. The following are the events that occur during each stage of labor and delivery:

The First Stage of Labor

The earliest signs of labor begin at home regardless of where you are planning to birth. During this phase, you can remain active if you have energy as long as you refrain from activities causing exertion. You can do anything that's fun, calming, and distracting. Double-check your hospital bag or birthing supplies or take a relaxing shower. You may eat foods that are light and easily digested. Rest when you need rest as you will need your energy later. It would be best to be with your partner or someone close to you at this time in case you need assistance.

One of the first ways you will know if you are in labor is if you have a *bloody show*, a small amount of bleeding as a result of the rapid stretching of the cervix. A bloody show can look like a watery discharge with some blood. If there is a lot of continuous blood, call your birthing professional. He or she will also want to know immediately if your water broke, which means you will deliver within twenty-four hours. You may also have diarrhea or develop a backache like one you may get around your menstruation cycle.

You will also have contractions, which at first will feel like menstrual cramps. These early contractions do not last very long and are spread apart (greater than eight minutes). Rest between contractions to save your energy for the more active parts of labor. During this time you can be utilizing all the restorative breathing tools you have learned. Particularly with first pregnancies, the first stage of labor will typically take a long time—anywhere between twelve and seventy-two hours—before you move into a more active phase of dilation. If the contractions are very mild and many hours have passed without them intensifying or growing closer in time, consider drinking raspberry leaf tea. This can help encourage uterine contractions.

As the contractions become more frequent, your cervix will continue to dilate. These contractions will feel more intense, will last longer, and will occur closer together. You can move around and try out a variety of positions that make you feel more comfortable (see page 316 in this chapter for suggestions). Your birthing professional will want to see you to get checked for dilation once contractions are five minutes apart consistently for one to two hours. Once you go to the hospital, or birthing center, your cervix will be measured. The first stage of labor ends when you are 10 centimeters dilated.

At the end of the first stage of labor, you may go through a transition stage, where your contractions will be very intense and often last 90 to 120 seconds with only 30 seconds of rest. It is often the time when new mothers feel the most tested. Just know that this pain will go away and be replaced with an uncontrollable urge to push. However, don't push until your birthing professional tells you that you are ready. In the meantime, hang in there, breathe, and ask your supporters (practitioners or partner) to help you cope with the height of the pain. Try to let your body release/relax into the moment and remember that any discomfort you are feeling should be short lived.

When to Go to the Hospital/Birthing Center

When your contractions occur about five minutes apart for two hours, get to the hospital or birthing center. This timing may indicate that your cervix is dilating, however, the only way to know this for sure is to get examined. Ask your physician or midwife well beforehand when they would want to you to come in for evaluation. For mothers who have already had a prior vaginal delivery, you may want to get examined a bit sooner as oftentimes the second or third delivery will progress more quickly.

The mindset of many nurses and doctors on a hospital's labor and delivery floor is to expect that labor should take place within twelve to twenty-four hours once the pregnant woman has been admitted. This is referred to as the *starting the clock phenomena*, which increases the chances of unnecessary interventions and reduces the chance of having a vaginal delivery. Many laboring women come to the hospital too early because they're either afraid of laboring at home or they're in too much pain, yet when they get admitted, this unspoken timer begins, and then the staff may start a series of interventions to try to hasten delivery if you are stalled. Keep this in mind as you are weighing your decision to leave home or to stay in the hospital if you are remote from delivering.

The Second Stage of Labor

The second stage of labor is when you will be actively pushing and pausing. When it first begins, your contractions may temporarily go away. If you are having a hospital birth, you may be given the medication Pitocin (a form of oxytocin) to increase your contractions.

You may vomit or feel like you need to have a bowel movement. This may mean that the baby is coming as the baby puts pressure on the rectum on its descent. If the baby is facing the wrong way with the back of the head on the sacrum instead of the face, then you may have intense back pain and rectal pressure. Keep yourself hydrated—take a sip or two of water, suck on an ice chip, or even take a sip of juice (or coconut water) if you feel you need something besides plain water.

By this point, the pelvic floor can stretch up to 250 percent, as can the tissues in the vaginal canal. We want the tissues to fan out and optimally stretch to adapt for the baby's exit. When your birth professional tells you to push, listen and follow their guidelines. You want to employ all the pushing techniques outlined in this chapter and allow yourself the freedom to change positions if something isn't working. Keep yourself relaxed. Do not tense against the contractions or feelings you are experiencing as the baby descends for its exit; instead, surrender and remember your wise body is doing everything it can to swiftly deliver your baby. The less you tense against it, the faster the process will be.

As you get deeper into labor, use the visualization tips in the Restorative Breathing section of Third Trimester (see page 190). With each contraction, whether light or intense, stay present and visualize your baby slowly descending. With each inhale and exhale, you are allowing the pelvic floor to open and release.

You may need to lie on one side or shift your position to assist your baby in rotating properly for its exit. As the baby descends into the pelvis, it tucks its chin in and rotates. The baby ideally turns to face the mother's back, which pushes the sacrum out of the way. The baby then passes through the pelvic floor. We call this position *engaged* with the pelvis. The suppleness in a balanced pelvic floor aids in the baby coming down and out. That is why all our exercises, stretches, and breathing up until this point are so important.

If the baby is in the right position, you will feel the baby *crowning*. This doesn't mean that the baby is going to make a quick exit; you may still be in for what is known as a slow birth. The baby generally has been mainly in flexion, a curled "fetal position" throughout pregnancy and earlier stages of labor. But as the baby is ready to come out, it extends the head back for its exit. The baby's head can get squished as it comes through. There may be a drop in heart rate, but usually after the final contraction, it comes back up again.

The head slides out of the vagina, and the *perineum*—the area between the anus and the vulva—softens, thins, and effaces to make room. If you don't have an epidural, you will feel a burning sensation as this is happening; this is caused by the fascia and tissues stretching. When you feel this sensation, it is time to stop pushing and allow for the baby to just ooze out (*slow birth*). Your breath can imitate softly blowing birthday candles out, or you can gently pant. By pausing and allowing the tissues to stretch, you are more likely to preserve the perineum and prevent tearing, which can cause incontinence, pelvic pain, or organ prolapse later on. If you do tear, ask your birthing professional if you can allow the tearing to happen naturally instead of them cutting the perineum, which is called an *episiotomy*. As Elizabeth Noble, natural birthing pioneer and physical therapist said, when we tear naturally, the tearing is jagged, and so the healing happens in various angles within the tissues, which allows for more functional support. An episiotomy involves cutting the perineum in a straight line. The reason that an episiotomy should be avoided if possible is because once you cut the perineum in a straight line, the tissues heal in one direction, and you have a greater chance of tearing further with your next delivery, even without an episiotomy.

After the baby's head is out, the shoulders need to be birthed, one at a time. The baby continues to rotate as it passes through you completely. You are given your baby to hold and welcome into our world!

The Pros and Cons of Receiving an Epidural

An epidural is the most common type of anesthetic used for pain relief during labor. An anesthesiologist inserts a needle and a tiny catheter in the lower part of your back. The needle is removed and the catheter left in place for delivery of medication through the tube. You can begin an epidural at any time during your labor.

This medication allows you to rest when you can and stay alert and can spare you discomfort if forceps or a vacuum are needed. If you need to deliver by C-section, an epidural allows you to stay present and awake during the procedure and provides pain relief during your recovery.

A common side effect of using an epidural is a sudden drop in blood pressure. If your blood pressure drops too low, this could reduce blood flow to the baby or cause you to feel very light headed and dizzy. This can often be treated with increased intravenous fluids and blood pressure stabilizing medications. Sometimes, the medications used in the epidural may cause shivering, fever, or itchiness.

Epidurals can also affect the birth experience. Pushing is more difficult with an epidural, and having one may increase your chance of needing other interventions, such as forceps or a C-section. Perineal tears are also more common in women who have epidurals. A laboring woman with an epidural is somewhat limited in the number of different positions she can try.

If you choose to have an epidural, make sure that you follow directions from the professionals in the room as they monitor your contractions. They will tell you when to push or slow down and when to blow/breathe/pant until the baby is out, as you will have less sensational feedback to know when to do it on your own.

The Third Stage of Labor

The next sixty minutes has been called the "Golden Hour."[1] This is a time of transition where you and your baby need to bond and have skin-to-skin contact. This bonding can occur with the umbilical cord intact. Once the baby is out, the umbilical cord may be delayed in clamping or immediately emptied by the practitioner. The World Health Organization (WHO) recommends that cord clamping should occur one to three minutes after delivery or longer for all births. This delay allows for more blood to transfer from the placenta to the baby, sometimes increasing the child's blood volume by up to a third. The iron in the cord blood increases the baby's iron stores in the moment, which is great for healthy brain development and reduces the risk of iron deficiency anemia.

While you are waiting for the cord to drain, WHO recommends that birthing facilities should "facilitate immediate and uninterrupted skin-to-skin contact and support mothers to initiate breastfeeding as soon as possible after birth, for at least sixty minutes."[2] You may want to request that the baby not be cleaned of its *vernix* before you touch it. The vernix is the waxy or cheese-like white substance that covers the baby. It can make baby's skin soft and protect it from drying out after birth. You can ask the nurse or birthing professional to lightly wipe any blood or fluids off the baby with a washcloth but to leave the vernix on the skin.

Once the blood is drained completely, the cord will be pale, and the placenta will separate on its own. This can happen naturally between five to thirty minutes after delivery. However, to reduce maternal blood loss, your doctor may massage your uterus to expedite the process if it is taking too long or if bleeding is moderate. Labor concludes once the placenta is completely outside of your body.

What Happens During a C-Section?

A cesarean section may be necessary due to a complication, may be planned ahead of time with your practitioner, or occur due to a delay in progress of labor/ dilation. During a C-section, the baby is surgically removed through an incision in the mother's abdomen and then a second incision in the uterus. Typically, the mother is given a regional anesthetic and a single horizontal cut is made, rupturing the amniotic sac surrounding the baby if your water has yet to break. The baby is removed from the uterus, the umbilical cord is cut, and the placenta is removed. The baby is then given back to the mother for skin-to-skin contact.

If you have a C-section you may need to stay in the hospital a bit longer, between two to four days. Afterward, you will have more restricted physical activity, and the recovery typically takes four to six weeks after the surgery.

The need to have a C-section can come as disappointing news. When Patricia was pregnant with her second child she was also expanding her practice and moving it to a new location. In hindsight, she may have taken on more than she should have because her water broke spontaneously at thirty-six weeks—four weeks before her due date. Since she had a completely natural, vaginal birth of a nine-pound baby before, she felt delivering a smaller baby would be easy. However, during labor the baby's heart rate was plummeting and not recovering as she got up to six centimeters dilation. Her obstetrician knew Patricia really wanted another natural vaginal birth, but that was not in the cards. After the C-section, her baby boy was born healthy, breathing on his own at six pounds. So while she was initially disappointed, Patricia realized that she didn't "fail" at delivering her baby—the experience was different, but the outcome was the same.

Anita always likes to tell her patients that they didn't get pregnant to have a vaginal delivery—they got pregnant to have a baby!

Am I Really a Candidate for a VBAC?

If you've had a C-section before, you may be a candidate for a vaginal delivery with this pregnancy. Your ob-gyn will determine if your uterus is strong enough. Your chances for a successful VBAC also increase the more time has passed between pregnancies.

Birth Positions and Options

Childbirth is truly miraculous, but it doesn't occur without your participation. You can choose the most effective position to give birth based on your body and the baby's location in it. Changing your position can decrease pain, increase maternal-fetal circulation, improve the quality of your contractions, decrease the length of labor, and facilitate the baby's descent.[3] Remember, you are working together with your baby and your birthing professional.

No matter what position you birth in, during labor you can connect with your baby. With every breath, every contraction, and every push, you want to visualize the baby descending. You can visualize your pelvic floor lengthening and relaxing so that you can get the most success with each contraction or push. When you feel something change or a resistance when you're connected with your baby, you will know innately what position to change into.

Each of the following positions are options for you to choose from. Some require additional tools. Most hospitals have birthing bars, physio balls, or peanut balls, but you may want to bring your own balls because you cannot reserve them, they may not be the right size for you, and there is typically limited availability:

- **Reclined on your back.** Bring your knees up toward your chest but keep your thighs inwardly rotated. As your knees drift toward each other, it widens the back of the pelvis making baby's exit easier.
- **All Fours:** You may find it more comfortable in a hands-and-knees position on the bed. This position can take pressure off your spine and help with a baby that is presenting "sunny-side up." Keep your knees close together in order to widen the back of the pelvis as well.
- **On left side with (or without) peanut ball between knees/legs.** This position can relieve pressure on the spine and guides the baby to rotate in order to descend downward. A peanut ball is shaped like a peanut shell, where the middle is smaller than the ends. It was created to optimally position the fetus in relation to the mother's pelvis.[4] A peanut ball can be placed between a woman's knees while she is on her side to increase pelvic diameter and allow more room for fetal descent. Turning your thighs inward helps to open the back of the pelvis to make more space for baby. It elongates the pelvic floor as the sitz bones widen. Keeping your top thigh on the peanut ball will help widen the pelvis to make space where baby needs it.
- **Squat position using a birthing bar.** Hospitals and birthing centers may have a birthing bar attachment to the delivery table/bed. The bar can be used for you to hang into the resting squat position to release the spine, using gravity to assist the descent of the baby and open the pelvic floor for baby's exit.

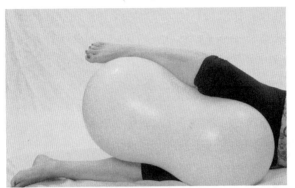

Photo courtesy of Chantal Traub

Balls Used Before and During Labor

Sitting on a physio ball right around your due date and during labor can help to open the cervix. Getting on a ball and rolling on your perineum around your due date helps improve the suppleness of the pelvic floor. You should only be sitting on the ball for twenty minutes at a time: it requires an enormous amount of abdominal and core support to balance on it in a seated position, and you may become fatigued if you sit on it for too long.

Our colleague Yamuna Zake is a massage therapist and a master teacher of body sustainability who has created a line of balls that have varying levels of firmness, varied shapes, and a level of buoyancy making them appropriate for releasing fascia throughout the body.

About a week before their due date, Yamuna has her pregnant clients massage their pelvic floor by sitting on a ball. This helps to improve the suppleness of the pelvic floor and also can help to open up the cervix. Partners can massage the perineum, but many do not feel comfortable doing so; the balls are a great option instead. The balls can be very helpful for releasing and lengthening the tissues and can help decrease perineal tearing during a vaginal birth. Yamuna also believes that you can increase your awareness of your perineum and vaginal region by rolling on the ball. Yamuna also recommends using her balls to stimulate the pubic bone, sacrum, and inner thigh muscles before the due date to further relax the pelvic floor to increase ease with delivery. There are videos on her website to help you self-release these various areas and tissues with the balls.

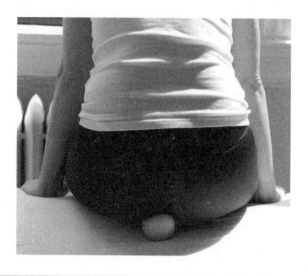

How Your Partner Can Help During Labor

There are also manual techniques your partner/friend/doula can help with to speed up dilation and prepare the pelvis for delivery. These include

- ◆ **Perineal massage.** Your partner can gently massage along the perineum/ pelvic floor around the vaginal opening with linear, front-to-back strokes, with or without a natural oil like olive oil or fractionated coconut oil. This massage is particularly helpful for women who feel tightness or gripping in the pelvic floor region. If you feel that it is hard for you to get into a deep squat, you may have gripping or tension in the pelvic floor.
- ◆ **Compressing the pelvis between contractions.** When you feel more supported with this compression, the contraction can be less painful. You can be sitting on a ball or the bed or even hanging in a squat. Your

partner puts their hands around your pelvis with their thumbs along your sacroiliac joints, which are on the back of each side of the pelvis. Gently pressing their hands together, they are simultaneously compressing the pelvis together. As this happens, the pelvic floor softens, and you are able to relax and let go to allow for a contraction to be more efficient in helping the baby descend.

There is an alternate position you can try. Your partner can press the pelvis down and in by placing hands above on the iliac crest—the top of the two pelvic bones. This pressure also opens the bottom of the pelvis and allows you to let go during the contraction.

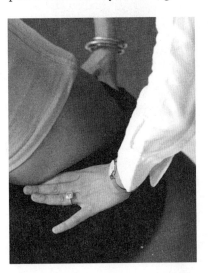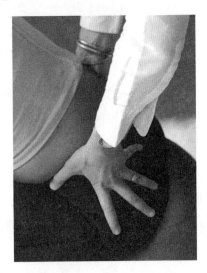

Try both and see which you prefer. If one feels good for a while and then doesn't, you can switch them up.

- ◆ Guided visualizations, breathing, and relaxation techniques. Your partner can make sure you are using breathing appropriately and remind you to do your visualizations in order to keep you in a relaxed state. When we remind our brain that we are in a safe place, pain can be better tolerated. They can also help with adjusting lights, temperature of the room, and background music—the subtle changes that make a big difference in an effort to keep you relaxed.

- **Butterfly Technique.** If labor is progressing slowly, you can get on all fours and have your partner gently press your sitz bones apart. This technique will widen the posterior pelvic floor and make more room for your baby to descend. Always coordinate your breathing as you rock back (almost going into child's pose). Inhale as your partner presses the sitz bones apart, then exhale as you return to the start position on all fours. Repeat 10 to 20 times every hour as needed. You may also do this if you are past your due date and want to facilitate labor.

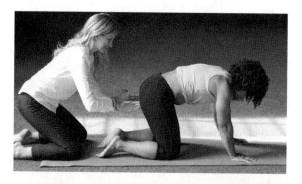

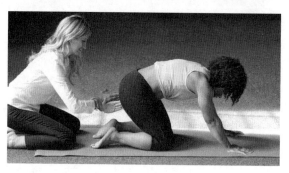

- **Hanging to release pressure.** You can do a hanging squat with your arms around the back of your partner's neck or shoulders. You can hang low or hang backwards, allowing the body to be like a relaxed hammock. This will help release tension in your spine and pressure in the abdomen or pelvic floor. This position will also lengthen the sides of your body and add space to the diaphragm so that you can breathe better and allow for a greater pelvic floor release.

Delivering a "Sunny-Side Up" (Posterior) Baby

Sometimes the baby is facing toward the pubic bone with the back of its head up against the sacrum. This is referred to as "sunny-side up baby" and can lead to a particular type of pain known as *back labor*. During the first stage of labor, placing soft balls against your lower back can help release tension by creating pressure points.

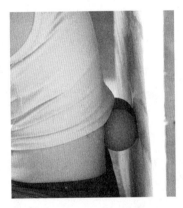

The all fours position can help labor and delivery when baby is sunny-side up. When you are on hands and knees, gravity can help turn the baby since the back of the head is heavier and the baby may be more inclined to rotate so that their face is facing your back.

Sometimes doing a "resistance push" is quite effective as you push back with your pelvis and firmly ground through your hands, pushing into a surface. This allows your sitz bones to widen as you make space for the baby to rotate and descend. You will have to work harder and breathe to drive the baby down and to help the baby rotate.

If you know your baby is in the sunny-side up position before labor begins, sitting on a round disc "stability or wobble cushion" can help change this position, as can some prenatal chiropractors. Sitting on the unstable circular surface can promote mobility of the baby in the womb. We like the AppleRound stability/ wobble cushion.

MOVEMENT

*We've heard many stories of women who have been told in the deliv-*ery room that pushing is just like going to the bathroom, and so they push from the pelvic floor downward. And that's not the right thing to do. The fact is, pushing requires strength and a coordinated effort using your entire body. For instance, pushing requires upper body strength. During labor, you will need to pull or push with your upper body, pull a leg inward perhaps, hang supporting yourself with your arms, or pull on a birthing bar. Don't worry! You are prepared because the exercise program has been strengthening your upper body, especially in the third trimester.

Some women are embarrassed and fearful, and once they start contracting, they literally hold back and pull up and in with their abdominal muscles, which actually prevents delivery. For instance, Anita was once working with her patient, Elizabeth, who was delivering her third baby. During labor, Elizabeth was stuck at seven centimeters. Anita spoke gently to her and asked, "What are you afraid of right now?"

Elizabeth was taken aback, but when she thought about it, she replied, "I don't think I'm ready to have a third baby. I'm overwhelmed—I can't do it." Anita realized that Elizabeth was working herself up, tightening her abdominals, and stalling her own delivery. The two women acknowledged Elizabeth's fears, and within a few minutes she was at ten centimeters, and pushed the baby out in fifteen minutes.

How to Push

Rehearsing the sequence of pushing can help you become familiar with the feeling and optimize the coordination of your breath and muscles to be more successful when it is time. Seven days or so before your due date, you can gently practice these pushing techniques. Then, when you are really in the moment, use what feels natural or go with how your body is responding. Remember to always allow for ultimate relaxation at the pelvic floor and, when needed, only engage upper abdominal muscles, never the lower abdominal region:

◆ **The Exhale Push.** On an exhale, use your upper abdominal muscles, relax the pelvic floor, and push downward. Some people like inhaling for four counts, filling the lungs, then exhaling for six counts and pushing with the upper abdominals compressing down and in on the extended exhale. Extending your exhale calms the nervous system, keeping you connected with the parasympathetic system so that you experience less pain.

◆ **J Position Push.** Similar to the exhale push above, use your upper abs pressing down and in from above to focus your downward push as you exhale. Allow the body to curl forward/around your baby as you perform this J push. Keep the neck soft and relax the pelvic floor. The lower abs remain relaxed throughout, with no transversus abdominis activity here.

◆ **Inhale Momentum.** Although it feels very natural to push hard upon exhaling, remember you need to use your inhale as momentum to get the exhale to be even more successful. Make sure to inflate your lungs, widening the lower ribs to accentuate the space as you inhale. Your pelvic floor relaxes and opens with each inhale naturally. Then allow for that momentum, like a pendulum swinging all the way to the extreme left only to rebound to the extreme right. Let the large inhale swing into a large exhale, increasing the power of your push (continuing to keep the pelvic floor relaxed the whole time).

◆ **Hold Your Breath and Push.** You may find yourself holding your breath with some intense contractions or urges to push. Get into a rhythm to take a few extra breaths first to prepare for a breath holding as you ride the wave at the top of the contraction and push. Chantal Traub, an experienced doula in New York City, explains that this push is analogous to preparing for swimming underwater: you take a few breaths, then hold your breath for that initial momentum (as you push with the top of the contraction) and then slowly let out the air as you move through the water. You may have feedback (either from the baby heartrate monitor you may be hooked up to, or that inner feeling) that a contraction is coming, and that is precisely when to take those quick few extra breaths, then hold your breath as you push at the top of the contraction's intensity (relaxing pelvic floor and lower tummy/abs), then exhale and coast through the remainder of the push.

◆ **Pant or Blow Out Candles and Push.** In the final moments of the second stage of labor, you will want to pause to avoid tearing the perineum. It is helpful at this time to gently pant or blow (like you are blowing out birthday candles) to keep your pelvic floor relaxed as baby's head oozes out.

◆ **Make Some Noise.** Sound can energize or calm the systems of the body and mind. Some women find it helpful to make low and long sounds when they are in labor and pushing. These sounds are calming and can intuitively feel helpful in the moment. A low *Om* or *oh* are good options, or anything low that feels good will work. Generally, a high screeching sound will tighten the pelvic floor and won't be helpful, so it should be avoided.

◆ **Using Resistance.** If you are having difficulty pushing, getting onto all fours, or kneeling or half standing (feet on floor with hands or forearms on a bed or table) can help. You can push with the upper body away from you as you widen the sitz bones and pelvis. Utilize your coordinated breath to push in this resisted position to direct your baby downward. You can push against the bed, a table or wall, or even your partner's shoulders or hips as you exhale. You want to use upper abs to push downward. As you push with the upper body, the pelvis will naturally move backward and widen more, giving more room for baby's exit.

Letting Go of Fear

As wise women we want to trust that our bodies know what to do during labor, and we need to remember to get out of its way. However, fear can cause you to literally tighten your grip during a contraction instead of releasing your muscles. One of the top causes of prolonged labor is when we allow fear and the pain response to take over.

Instead, we want you to go into a state of deep relaxation so that we feel free enough to let go. The more we can visualize the baby descending and use breath and imagery to relax the pelvic floor, the more successful we will be during labor and delivery.

The breathing techniques you have learned throughout the book will help immensely. Just being aware when you're going into a fearful state, taking a pause and thinking of something positive, and really relaxing on an extended exhale can bring back the parasympathetic system to help you relax.

WISDOM

You can finalize your birth preferences and create the ambiance you want for the labor/delivery room, wherever that may be located. Music is a vehicle that can transport you to another place and a different state of mind and provide essential calm. You may think that a softer genre of music may be helpful, or listening to nature sounds, or meditative spa-like tunes. But in the moment, you may want to hear George Michael and bop to *Faith.* So while you're waiting for baby to arrive, make a couple of different playlists. Then, during labor, your partner can be the DJ. What's most important is that you choose the songs, vibrations, or sounds you may need to stay in parasympathetic mode. After the delivery, your baby will need some quiet time as an immature nervous system is easily frazzled. Baby will need to focus on you, hear your familiar voice, smell you, and look to feed. Limit sounds in the room to gentle voices, very light classical music, or nature sounds.

You may want soft lighting as well. Dimmed lights or candles (organic, unscented) may be what you prefer, if they are an option. The weather on the day of birthing may be sunny so you lift the shades and bask in the sun—or you black out the windows and stick with soft lighting options.

Scented essential oils can help to calm your nervous system. Diffusing them in the labor/delivery room is not recommended because the baby may be overwhelmed by the scent. However, placing a couple of drops of essential oil on a cotton ball or tissue and breathing in from there is all you'll need to get the desired effects. Choose from any of the following:

- Peppermint oil can give you a much-needed boost of energy and can ease nausea.
- Clary sage can help promote regular, strong contractions to keep labor progressing.
- Bergamot is helpful to ease with the overall anxiety of labor.
- Lavender can help you rest between contractions and through the varying stages of labor.

Yet even with lots of planning, you may change your mind or want something different in the moment. For instance, you usually love massages, but as your partner tries to relax you with a massage, you find that in the moment it is not pleasing to you. Be patient and kind with yourself and feel free to deviate from your plan.

Choosing a Birthing Location

By the beginning of the third trimester, you need to lock in on where you intend to give birth and who you want to be there for support. We believe that having more support throughout labor and during delivery can make all the difference in preventing unnecessary medical interventions and unnecessary perineal tearing.

Home births are considered to be a safe option if you are past thirty-seven weeks of your pregnancy and it's been a healthy pregnancy of a single baby.[5] If that's the case, the first decision you need to make is to find experienced birthing professionals who will come to your home. A good midwife will be able to help you through the birth and assess any problems early on in case you have to transfer to a hospital. A doula will then assist you and the midwife.

One of the great things about home birth is that you may have more choices in terms of movement and birthing positions during labor. This is particularly true if you want to have a water birth.

Hospital births will vary greatly depending on the hospital you choose and how your obstetrician works. Every doctor practices a little differently. Hospital births are necessary if there are any expected complications, and the majority of women choose a hospital setting to mitigate the risk of unexpected issues. However, because they all have their own procedures, you will have to advocate for your own preferences, although we have many clients that give birth in the hospital and have very positive experiences.

A birthing center is a great compromise between a home birth and a hospital birth. Some birthing centers are actually within hospitals, and some are separate but only a short distance away, close enough to transfer. For women who are not 100 percent comfortable birthing in their own home but still want options for water and a more natural birth, then a birthing center is a great choice.

You Have Everything You Need

At this point you're ready to welcome your baby into the world! You're prepared, you're strong, and you're wise. You have all the tools you need to start this journey from a place of abundance: an abundance of knowledge, support, and a deeper connection to yourself. You have prepared yourself with the tools that you need around you, from packing your hospital bag to how you're going to talk with your partner and your provider. You know what to say, how to guide everyone so that you can let go and actually rejoice in that abundance.

And because you have been nourishing yourself, exercising, centering your mind, keeping your body calm, and staying in a parasympathetic mode, there is nothing to fear. You can move forward right into the birth from this very positive place that gives you the wisdom and the confidence that you need to succeed.

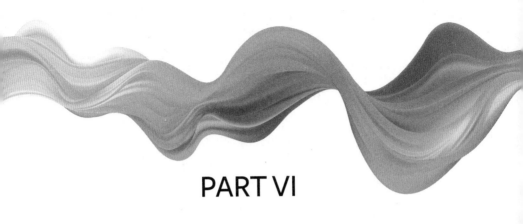

PART VI

The First Forty Days: A Rest and Recovery Protocol

The moment you get to hold your baby for the first time is nothing short of life-changing. Looking at how beautiful your baby is and thinking of the wonders that are ahead for your new family can be almost too much to take in all at once. That's why we believe that the first forty days after birth are a very special time. We want to create a sacred, safe, and secure space for you to take the time to rest, recover, and get to know your new baby.

We like to think of these first forty days as a much-needed transitionary process. For the next few weeks, you and your baby should be living as if you were inside a cocoon, where you have everything you need—including time—to change into a beautiful butterfly. While you may think that you are ready to spread your wings and fly, the truth is, both you and your baby cannot. He or she is just learning to adapt to reflexes and muscular coordination. You need time to heal as well as you begin your matrescence journey, becoming the mother you've always wanted to be.

Use this image of being inside a cocoon as a guide to help you make decisions as to what you should or should not do. Stay in your home, with your baby, and look inward. It's your special time to be quiet, peaceful, shut the outside world out, and just relax. It's completely normal for you to feel exhausted and want to rest. Luckily, as a wise woman, you have planned well for the opportunity, and you've surrounded yourself with people who can help you out with the mundane daily tasks. In the same way that you are caring for a baby that can't care for themselves, you also need to be cared for. If you've never had this opportunity before, allow yourself the privilege to be able to take time for yourself. Let others take care of you so that you can take care of your baby and look forward to what's to come.

YOUR BODY:

MOVEMENT:

NOURISHMENT:

WISDOM:

YOUR BODY

The idea for separating out the first forty days from the rest of your life is grounded in the traditions of many cultures. In fact, the English word *quarantine* originates from the mid-seventeenth century Italian *quarantina* or "forty days," which comes from the Latin *quadrãgintã*, meaning "forty." Yet this idea has much deeper roots. In fact, many cultures all over the world have some form of a forty-day practice that includes the belief that the body needs a period of time to reset, especially during vulnerable periods such as childbirth. The ancient Greeks believed that if a woman took great care of herself during the first forty days, she could reset her health for the rest of her life. We now know that this practice has real epigenetic influences. As you've learned, your lifestyle choices are what allow you to express positive (or negative) genes. Your ability to rest and heal well will help you feel great potentially for many years to come, so use this time as a springboard for positive change. Some women have been able to transform their bodies for the better *after* pregnancy—we know that it's hard to believe, but it is true.

We also know that if you don't take care of yourself now, there can be real health consequences later. After childbirth, you can expect an overall feeling of depletion. If you go against it and push through your fatigue with lots of activity your body just isn't ready for, something will fail or not heal appropriately. That could mean that you bleed for a longer period of time, that you heal poorly at an incision point or at the perineum, or that your mental health suffers.

Even if you're a second- or third-time mom, this baby is new and has its own energy and its own needs. Creating a unique connection at this early stage will actually bring calmness to your whole family because you will be boosting your oxytocin so that you have plenty of love to go around as you rest.

Setting Reasonable Expectations for Recovery

You may not be feeling right in your body for some time, and your recovery will vary depending on the type of delivery that you had, how big the baby was, and how many years it has been between births.

+ A vaginal birth. The experience can be quite depleting. All births have a period of bleeding as the uterus heals and sheds lining that it hasn't shed for ten months, but a vaginal birth may lead to additional blood loss caused by the dilation of your cervix, the separation of the placenta from the uterine lining, uterine contractions, and healing any tears or sutures. You may have localized soreness at the epidural site in your lower back, or tenderness at the swollen vaginal and vulvar tissues, the pelvic floor/perineum, sites of tears, and your breasts as your milk comes in. The perineum may be completely intact, it may have torn, or you may have had an episiotomy.

+ An unscheduled C-section. You may have experienced labor, dilation, or even pushing and have had many of the same experiences as a vaginal birth, leading to the same issues afterward. In addition to pelvic and pelvic floor soreness, you will also have an abdominal scar and tenderness across the abdomen, causing soreness. You may have gas and bloating, and general pain, making moving around more difficult.

+ A scheduled C-section. While you will have a scar and tenderness across the abdomen, because you didn't go through labor, you may feel a little less depleted by comparison. Even if you find yourself with a little more energy than expected, you still need to stick with your forty-day rest period. You will need to rest to heal your body, allow for proper scar healing, and be quiet to connect with baby. Your pelvic floor wasn't stretched, and the perineum remained intact. You may have gas and abdominal pressure and need to brace yourself when sneezing/coughing or transitioning between positions. You can brace yourself by hugging a pillow against your abdomen for support. You will be limited in how you can move.

- **A vaginal birth after Caesarean (VBAC).** Just the fact that you've had a baby prior puts you in a position to know what to expect, which may in itself give you a little bit more resiliency. However, you will have the same soreness, depletion, and blood loss as a regular vaginal birth.

On top of these changes, many new moms experience other similar aspects of recovery:

- You will have a surge of new hormones, like prolactin, which is responsible for breast milk production. The hormones that increased during pregnancy are now on the decline, and your body may have a hard time regulating these shifts. Estrogen and progesterone fall precipitously, which can lead to hair loss, vaginal dryness, depressed mood, and irritability. Your thyroid hormones shift, and adrenal hormones like cortisol can be imbalanced because your body has been through a great deal of physical stress and sleep deprivation. The most influential thing you can do for that regulation is rest. If you are noticing significant hair loss, consider an iron supplement (like Ferrasorb by Thorne).
- Your breasts are going to swell, or *engorge*, as milk production increases. Whether you decide to breastfeed or not, you will produce colostrum for the baby's first few feedings. You will experience larger breasts, tenderness, often darkened nipples, and potentially leak milk even when not feeding. If you will not be breastfeeding, the engorgement will

eventually pass within two weeks. You can minimize the discomfort and pain related to not emptying the breast with cold compresses, wearing a snug sports bra, and avoiding nipple stimulation. It is no longer recommended to take medications to "dry up" your milk supply.

- Your belly will slowly shrink back to its pre-baby size. Your uterus has been stretched significantly, and it's going to take a while before your belly returns to its previous state. A pregnancy belly isn't just about the uterus, but the laxity in the abdominal wall. The muscles of the abdominal wall have been stretched and will take time to regain tone and support. What's more, your organs and connective tissues need to move back into place, which can take as much as twelve months. So, if your belly isn't changing much in a week or two, don't fall into thinking that you're doomed. You are going to slowly see the change. Breastfeeding can speed the process along because the uterus contracts during feedings and you can feel this actually happening. These contractions can feel like menstrual cramps and can sometimes be painful. If you can stay relaxed about your body and not have high expectations early on, you can amplify your chances of returning to pre-baby or even better than pre-baby weight and shape. If you stress about your appearance, lose hope, or have an unattainable timeline for your goals, you may unintentionally create a cortisol stress response, which will slow your metabolism and put you in a fight/flight/freeze mode that goes against healing. Cortisol impacts blood sugar levels for your body to use as energy. However, constant cortisol production can lead to increases in insulin, a fat storage hormone. The more insulin that is around, the more likely you are to gain weight or resist losing weight. If you rush to exercise, you risk stressing your cortisol response even more, making weight loss even more difficult.

Belly Wrapping

Imagine a balloon that's filled to its maximal capacity, where the elastic of that balloon has reached its tensegrity, or most tense status. That balloon was your belly during your third trimester: a fully taut set of tissues providing support through tensegrity. Once you have given birth, that formerly tight space has softened and emptied. It will take time to properly restore tone and support from your muscles, tendons, ligaments, skin, and fascia/connective tissues to regain tensegrity. You cannot expect to gain that tightness, tone, and stability right away, so be patient because it will happen.

Remember, this early postpartum lax state is just a temporary phase. You have lost your connection to your core stabilizing muscles because your body just went through delivery. During this time, some of these lower abdominal muscles or pelvic floor muscles became inhibited, less active, or completely dormant in order to allow for the baby to exit. After the first forty days, you will have to reactivate your lower tummy and start to wake up the deep supportive muscles again. However, if you try too fast to do that because you can't stand what you look like, you will actually fire the wrong muscles and perhaps increase your chances of developing a diastasis. This is why we don't want you working on these muscles just yet because you're more likely to recruit them in an improper fashion. The last thing you want is to start activating the wrong superficial muscle groups by exercising them too soon, which will lead to inefficient support, superficial tension, and possibly pain.

While you are recovering, you can brace your belly with a belly wrap to help guide the tissues where you want them to go. This device will support you during functional tasks like feeding, changing, and dressing/bathing baby and yourself. The wrap provides the same support as your muscles by *approximating*, or bringing together, the connective tissues of the abdomen. This will allow your tissue's collagen to organize itself back to being close together and tight through the middle. The one we like is the Abwrap from Bellies Inc.

You can wear the wrap every day during daylight hours and take it off after dinner. Don't make it too tight where you feel like you're compressing your belly. If it is too tight, you might end up slowing down your bowel movements and the intestinal system. If you have an adverse skin reaction, like hives, or if the compression doesn't feel good, take it off. You can also wear yoga pants that come up high enough to give you a bit of support through the lower belly.

Common Postpartum Complaints

According to the American College of Obstetricians and Gynecologists, women should have contact with a maternal care provider within the first three weeks after childbirth. If you gave birth at a hospital, your ob-gyn examined you after birth and before discharge. However, most women will not see their ob-gyn again until six to eight weeks after birth. The following are common complaints you can discuss with your doctor or try to resolve on your own.

Constipation

After childbirth, you may feel reluctant to release your bowels. You may be holding back because you're scared of going to the bathroom, yet that fear only exacerbates the problem. Some women are afraid that they will tear the perineum more or increase their soreness. If you had a vaginal birth and you did have tearing, you might have a decrease in sensation in the perineum, causing you to feel an urge to push and this may cause pressure on the healing tissues or even cause the development of a hemorrhoid. However, the truth is you won't tear or harm yourself by allowing yourself to poop. More important, it will only cause problems if you become constipated and don't address it quickly.

Some women believe that breastfeeding makes one constipated, but this isn't the truth. As long as you don't allow yourself to get dehydrated (which you may be at higher risk of because of producing milk all day long) and eat foods that will naturally soften your stool, you'll be fine. The foods you will be focusing on over the next forty days are exactly what you need to keep your bowels soft so that you can move them with more ease.

The key here is not to aggressively strain or be overly forceful in the bathroom. By following the instructions below, you can soften your stool, reducing the need to bear down. Remember, if you strain when you are going to the bathroom, you're putting pressure on an area of your body that's just been significantly overstretched is and currently healing. If you've had a C-section or you're compressing into a Valsalva maneuver, you're increasing internal abdominal pressure, and you're actually putting more pressure on the scar.

Instead, try any of these tips for relieving constipation:

- Drink more water.
- Increase your vegetable intake, preferably cooked or in soups.
- Massage your abdomen: This massage can be done either lying down on your back or in a seated position. The massage follows the path of your large intestine in a clockwise fashion. Start on the lower right side of your belly and massage in small circular strokes. Slowly work your way to the upper right abdomen. Move from the upper right to the upper left abdomen, just below the rib cage. Progress from the upper left abdomen to the lower left abdomen. Finally, move from the left lower abdomen to the right lower abdomen where you started. You can perform this clockwise path ten times and repeat several times a day as needed.
- Sit on the toilet with optimal positioning. Consider purchasing a Squatty Potty or placing a tall stack of books or a bench under your feet for optimal elimination posture. If you angle your legs almost like you are squatting, you are in a more sound anatomical position, which allows for ease in elimination.
- Practice releasing your pelvic floor through breathing. Use diaphragm breathing and notice how each inhalation helps the elimination process.

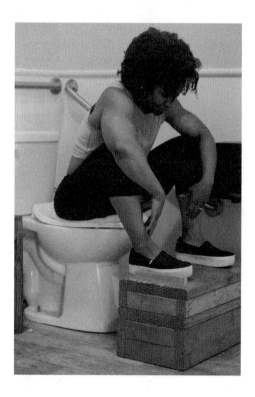

When you inhale, your pelvic floor relaxes, and when you exhale, it contracts and lifts gently. When you are constipated, allow for a nice full inhale, widening the sides and back of your lower ribs to open up and relax the pelvic floor as you try to pass a bowel movement. You can visualize the pelvic floor descending and opening as you inhale.

- Supplement support: Consider the following measures that can be taken daily or as needed:
  - Magnesium oxide or citrate to promote easier bowel movements
  - Vitamin C
  - Coconut or medium-chain triglyceride (MCT) oil
- An enema.
- Smooth Move tea.

Incontinence

There are two main types of incontinence: stress and urge. Stress incontinence occurs when the pelvic muscles are weak and sensation is dulled. Leaking happens when the body is exerting force, like coughing or sneezing. Urge incontinence occurs when the bladder becomes oversensitive and the brain sends signals of unnecessary urge. Many women experience either type of incontinence following a vaginal birth. You may have stitches in the perineum or regional inflammation from birthing the baby. These inhibit the muscular control of the pelvic floor that normally helps with continence. What's more, your bladder may not be in the most opportune position to be able to be controlled. If you've had a C-section, the scarring, abdominal inflammation, and the fact that you can't fully connect with your deeper abdominal muscles right away may affect your continence.

It is very common to experience urine leakage with exertion after pregnancy. However, if it continues beyond the first forty days bring this to the attention of your doctor. You may need to see a physical therapist or urogynecologist. In some cases it is a matter of rebuilding the muscles around the urinary sphincter—in other cases there may be actual breaks in the supporting ligament as a result of pregnancy and childbirth that may need to be repaired.

In the very short term, you may want to remain close to a bathroom and use it whenever you get the urge to urinate. The gentle pelvic floor activation and breathing exercises in this chapter should be able to help. Keeping your thorax at the right level will also help. With breastfeeding and bottle feeding, it's very common to hunch over a bit. As we've discussed, holding a forward posture compresses the abdomen, forcing more of a downward pressure on the pelvic floor, which can lead to incontinence. Be aware of your thorax, keeping your ribs over your pelvis, and lengthen the side body, keeping your waist long. If you get that urge, lift the thorax (rib cage region) and lengthen the side of your body until you get to the toilet.

When you are lying down and resting, you are giving your diaphragm more room to activate, and you don't have the pressure of gravity on your pelvic floor or bladder. This is why you naturally have better continence in bed, so allow for extra time in bed or on a recliner or couch to decrease any urgency.

Limit Climbing Stairs

In many cultures, postpartum women are told to limit climbing stairs because it is thought to lead to prolonged bleeding. We recommend limiting stair climbing during this period. For example, for each of Patricia's three pregnancies, she restricted her stair climbing to only once a day. Every day for forty days, she only went up and down the stairs once. Yet after her third pregnancy, by the last couple weeks of the forty-day period, she was not as diligent, and she bled the longest. Her bleeding was so excessive that her iron levels got very low, and her hair was falling out in clumps.

Whole Body Laxity Continues

During the last months of pregnancy, the hormone relaxin creates looseness in your tissues and ligaments—the structures that hold your joints together. Once the baby is out and you no longer have tensegrity in the body, these overstretched ligaments don't provide much support. You may not feel as loose in your joints as you did during pregnancy, but you may feel a little wobbly through your pelvis, especially when you transition from sitting to standing. This is one of the reasons why it is so important to take it easy during the first forty days: we want you to decrease activity because your body is not actually fit enough to take on too much right now. What's more, that stability and tensile strength in your ligaments does not get fully restored until about ten months after you stop breastfeeding.

Maintaining good seated and standing posture will put you on more solid footing. Good sitting posture is especially important when you're breastfeeding so that you avoid developing a dowager's hump, which is a bump that forms at the base of the neck before the midback. The Cooper's ligament runs from the clavicle (collar bone) through and around the breast tissue and connects to the tissue surrounding the chest muscles. As your breasts enlarge, this ligament stretches, causing the breasts to sag for easier letdown of milk. There are cardiac ligaments that run from the neck to around the breast that will also elongate during this time and may pull down on the nape of your neck. If these pulls are not matched by deep stabilizer muscle activity in the neck and thorax, over time you can develop the dowager's hump and neck pain. To prevent this, make sure that when you are breastfeeding, you are maintaining good posture and not looking down the whole time. Hold your shoulders back so they don't roll forward, and keep your head aligned with your spine, instead of holding a forward head posture. In the Movement section you will find clear instructions to prevent this from happening, as well as optimal breastfeeding positioning.

If you have a tendency toward double-jointedness or hypermobility, be even more careful with how you hold and support your body, especially when you are sitting or standing still. While you may feel comfortable lying on the couch, you may unintentionally be putting a joint into an extreme angle where it can't rebound back to center. So when you're resting, stay in a very square position, with shoulders and hips aligned, chest open, head supported, legs straight, and not leaning into one side or rotating to another. Use pillows so that you are fully supported in the most aligned position possible. A supportive, well-fitted breastfeeding bra can also help support larger breasts and decrease the amount of tugging on your neck, thorax, and upper body. We do not recommend wearing an underwire bra or sports bra if you are breastfeeding.

Post Epidural Issues

Some women complain that they feel the injection site for months after delivery. You may have back pain and soreness where the epidural needle was inserted and removed. Less than 1 percent of women will experience a severe headache caused by leakage of spinal fluid following an inadvertent puncture of the spinal sac. This can be treated with a procedure called a *blood patch*, which involves injecting some of your own blood into the epidural space. The blood patch hardens and blocks the fluid leakage, which relieves the headache.

Once you are home, you may have continued numbness or weakness in your legs or feet if the epidural encroached on a nerve. This will eventually resolve as you rest and recuperate. However, be careful that you're not compressing the nerve by sitting on very hard chairs. And while you may feel the urge to stretch to resolve the numbness or tingling, it's actually the opposite of what you need to do. You want to avoid any sort of stretching, as this can make the nerve more sensitive and keep the numbness and tingling around for a longer period of time. You can do the pelvic tilting exercise (see page 354), or you could do a modified version of nerve flossing (page 174), where you extend a leg and round the body in a small range of motion very gently.

Skin Care and Stretch Marks

During the first forty days, the skin on both your face and the rest of your body may look and feel different. You may develop either hyperpigmentation or dry skin caused by shifting hormonal levels.

You can replenish dry skin by keeping your daily routine simple:

- Cleanser
- Exfoliating cleanser three nights per week to gently remove dehydrated dead skin cells
- Night cream in the morning and again at night
- Hydration mist

Hyperpigmentation or melasma are dark spots that appear on the face or body, almost like sunspots. Sometimes they are only temporary. While there are products on the market that can address them, you don't necessarily need them, as they typically go away within six months on their own, and many products for hyperpigmentation are bleaching creams that often have very toxic chemicals (like hydroquinone). There are some natural alternatives like a brightening vitamin C serum, or an organic product with either kojic acid, aloe vera, or green tea extract. Sun avoidance, wearing hats, and keeping your face in the shade may help the spots from getting darker.

You may have also developed stretch marks as a result of tissue stretching and cortisol levels that increase in pregnancy. Avoiding quick weight loss is a great prevention strategy, but stretch marks do seem to be a result of your genetics than anything else. They typically will fade to white or silver toned stripes with time. While there's not much you can do to avoid them during pregnancy, once you have them you can reduce their appearance and reinvigorate your skin by massaging the areas with pure sesame oil. Sesame oil is preferred because it is warming, as opposed to other oils, like coconut oil, which has cooling properties. Rub a thin layer of sesame oil in a clockwise fashion, which can also help digestion and elimination.

While there are no scientific studies that show strong benefits, you can try the following products: topical retinol creams (not to be used during pregnancy but after), laser therapy (after), and platelet-rich plasma (PRP) injections may help. Collagen supplements are thought to reduce stretch marks,[1] increase skin elasticity, and potentially reduce diastasis. It can be taken as a powder added to water or tea, or in pill form. The products we prefer are CollaGEN from Ortho Molecular Products, Vital Proteins Collagen Peptides, and Truvani Marine Collagen.

Lastly, the darkened stripe that runs along the lower abdomen from around your belly button down to the pubic symphysis is called the *linea negra*. This occurs as a result of high estrogen levels during pregnancy and may take up to six months to fade.

Perineum Repair

Even if you didn't have vaginal tearing, you may have sensitivity around the perineum. Sitting on an inflatable donut cushion can take the pressure off this area. If you had a hospital birth, you may have been sent home with one, or you can buy one on the internet.

The Importance and Ease of Breastfeeding

We support every mother's choice on how she wants to feed her baby, yet we also know that breastfeeding is best. The world's leading health agencies, including the World Health Organization (WHO) and the American Academy of Pediatrics (AAP), recommend that babies are fed only breast milk for the first six months. Breast milk contains a variety of nutrients, growth factors, and hormones that are vital for early brain development. In 2013, scientists determined that children who were exclusively breastfed for at least three months had increased development in several brain regions.[2] Breastfeeding for twelve months or more is associated with higher IQ scores as well as higher educational attainment.[3]

Breastfeeding also fuels physical growth and overall health and protects babies from infection and illness.[4] Breastfed infants are less likely than those consuming formula to develop respiratory and/or gastrointestinal infections and allergies as well as chronic diseases like diabetes, obesity, and inflammatory bowel disease. The microbiome of breastfed infants is thought to have a substantially higher abundance of bacteria that supports optimal immune functioning.[5] Breastfeeding is the best and safest way to expose babies to their mother's beneficial bacteria after delivery, as breast milk contains many of the same bacteria found in a woman's vagina. In a study published in *JAMA Pediatrics*, researchers reported that babies who got all or most of their milk from the breast had microbiota most like their mothers.[6] And it's not just babies' health that benefits from breastfeeding. For every year a mother breastfeeds, she significantly reduces her risk of developing ovarian cancer, invasive breast cancer, and heart disease.[7]

It appears that the benefits of breastfeeding come both from the breast milk itself as well as the overall experience. The physical act of breastfeeding involves direct mother-child interaction and nurturing, and plays an important role in strengthening the baby's sensory and emotional brain circuitry. Breastfeeding also facilitates a naturally responsive style of parenting because

you are meeting your babies' needs instead of feeding him or her on a schedule.[8] Both mother and baby learn how to regulate intake of food and to stop
eating when full—a skill that is important throughout life.

For the first few days until your milk comes in, you will produce *colostrum*, which is extremely rich in nutrients. It is highly recommended to be
your baby's first food even if you are not planning to breastfeed. According to
colostrum expert Douglas Wyatt, the newborn gut is unique in that it is not
fully mature at the time of birth and needs colostrum to complete its development. Nutrients in colostrum also bind to disease-causing pathogens in
the gastrointestinal (GI) tract, preventing them from colonizing and causing
infection. What's more, colostrum helps seed the newborn's GI tract with
beneficial bacteria. If you choose not to breastfeed, consider just feeding baby
your colostrum or supplementing with bovine colostrum, either on its own or
with formula. Studies with bovine colostrum have demonstrated its antiviral
properties[9] and ability to increase immunity.[10]

Simple Breastfeeding Rituals

- **Keep a diary.** Use time as a measure to determine how much breast
  milk your baby is getting. Record how many minutes your baby suck-
  les on each breast. This will help you remember the last time they ate
  and which breast they fed from. Your baby's pediatrician will want to
  know how the breastfeeding is going, and a journal is an excellent way
  to give that feedback. There are specific breastfeeding journals, or use
  a regular notepad.

- **Wear a reminder bracelet.** Use an easily removable bracelet if you want a
  physical reminder of which breast you fed your baby last with. Place the
  bracelet on the hand that corresponds to the breast you begin to nurse
  from. When it is time for the next feeding, you can look at your wrist
  to see which breast you began the last feeding with. Take the bracelet
  off and place on the opposite side and begin feeding from that breast.
  Continue this ritual and even say a little intention as you switch the

bracelet to the new side to feed on, allowing you to confidently breast-feed with balance so the focus can be on connecting with your baby. Keeping track like this helps to avoid milk duct clogs because you are ensuring that you are nursing from both breasts equally. We like the BuDhaGirl brand because it is lightweight, fun to wear, and made of 100 percent medical grade polycarbonate tubing so it is hypoallergenic.

◆ **Try a nursing pillow.** We like The Breast Friend for newborns because it wraps around your body and provides an elevated, supportive shelf to place the baby on so that you are not bending over to meet the baby. A firm sofa pillow or a pregnancy/body pillow rolled up around you is another good choice.

The Surprises of Breastfeeding

Breastfeeding can be a beautiful experience, and while you're in the privacy of your own home, as you will be in these first forty days, you can really relax and enjoy it. However, it can also be somewhat annoying. Feeding the baby on demand means meeting their needs, which can come at any time of the day or night. Breastfeeding can also be physically challenging and uncomfortable, especially in the first few weeks. Your breasts may become engorged, you can develop clogged milk ducts that can lead to an infection, or you can have soreness resulting from blisters and even minor cuts. Your baby may tug or bite a nipple causing a break in the skin, or your nipples can become raw due to the frequency of feedings early on. Applying nipple cream preventatively after every feeding is an effective way to protect your nipples. You can also apply some expressed breast milk straight onto the nipple to amplify healing.

As you are breastfeeding or pumping, you want to gently massage your breasts from the armpit toward the nipple to keep the milk flowing. If you feel feverish or notice tenderness or a hardening at an area of the breast, you may have a clogged milk duct. Take a warm shower and self-massage that area with the warm water hitting directly on the breasts to release the trapped milk.

Don't worry; you're not wasting the milk! Then, after the next feed, place a cool compress over the tender area to ensure that it doesn't get backed up again right away.

Some women produce an abundance of breast milk, which can increase the chances of having clogged milk ducts. If you feel that you are overproducing, you can pump after a feeding and store the breast milk in the freezer. However, breast milk is produced like supply and demand, so the more you pump, the more you will produce. You'll find that in a few weeks your milk production will level off to meet only your baby's needs.

There are also mothers who worry they are not producing enough. If this is a concern, keep track of how much water you are drinking. Oftentimes, we are not drinking enough, and that can slow milk production. Also, skipping a feed or supplementing with formula early on will stall your production. Again, it is supply and demand, and if the demand decreases because you slept through a feed or you supplemented and didn't pump, you will drop production. Drinking a mother's milk tea, like the one from Traditional Medicinals, may help increase your milk production. They typically contain spices and herbs that are thought to promote lactation, such as fenugreek, fennel, cumin, cinnamon, holy basil, and garlic.

Your Environment Is Baby's Environment

Everything in your environment will affect what gets into your breast milk and eventually, your baby. There are thousands of chemicals produced and used each year in the US, and hundreds can be found in your home.[11] A child's liver is not fully able to detoxify what enters their body, including the air they breathe and what they absorb through the skin, until they are about three years old. And there have been many studies showing how toxic chemicals from plastics, flame retardants, cleaning products, and heavy metals remain in breast milk.[12, 13]

The current environmental laws are over forty years old and still include asbestos as a substance that is NOT banned.[14] These laws are industry driven, and it takes a long time for them to catch up to the potential harmful effects of a substance. We have to do our own research; we have to be our own advocate. So starting now, you want to be very diligent about controlling the environment that your baby is growing up in. While you're breastfeeding, keep eating organic foods to minimize your exposure to pesticides and herbicides. While plasticizers like BPA have gotten a lot of press, there are also BPB, C, D, E, all the way to Z. The more natural materials you can use, the less likely that your child will be exposed to chemicals. And just because you received a baby gift doesn't mean you have to use it. Don't feel pressured to expose your child to products and materials that may not be safe.

The following tips will help you get as close as possible to eliminating your baby's exposure to harmful chemicals:

- Buy all-natural cleaners, especially for all the surfaces that baby comes in contact with. Or make your own (see page 41).
- Choose baby furniture that is made of wood or iron instead of plastic.
- Choose glass baby bottles over plastic ones. Many now have a rubber outer coating that helps to decrease their likelihood of shattering.
- Clothing and bedding should be made of 100 percent organic materials without flame retardants for both you and your baby.
- When visitors handle baby, place an organic burp cloth or blanket over their clothes to protect the baby.
- Cover crib mattresses with a Tencel covering to reduce off-gassing. We like Perlux brand.
- Keep an air purification system, like Intellipure, going to promote healthier indoor air.
- Stay off the grass at a public park, as it may be sprayed.
- When washing baby's clothes, skip the fabric softener, which will limit the amount of chemical dyes or scents on their skin.

Keep Baby Safe from EMFs

Your baby will be highly sensitive to EMFs, especially during the first two years of life. While there are no peer-reviewed studies to date to show that Wi-Fi and cell phone radiation is safe for baby—or that 5G is safe for *any-one*—we do know that a child's EMF absorption can be over two times greater than adults, and their skull's bone marrow can absorb ten times as much as an adult.[15] Remember, if it is wired, it is safer.

As we discussed earlier, keeping wireless devices away from your body and on airplane mode will decrease your exposure. Now that baby has arrived, you will want to be even more careful:

- Facetime or have video conferencing calls away from your baby.
- If you are using a baby monitor, use a wired one that has *sound only*, and place it as far as possible from the baby's head. Video monitors have more exposure.
- Use a regular camera whenever possible to take photos and videos of your baby. Or if you do periodically use your phone or tablet, keep it on airplane mode when not in use.
- Never take a phone call when holding baby, and remind others not to do so either.
- Never use your cell phone to play music for baby, unless it is away from baby's head and on airplane mode.
- There are EMF-reducing paints you can use for bedrooms, electromagnetic cage/shields for over bassinet/crib, and copper shields to place over wireless routers to decrease EMF exposures in the home.
- When carrying baby, do not have a cell phone or wireless devices near you.

Maintaining Calmness Helps Your Brain and Body

The word postpartum does not have to be synonymous with depression, although we know that many women will experience a wide range of emotions and psychological stressors following childbirth. According to Postpartum

Support International, one in seven moms and one in ten dads experience postpartum depression.[16] Without a doubt, the next few weeks will include disrupted sleep, a crying baby, and possibly even some physical discomfort. All of these things can agitate you. However, we believe that if you maintain a strict forty-day rest period, you're less likely to fall into postpartum depression.

When we are doing more than we should, when we're not carving out the time to rest or sleep, we can create a stress response, which elevates cortisol production. This is inflammatory to your system and reduces your ability to stay in the parasympathetic mode where you want to be in order to amplify healing and ultimately lose those pregnancy pounds. That's why it's critically important to prevent the cortisol stress response. The more you can stay in a calm state, give yourself rest and self-care, the better you will feel.

For instance, Dawn came to see Patricia during her third trimester to share her frustration about her inability to lose the baby weight between her pregnancies. She was worried it would get worse after the delivery of her third child. Patricia gave her strict instructions for after the delivery: to stick with warming foods for the first forty days, to rest as much as possible, to relax her mind and body, and to not ascend/descend stairs more than once a day. Dawn took the advice and focused on rest and her baby. By allowing her body to be free from stress and quieting things at home, her cortisol levels most likely never spiked. Because of this, her metabolism rebounded nicely, and her energy was restored. Over the next six months, she lost all of her baby weight and felt great!

Some women are genetically predisposed to postpartum depression, especially if they have experienced depression before they were pregnant. A hormonal shift may lead to you feeling a little bit of those "mommy blues." However, we're hopeful that because you have improved your microbiome, built your support network, and adopted all of the wonderful calming tools in this book, then maybe you can prevent it entirely, or the blues will pass quickly. If you are feeling depressed or feeling like your judgment may be off, reach out for support. There is a wide range of mental health experts and hotlines (like the one from Postpartum Support International) that can help you improve your mental health during this time.

Get Plenty of Sleep—Really

According to the *New York Times,* sleep is particularly important to maintaining good mental health. Studies have shown that the early weeks after a baby is born can give rise to a vicious cycle, where poor sleep increases the risk of developing postpartum depression, and women who have postpartum depression are more likely to have trouble sleeping.[17]

Create the right environment to get the sleep you need, both during the day and at night. Blackout shades, a quick meditation, avoiding bright light around key naptimes, minimizing screen time in general, and listening to calming music will help you nap when the baby naps. Even a brief five to ten minutes of shut-eye can make a world of difference.

Prevent Your Stress from Transferring to Baby

According to Jennifer Lansford, PhD, stress transfers from parent to child, which is another important reason for you to stay calm and rested during the first forty days. Babies are extremely sensitive to their mother's/father's stress and anxiety. Feeling anxious and pressured can also impact how you care for your baby. Stressed parents are less responsive to their infant's cues, and less-sensitive caregiving is stressful to babies.

You need to be calm and resilient to reduce stressors. Every day is an opportunity to shift what you're doing to amplify feeling good. Remember what helped you feel calm during pregnancy and stick to those activities. Maybe it was reading a book, listening to a guided mediation, or going outside. These forty days of rest offer the perfect opportunity to reconnect with good friends on the phone or quietly pick up an old hobby. As you incorporate these practices into your day, pay attention to how you feel and how you responded to your baby.

There will always be days when you won't feel great because you're totally sleep deprived, and those are the days that you want to lean on your partner or others in your support system so that you can let them take care of baby for a little while. In one 2009 study, social support was shown to be effective in helping women cope with postpartum stressors.[18] However, if you're finding that your support system is actually stressing you out, speak up. If you are noticing that you are not looking forward to a visitor coming—even with the aim of helping you—then the support they are trying to give you isn't additive. Be honest, and let them know that, while you appreciate the gesture, you really don't need their help at this time. If you don't, you run the risk of creating another stress response, which is what you are working so hard to avoid!

MOVEMENT

Every exercise that we suggest for postpartum can be performed in the home. There is no rushing back to the gym. The goal for the next forty days is to gently activate the deep hip and pelvic muscles and connect with postural muscles to support feeding and holding your baby. These few exercises will create the right foundation that we will later build upon.

For now, put the 30-plus minute walk on hold. Be mindful when walking around the house: exercise tall posture, and grow tall from the crown of the head.

Equipment Needed

- Sturdy chair
- Towel
- Pillow

The First Forty Days Exercise Routine

Ten Minutes of Muscle Activation/Coordination

Continue with the Pelvic Self-Correction in bed page 197), Diaphragm Breathing in the inverted position (page 47), and Book Opening (page 152) 2 to 3 times per day. Then, add the following exercises:

Exercise: Pelvic Tilts

PURPOSE: To gently reduce pressure and tension in the pelvis, sacrum, and lower back [Lumbar Core].

START POSITION: Lie on your back with knees bent and feet on the bed. Arms can be comfortably by your sides or put your hands on your pelvic bones.

SEQUENCE:

STEP 1. Exhale and roll your pubic bone up toward the ceiling, using your gluteal muscles. Your lower back will naturally press into the bed.

STEP 2. Put your hands at the front of your pelvic bones. Inhale and let your tailbone move down toward the bed, allowing the pelvis to tip forward. Your lower back will naturally lift off the bed.

STEP 3. Perform 10 reps, tilting/rocking the pelvis with ease. Coordinate your breath and keep the abdominal muscles relaxed the whole time. You can do 1 to 2 sets.

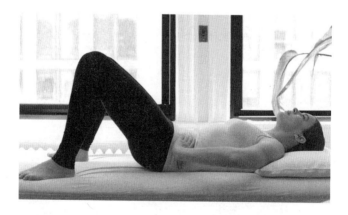

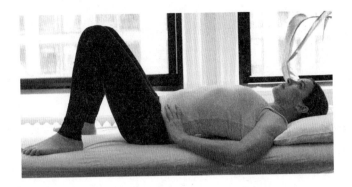

Exercise: Gluteal Activation

EQUIPMENT: Towel or pillow.

PURPOSE: To begin engaging the gluteals for pelvic, hip, and low back support. [Lumbar Core].

START POSITION: Lie on your back with knees bent and feet on the bed with towel roll or pillow between the knees. Place your hands under and at the sides of your buttocks.

SEQUENCE:

STEP 1. Exhale, and squeeze the pillow between the knees softly from the hip muscles.

STEP 2. Press through both heels to target the lower region of the glutes while maintaining the pillow squeeze for 10 seconds. Perform 10 reps.

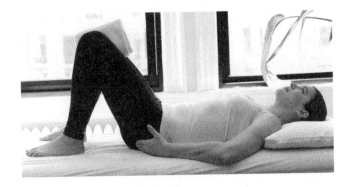

Exercise: Pelvic Floor and Diaphragm Breathing Coordination

EQUIPMENT: Pillow.

PURPOSE: To coordinate the diaphragm and pelvic floor to gain pelvic floor strength [Thoracic and Lumbar Cores].

START POSITION: Lie on your back with a pillow under your head, both knees bent, and feet on the bed. You may also use the inverted position as previously described if it is more comfortable.

SEQUENCE:

STEP 1. Gently inhale through the nose, quietly and softly, feeling the back and sides of your lower ribs expand. Consciously allow the pelvic floor to relax. Imagine a piston action: as you inhale, the diaphragm descends and expands, and the pelvic floor also gently descends and releases.

STEP 2. As you slowly exhale and the ribs come together, gently activate your pelvic floor: feel all four corners of the pelvic floor (from pubic bone to sacrum and to the left and right sitz bones) coming together as if an internal vacuum is lifting them up through the middle of your pelvis/abdomen.

STEP 3. Regardless of what type of birth you have had, only perform this gentle pelvic floor lift on each exhale. Similar to how an elevator lift operates, feel that you are only lifting to the first or second floor of the elevator, not maximally to the fifth floor. Perform 10 repetitions coordinating the diaphragm breath through the nose quietly with each rep.

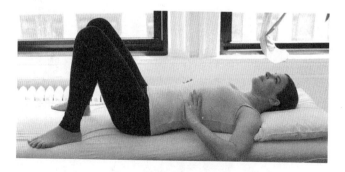

Exercise: Flat Back Squat

EQUIPMENT: Chair, optional.

PURPOSE: To strengthen legs and core, and to practice neutral spine mechanics. You will be utilizing this flat back squat with functional activities with and without baby [All Cores].

START POSITION: Stand tall with your hands by your sides or on a countertop or chair back for balance.

SEQUENCE:

STEP 1. Inhale and gently bow forward with a flat straight spine as your knees bend over your second toes. Allow the front of your hips to crease and fold backward.

STEP 2. Keep your chin down as if you are holding an apple at your chest, and look out at the floor in front of you. This should keep your head in-line with the rest of your body, and your ears in-line with your shoulders. Hold this position for an exhale and another inhale, feeling your legs carrying your weight.

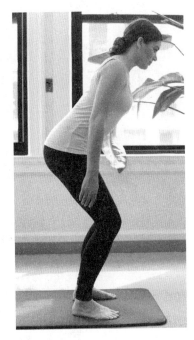

STEP 3. On the exhale, press gently through the legs and rise up to standing. Perform 5 to 10 repetitions as tolerated with your breath coordinated.

Body Mechanics for Parenting

It's easy to put your baby first without thinking about your own body. However, it is absolutely crucial to practice good body mechanics while parenting—it could save you lots of discomfort, prevent injuries, and help you be a much happier, more present parent.

Every time you transition from one activity to another, no matter how routine, think about your movements. How are you lifting, cleaning, and changing the baby? How are you getting up and down from the toilet? All of these motions matter because you can actually use them to guide your body's healing. All of the functional movements you do in your day are opportunities to exercise. When you move your body in a neutral way with daily activities, you are actually engaging that foundational, deep muscle system and strengthening your legs and hips.

The basic rules of good body mechanics are

- Always favor pushing an object (e.g., carrier, stroller, etc.) instead of pulling it toward your body. Try practicing without your baby at first, then practice with your baby when you aren't rushed.
- Avoid twisting. Face your baby straight on when at the changing table or playing with him or her.
- Bend from the knees and hips and keep your spine in neutral. Engage the legs with a flat back when bending to pick up your baby. Be mindful not to curve your spine or jut your head forward! When bending and lifting, keep your feet wider than your hips—this will give your body a wider base of support and provide more low back and pelvic stability.
- Hold everything near, not far. Hold your baby (or anything, including baby gear) as close to the center of your body as possible. Think of having short dinosaur arms that can't reach. Get your body close to objects requiring lifting/pushing and utilize your center and extremities in good alignment.

Body Mechanics Modifications Post C-Section

If you have had a cesarean section, don't lift anything for at least two weeks. Your partner or other supporter can help you with baby so that you do not have to lift, bend, or reach too much or too often.

When you are comfortable, use the same body mechanics instructions outlined in the chapter. You should feel confident in your arms and legs to support you with these tasks as your abdominal scar is healing. You may also feel stronger using your belly wrap or pregnancy pelvic baby belt for extra support.

Body Mechanics Exercises

Stroller Mechanics

STEP 1. Lock the stroller wheels so that it doesn't slide away from you.

STEP 2. Standing close to the stroller, hold baby close to you and perform the flat back squat.

STEP 3. Keeping your spine neutral/straight, allow your buttocks to move backwards, and hips to crease farther. Place the baby in the stroller when you and baby are both at the seat level. Maintain flat back posture as you buckle your baby in.

STEP 4. Walk around to the back and push baby with the handlebars at a comfortable height, where elbows are roughly at 90 degrees and your shoulders are relaxed.

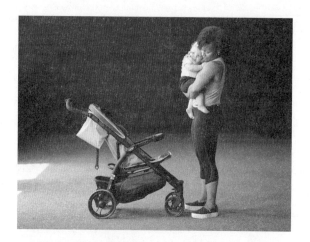

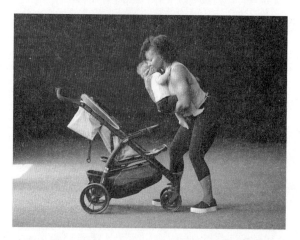

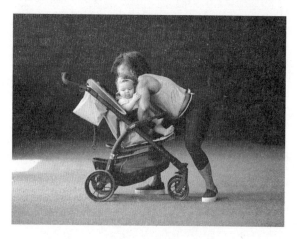

Car Seat Mechanics

We see many new moms hold the baby in the car seat with a straight arm by their side. This is not ergonomic and can strain muscles and/or joints. For the first forty days, it would be best if your partner or your support person accompanies you out of the home to deal with baby and the car seat. These are the proper mechanics we want you and your partner to adopt.

STEP 1. Perform a flat back squat to pick up an *empty* car seat from the floor.

STEP 2. When arms are at the level of the car seat, grab the handle and lift the car seat by bending your elbows, using your arm strength. Use short dinosaur arms and carry the seat close to you.

STEP 3. Press into the legs and rise up, using your lower glute muscles and keeping the car seat close to your center, elbows bent the whole time.

STEP 4. Place the empty car seat on a high, stable surface like a table or countertop. Get the baby and keep him or her close to your center, up against your chest and belly.

STEP 5. Bend your knees with baby close to your chest to place the child in the car seat. You may need to stagger your stance by almost straddling the corner of the table to get baby in the car seat more easily. Buckle baby safely into the car seat.

STEP 6. Pick up the car seat with baby in it by bending your knees and lifting from your legs and arms. Place one hand on the handlebar and the other underneath the car seat. Cradle the car seat close to your center as you walk toward the car.

STEP 7. Clip the car seat into the car base. Make sure to face your shoulders and hips in-line, straight ahead, and bow forward with a flat back squat, even if you have an SUV. Bending the knees, grounding the legs, and keeping the chin tucked down will help to protect your spine, which often gets strained with these repeated movements.

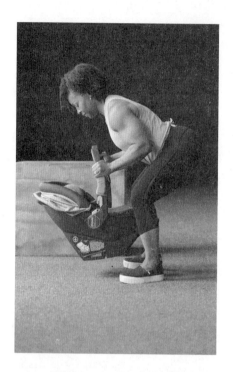

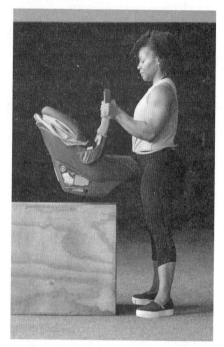

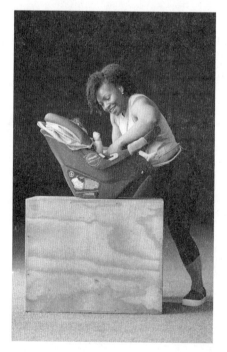

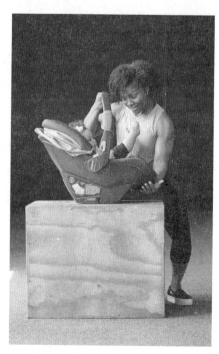

Dishwasher Mechanics

Although your support network can be taking care of your chores, you may have to put a dish away or do something in the home. It is best to create good habits for safe and supportive body mechanics early on. Once again, you will maintain a flat back squat even when placing the lightest dishes and silverware in and out of a dishwasher.

STEP 1. Stand in front of the dishwasher with feet shoulder width apart. Use the flat back (neutral spine) squat to open the dishwasher door and roll the bottom or top rack out.

STEP 2. Standing up, hold the dish with a nice, upright posture and get close to the dishwasher.

STEP 3. Stand in front of the dishwasher tray and place the dish in the compartment. Never twist when you are bring dishes in and out of the dish-washer, although it may be a tempting shortcut.

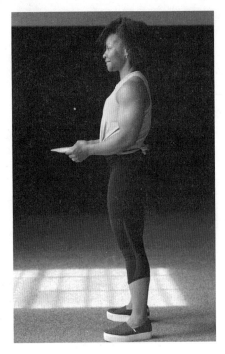

You run the risk of a strain, but you also miss out on an opportunity to do your flat back/neutral spine squat exercise.

STEP 4. Stay in your flat back squat as you roll the rack back in and close the dishwasher door.

STEP 5. Stand tall, with side body long and the crown of your head lifting to leave the kitchen.

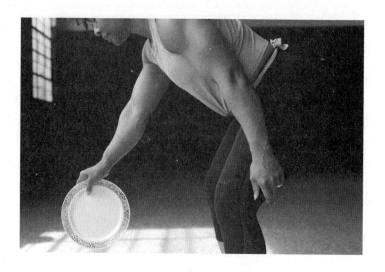

Getting Out of Bed Safely

You may find yourself sleeping on your back again or staying on your side. Either way, we want to still avoid putting any compression through the central abdominal seam (*linea alba*) over the first forty days. The following directions are slightly different than what you were following in the third trimester, so please read carefully.

STEP 1. If you are on your back, bend the knee farthest from the edge of the bed.

STEP 2. Push through that foot firmly to assist the whole body to logroll to your side so your body is facing the edge of the bed closest to you.

STEP 3. Rest the top arm onto the surface of the bed as the top thigh comes in-line with the bottom thigh.

STEP 4. Bend both knees and dangle the legs over the edge of the bed.

STEP 5. Push with your hands to come up to a sitting position on the edge of the bed. Use flat back squat to get up from there.

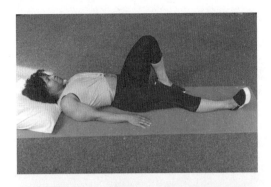

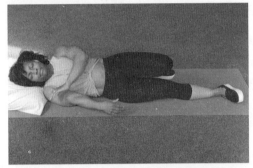

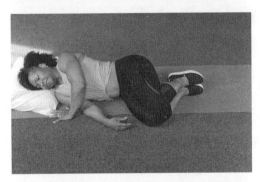

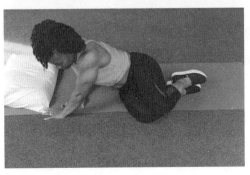

Golfer's Lift

Try to limit lifting anything during the first forty days. However, if you must lift anything light off the floor, using this lift can prevent injury. If the object you want to pick up is too heavy for this motion, you may not want to lift it at all. Later on in your postpartum recovery, you should safely be able to lift more again utilizing your flat back squat.

STEP 1. Stand tall, close to the item you want to pick up.

STEP 2. Swing one leg back behind you as you bow forward with a flat back. Your body will swing like a pendulum so that your hand effortlessly comes forward to the object.

STEP 3. Grasp the object and allow for momentum to swing you right back up to an upright standing position.

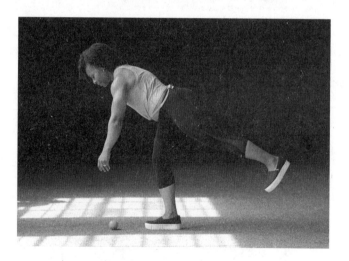

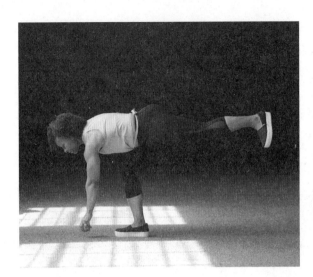
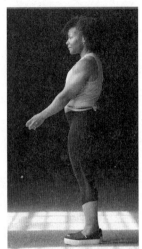

Carrying a Diaper Bag and a Baby

Always hold your newborn baby right in front of you: do not ever keep your baby at your side. Your ligaments still have laxity. If you lean into your hip/pelvis when you position your baby on your hip to the side, you are predisposing yourself to potential injury or ligament strain, or you may overstretch the side of the hip muscles—the very same muscles we need to strengthen to restore proper spine and pelvic control. By leaning into them/stretching them, you are making it harder for them to be trained to support you again.

When you need to leave the house, hug baby close to your chest and abdomen and cradle under their buttocks and back or neck/head. The closer the baby is to your center of mass, the less pressure you will feel on your body, especially as it grows and gains weight. Having the baby in a carrier strapped to your center is another option that can help free up your hands. Once your baby is in the proper position, you can then lift up your diaper bag. Get into the habit of keeping the bag on a high surface or chair seat so you don't need to bend to get it.

Most diaper bags have shoulder straps; some have cross-body straps. A backpack is another option, but it is not a popular one. Keep the diaper bag straps short and the bulk of the bag at your side, close to your center of mass. Do not let the bag hang to land below your pelvis. This will cause unnecessary strain on the spine and pelvis. If you still feel the bag's weight on your body, the bag is simply too heavy, and you should lighten your load.

Proper carrying technique

Improper carrying technique

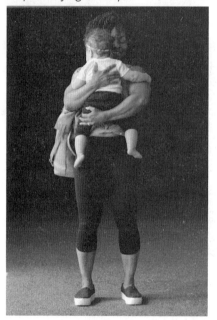
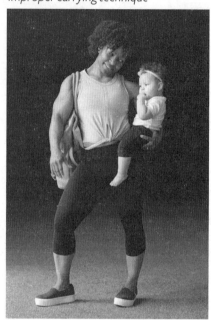

Breastfeeding Mechanics

Getting yourself into a comfortable position for breastfeeding is the key to a pleasurable experience. When you are more comfortable, your baby is comfortable. When you are comfortable, you can also enjoy this wonderful bonding experience more.

There are many options for positions to breastfeed your baby. The key is having many pillows available. Before you are ready to feed, place as many pillows as you need behind you to support your spine in an upright or semi-reclined posture. Make sure the pillows support you from the head all the way to the tailbone. When using a rocking chair/glider, we recommend using the paired ottoman glider for your legs to get the full benefit of decompressing the spine in a reclined position. The glider allows you to rock baby to sleep straight after the feed. Some women lie on their side and allow baby to breastfeed in that position, where baby is also supported by the bed. Do not lie on your back completely flat, as this may not allow for proper "let down" or flow of your milk.

Once you and your pillows are in position, place the baby on top of another firm, supportive pillow (like the Breast Friend) so that you do not have to hold/support the baby. Bring the baby toward your breast, helping him or her find your nipple. Your baby should latch on quickly and begin to suckle.

You may need to look down at baby periodically, but once baby is nursing, relax your head back on the pillow behind you. The more forward you allow your head to be, the more prone you are to developing the dowager's hump on the back of the neck/upper back.

Make sure the pillow is supporting your head with your ears back in-line with the shoulders.

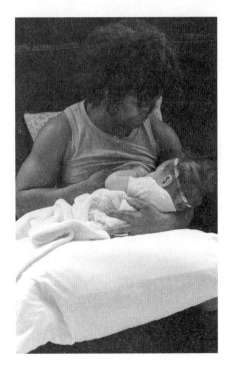

Although it is tempting, do not use this time to scroll on your phone, take pictures, or be on a computer or tablet. This is quiet time for you and baby to bond together and not have exposure to EMFs.

If you have trouble breastfeeding, there are lactation specialists your ob-gyn can refer. Most doulas can also help.

NOURISHMENT

Remember all those warming, anti-inflammatory foods that you made and froze back in the third trimester? They are ready to be eaten and are the best foods to support both mother and baby. An anti-inflammatory diet will help your body heal faster, regardless of the type of birth you had. Your body is recovering from an inflammatory episode, and staying away from inflammatory foods is going to make you feel and look a lot better. Cooked vegetables are the most digestible. Cooked meats, healthy fats, fruits, and filtered water are important and can reduce inflammation. High-fiber fruits and vegetables will help to keep your stool soft.

We recommend sticking with the same prenatal vitamin with iron and DHA, which is appropriate for breastfeeding and non-breastfeeding moms, and sticking with a gluten-free, dairy-free diet for the first forty days. There is a myriad of alternatives we recommend: goat milk, coconut milk, nut milks, and hemp milk. We also recommend staying away from coffee and other caffeinated beverages, even though you're going to be awake at night. If you have too much caffeine, you may throw off your sleep cycle, and the caffeine may be stimulating to baby as well. Lastly, if you've lost a lot of blood, you may need to either supplement with iron or liver pills or eat organ meats like liver.

If your stomach is feeling unsettled, have a few extra carbs, focusing on whole grains like rice or quinoa. Stay away from gas-producing foods like beans and cruciferous vegetables, especially if you are recovering from a C-section. These include the following:

- Bok choy
- Broccoli, all varieties
- Brussel sprouts
- Cabbage, all varieties
- Cauliflower
- Collard greens
- Daikon
- Horseradish
- Kale
- Kohlrabi
- Mizuna
- Mustard—seeds and leaves
- Radish
- Rutabaga
- Turnips—root and greens
- Wasabi
- Watercress

Stay well hydrated to flush out the extra fluids you held onto toward the end of pregnancy. The more water you drink, the more you can flush out. If you have a hard time drinking plain water, squeeze in some lemon or add a splash of organic fruit juice.

Foods to Choose While Breastfeeding

Experts recommend that you add 300 to 500 additional calories a day when you are breastfeeding. To get these extra calories, opt for nutrient-rich choices, such as a medium banana or apple with a tablespoon or two of almond butter. Many breastfeeding moms also find it beneficial to take a multivitamin, as it offers some security that they are getting a sufficient amount of nutrients to protect their health and produce quality breast milk.

Everything you eat transfers to your baby via your breast milk, so eat a wide variety of colorful foods rich in proteins, fats, and complex carbohydrates (organic, when possible). Each type of food will change the flavor of your breast milk. This will expose your baby to different tastes, which might help him or her more easily accept solid foods later.

As you are eating, record your meals in your journal, and watch how your baby is reacting to the foods you are eating. Sometimes their behavior can be related to the stimuli and what's happened in the day or perhaps a diaper rash, but it can also be a reaction to the foods you choose. Look for physical changes as well. Is he developing a rash? Is she having more difficulty going to the bathroom, or does she seem to generally be cranky? Is he having a harder time getting to sleep and staying asleep? Does she arouse more easily? For instance, we have found that babies negatively react to dairy that transfers into breast milk because it is inflammatory and hard to digest. Our new mothers who go completely dairy-free while they are nursing report that their babies sleep better and are generally more peaceful.

There are a few types of foods that can typically cause baby's distress. Avoid highly acidic foods, which may have caused acid reflux during your pregnancy. These could promote gastroesophageal reflux disease (GERD), not only in you, but also in your baby. And avoid eating the cruciferous vegetables previously listed, as they tend to promote gas, which will not be good for you or your baby.

Nursing mothers must also increase their water intake to twelve, ten-ounce glasses spread out over the course of a day. We also recommend abstaining from caffeine and alcohol during the first forty days that you are breastfeeding because both contain chemicals that end up in breast milk. A newborn is more sensitive to these substances. What's more, both are inflammatory and can decrease your overall milk production at a time when you are trying to increase your output.

WISDOM

Many women go through pregnancy excited and full of anticipation. Yet once they are home with their new baby, they fall prey to their fears and insecurities. Used to seeing their doctor every few weeks, they now feel abandoned, alone with their baby. If this is how you feel right now, don't panic; there truly is a maternal instinct, a powerful intuition of how to best be with your new baby and your family, and it is going to kick in. Every mother is innately blessed with this ability, even if you don't feel it right now.

Your intuition will guide you like a guardian angel. However, you need to be quiet in order to find your intuition and learn how to use it. The first forty days can provide this exact opportunity. As you recover and get back on your feet, you will also be creating deep connections with your baby, to getting to know this extraordinary new being who chose *you* to be their mom. As you learn her likes and dislikes, respond to her needs, and shower her with love, you're now becoming not only a wise woman but a wise mother.

Relying on others to help you through this transition will allow you to regain your energy, to feel that you are of sound body, of sound mind, and of sound heart. In your motherhood cocoon, you can focus your energy and educate the heart. What your baby needs most is to feel your love, to feel your presence. When you are strong enough, you will connect with your motherly intuition.

In ancient cultures, new mothers were never left alone. At home, the other women in her support network would each take a chore, cooking and cleaning as she healed. Her only responsibility was to feed and take care of the baby. In her book, *The First Forty Days*, writer Heng Ou explores her heritage and the ancient Chinese practice of postpartum care known as *zuo yuezi*, which lasts for a full lunar cycle. Today, your support can set up diaper-changing stations at multiple points in the home, clean the house, do your laundry, sterilize bottles or breast pump parts, prepare meals for you and the rest of the family, shop, organize all the gifts that have arrived, and perhaps take a turn watching the baby to give you an extra nap or a much needed break.

If you feel like you're still doing too much, or that you aren't able to tap into your intuition, a postpartum doula might provide the additional support you need. For example, our colleague Chantal Traub is a doula who works with women from pregnancy to delivery and beyond, offering guidance during the transition to motherhood. Doulas can help you master the art of breastfeeding and can provide both physical and mental support, mitigating postpartum depression. In this way, new moms feel like someone outside their family is checking in, attending to their adult needs. So many other people want to come and play with the baby; a doula is all for you.

What's Best for Mom

Ayurvedic medicine teaches that the forty days following childbirth is a time when new mothers are nurtured by their families, who provide foods that are good for breast milk production, for the baby's health/digestive system, and to balance the elements of her nature to achieve wellness. Of the five possible elements, all new mothers take on the element of ether, which is the essence of space, of emptiness. Ether represents the absence or loss of what had been growing and taking up space within the body, as the baby is no longer in the belly. So if you are feeling a sense of loss even in the midst of being with your newborn, we want you to know that it's not only okay to respond this way; it's expected.

You can balance your ether nature by making choices that will lead to a more grounded, earthy state. These are the same practices that we preach: looking inward, resting, and connecting to your baby with your heart and feelings of love. When you place your attention on yourself and your baby, you will be flooded with oxytocin, the hug you need to fill the void. The warming foods we recommend are grounding because they are earthy by nature: heavy and moist root vegetables and meats deliver the density of earth. Then keeping a consistent routine is grounding, even if it's as simple as intentionally waking up and going to sleep at the same time.

There is a very easy exercise to help you directly connect with the earth. Wearing minimal footwear or no shoes at all, stand on the earth, put your left foot in front of the right and face toward the sun, with your palms facing forward.

What's Best for Baby

As your intuition gets stronger, you'll see that many of the same things that keep you calm will positively affect your baby. We have found that the following three sensory practices offer the easiest and most effective ways of calming and connecting with newborns.

First, your baby may respond to the same music he or she has been hearing throughout your pregnancy. We have also found that babies respond to classical music, which is thought to improve brain development. Dr. Sergio Pecorelli, creator and co-founder of the educational platform The First 1000 Days of Wellness, believes that classical music like Mozart's Piano Sonata No.16 in C Major is an excellent place to start.

Your baby has committed your scent to memory, which will soothe and calm his nervous system, reminding him that he is in a safe place whenever you are around. If you place the swaddle blanket on your body when baby is not in it, he will be wrapped in your scent all of the time.

Lastly, connect with your baby by giving her a gentle massage when you change her or after a bath. Infant massage promotes digestion and better sleeping patterns. It automatically reduces cortisol levels and allows more oxytocin to be released. In many ways, it's a form of communication and sets the groundwork for a solid relationship.

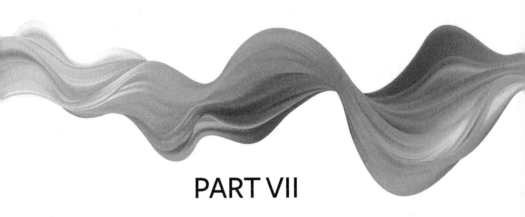

PART VII

Beyond Forty Days: Getting Your Body Back

Passing the first forty days means that you can slowly transition back into real life. But that doesn't mean that your body will be exactly the way it was before pregnancy. It may take up to a year for you to look and feel like your old self, especially if you're nursing. This last phase of the program is going to help you get your body back, and you'll be happy with the results as long as you understand that it's going to take time.

The biggest problem we see is when postpartum women get nervous about their body, usually about six months following delivery. They start to aggressively diet and exercise, yet nothing moves the needle. Essentially, they are creating a whole new stress response because of this approach. While they do double the work needed, they get poor results when they could have done way less and the weight would have melted away.

The truth is, every day it's possible to get closer to your goal when you put your attention on eating the right foods, making time for self-care, and making time to rest. And of course, moving well, with good form and alignment, and activating the right muscles that are all helpful for creating a tall, lean stature. As a wise woman, you know that everything's working in your favor because you've done such great work along the way. So relax, enjoy your time with your baby, and let's get back to work.

YOUR BODY:

MOVEMENT:

WISDOM:

YOUR BODY

With your doctor's permission, you should be ready to return to your previous level of sexual activity. Not only is sex an important part of your relationship with your partner, having an active sex life is also good for your baby. Sex can elevate both partners' health, and we know that the baby thrives when both parents are healthy and less stressed.

Immediately following orgasm, you should be resting quietly in the dark or with closed eyes. This will allow for a complete parasympathetic effect.

The Healthiest Food to Put You Back in the Mood

According to Greek culture, the apple represented abundance and fertility. It was customary for a bride to eat an apple on her wedding night, which was believed to ensure sexual desire as well as fertility. Today's medicine confirms this ancient ritual: Italian researchers recently discovered that women who eat an apple a day may in fact enjoy better sexual function.[1] Apples have an abundance of phytoestrogens, polyphenols, and antioxidants, all of which promote women's sexual health.

Later Postpartum Complaints

Painful Sex

Now is the time to have sex, but you might find it will be painful. This is a result of reduced estrogen exposure for the vaginal tissues. For many women, this results in painful intercourse, right at the time when they should be resuming normal sexual activity. In one study, nearly half of postpartum women reported a lack of interest in sexual activity, which may be related to dissatisfaction with body image, a lack of vaginal lubrication associated with breastfeeding, and previous experiences with painful sexual intercourse (dyspareunia).[2]

Over-the-counter vaginal lubricants may be enough to make sex more enjoyable. There are also other nonhormonal and hormonal options to address this issue. Your doctor can prescribe a compounded hyaluronic acid to apply to the vagina to improve moisture retention, or a topical bioidentical estrogen therapy that may restore the tissue to become more elastic, moisturized, and lubricated. You can also consult a pelvic floor physical therapist who can determine if there is a biomechanical issue causing pain during sex.

Pelvic Organ Prolapse

Following pregnancy and childbirth, the muscles and tissues of the pelvic floor can become so stretched and lax that they drop, allowing the bladder, rectum, uterus, and/or cervix to lower as well. In some cases, these organs may even protrude out of the vagina. This is referred to as *pelvic organ prolapse* (POP). These issues can be noticed immediately after childbirth. However, some women are significantly swollen, and they may not notice a prolapse for a few weeks following delivery.

Symptoms of POP can include

- Bladder urgency
- Chronic backache
- Feeling like something is "falling out" of the vagina

- Feeling of fullness, heaviness, or pressure in the vagina
- Painful sex

Many women only experience symptoms after doing specific activities. For instance, if they've been standing or sitting for long periods of time, if they've gone on a walk and pushed a stroller up a hill, if they've been coughing or sneezing, or if they have had a poor night's sleep. They also find that symptoms go away after sleeping or resting lying down, as the organs will temporarily go back into the correct position. However, the POP can reactivate when you're standing up the next day.

POPs can be evaluated by your doctor or a physical therapist. In fact, in other parts of the world, like France, this evaluation is part of the normal healthcare post childbirth. Liz Simons, DPT, a physical therapist who specializes in women's health and pelvic floor dysfunction, believes as we do that if you get a professional evaluation early, you can probably prevent a POP from getting worse.

A minor prolapse can clear up on its own within a year of giving birth. The tissue integrity just takes time to heal, especially if you are breastfeeding. Eventually, the organs will work their way back up to the proper position.

Having awareness of how you are using your muscles can help. Practicing good body mechanics, good posture standing and sitting, practicing good breathing, and avoiding bearing down or straining can help prevent existing prolapses from getting worse.

Practicing the pelvic floor or strengthening exercises that you have been doing can relieve the pressure from your pelvic floor and eliminate the effects of gravity, therefore reducing the stress on the prolapse. If you can elevate yourself into a gravity minimized position, like the inverted breathing positions (see page 46), then you can positively influence the tissues to return to their normal position, but it may be only temporary.

Some of the exercises in this chapter will help make significant changes if you have a prolapse. These include

- ◆ Ball Squeeze Pelvic Floor/Transversus Coordination (page 399)
- ◆ Transversus Abdominis Activation Series (page 400)
- ◆ Pelvic Floor and Diaphragm Breathing Coordination (page 356)

The Pelvic Floor and Diaphragm Breathing Coordination is a gentle Kegel exercise that will provide the lift you need to address a prolapse. However, we do not recommend doing forceful Kegels postpartum unless a doctor or PT has told you to do so. Some women subconsciously hold their pelvic floor tight all the time, and if they are doing so and then doing Kegel exercises forcefully, tightening the muscle in that way can actually makes things worse. However, Kegels are helpful because they engage the pelvic floor in a lifting fashion that then allows for more support for the internal organs. In this instance, it is very important to keep the contraction gentle and to rest and fully release the pelvic floor muscles between reps.

You may have more difficulty recovering naturally if this was your second or third baby, and even after you have tried all of these exercises and worked with a physical therapist, you may need a surgical intervention. However, physical therapy is always recommended before surgery: if you don't change the mechanics of how you're using your body, you can reinjure it and re-prolapse it.

Products That Can Help a Prolapse

- ◆ **Belly wrap:** This is a compression sleeve for your belly to help you feel supported. It's not necessarily for prolapse rehab, and while we don't recommend that you become dependent on it, it can help you as a reminder to reestablish a connection to your muscles. Having an upper compression through your belly can give you some awareness to not bear down as much.

> ◆ **Pessary:** A small silicone cup, similar to a diaphragm, that is usually fitted, inserted, and removed by a gynecologist. Once inserted into the vaginal canal, it creates a barrier that prevents prolapsed tissue from descending out of the vagina. It does not retrain the muscles; it's a passive instrument, more like a sling inside the vaginal wall.

Prevent a Pressure Belly

Oftentimes, postpartum women tend to grip/contract the lower chest with their external oblique abdominal muscles, which can create divots you can see on your upper abdomen. This maladaptive movement increases intra-abdominal pressure, creating a bulging at the lower abdomen known as a *pressure belly*, a term coined by Diane Lee, a women's health researcher, author, and physiotherapist. If you notice divots or a pooch at your lower abdomen when you are standing, handling your baby, or during the exercise program, don't brush it off as stubborn baby weight; it's due to using your body poorly to compensate for weakness. These divots will go away when you focus on your breathing, strengthen the deeper core muscles, and adopt the body mechanics strategies highlighted in both postpartum chapters. These will help you engage your core in an improved way.

Treating a Diastasis

Earlier we learned that all pregnant women develop some form of a diastasis. After childbirth, this separation can fully close over time, and as early as twelve weeks. Sometimes this separation does not fully close, and you may develop a small gap (about one finger's width) or a large gap (up to four fingers' width). You may notice a bulging or a large cone forming at the center of your abdomen when you are exercising, or with certain activities of daily life, like pushing or lifting your baby, or even getting up from bed. The larger the diastasis, the longer it will take to repair, the harder it will be to repair on its own, and the more symptoms you may have that accompany it.

Following childbirth, the symptoms often associated with diastasis include

- Back pain
- Pelvic pain
- Abdominal pressure with bulging
- Pelvic floor dysfunction
- Constipation
- Incontinence
- Pelvic organ prolapse

It's never too late to reverse a diastasis. An abdominal binder, like the belly bands we've mentioned, will *not* heal or close a diastasis. Instead, adapting better core function, along with correct diaphragmatic breathing, will help you resolve a diastasis as well as these accompanying symptoms. The Ball Squeeze Pelvic Floor/Transversus Coordination (page 399) and the Transversus Abdominis Activation Series (page 400) will help you resolve a diastasis. You will have to stick with the program in order to make an impact; you're not going to see real results immediately.

If you follow the program and do not see a significant change in four months, it's time to see a physical therapist specializing in postpartum women's health. This type of PT will assess your diastasis and your breathing and develop an individualized strategy for you to engage your abdomen. For example, in Patricia's practice she uses real-time ultrasound, like the one used to image your baby, to image the deep muscles of the abdomen. She works with her patients to create positive tension to close a diastasis.

If you cannot produce good abdominal tension to support your back and pelvis, you may need to consider surgery, especially if the diastasis remains larger than three fingers in width. Note that it may take up to eighteen months for your collagen to realign to close the gap. So be patient and stick with the program and your PT before rushing to surgical repair. In fact, surgery is only recommended when you are at least one year postpartum and are finished having children.

Identifying and Measuring a Diastasis

- Lie on your back with knees bent and feet on the floor, head supported with a pillow. Use two fingers on the center of your abdomen and poke from the top of the abdomen, descending slowly to the pubic bone. Feel for softness or soft patches along the central abdominal seam. You may feel areas of firmness and areas of softness or divots. Usually the tissue around the navel is the most lax.

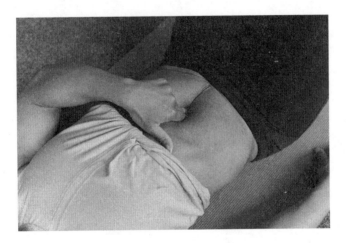

- With fingers on the softer portions, or right above your navel (if no softness was felt), lift your head off the floor and look at your navel. Use your fingers to determine which areas remain soft and if there is tension improving in any area. If there is a soft area that does not get tense with the head lifted, you have developed an inefficient strategy to support lifting the head that is creating some separation at the abdomen. This may be a sign of a diastasis.

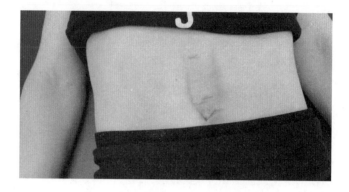

♦ Next, determine its size by feeling for a gap. Lift your head again and
   measure how wide the gap is by placing your fingers side by side inside
   the gap (can be 0–5+ fingers). If the depth is more pronounced than the
   width, it may be a signal to consult with a physical therapist trained in
   diastasis and postpartum management.

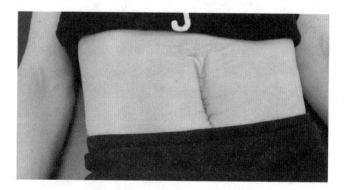

♦ Lastly, see if you create a cone or bulge during movements. Lie down
   with knees bent and head supported on two pillows to observe your
   navel. Straighten your right leg and lift it off the ground 45 to 60 degrees.
   Notice if there is a bulge or a cone that forms in the center of your abdomen; again, this is evidence of a poor strategy that may be a sign of a
   diastasis. Repeat this test with the left leg to see if there is a difference.

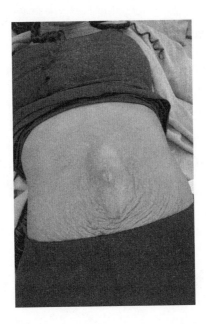

Postpartum Umbilical Hernia

This condition is characterized by the outward protrusion of the belly button through an opening in the abdominal muscles, post-delivery. The soft and tender bulge is generally small in size and, over time, may heal on its own. If the hernia is large, the skin around the protrusion may appear reddish blue. You may notice pressure or sensitivity at the navel that feels worse when lifting baby, coughing, or sneezing. You may also feel stiffness or pain, nausea, and vomiting. Any of these symptoms should be immediately addressed by your doctor.

You can brace your central abdominal region by putting pressure with your hands directly over the navel to prevent further herniation. Some women feel confident enough to poke the tissues "back in" to decrease the herniation tenderness or pain after sneezing, lifting, or coughing.

Simple Self-Balancing Techniques

It is very common to feel overwhelmed postpartum. And no wonder: you've just gone through an enormous change, and now you are responsible for a whole new person! Stressors create inflammation that lasts for a while, which is why it is so important to reduce your stress in the postpartum months. What's more, your stress can transfer to your child. Feeling pressured or stressed can cause you to be less attentive to your baby's cues, which can cause further stress.

Yet as a wise woman, you have the tools to rein in your worries so that you can feel like you are in control, even temporarily. Take time every day to dismantle your inner pressure. Even with all the chaos that can be motherhood, you can make a few adjustments to your day or evening to keep you feeling good:

- When anxiety, emotions, or feelings of imbalance arise, something as simple as smelling your favorite essential oil can bring you back to center. Orange essential oil is thought to bring joy, and lavender calmness.
- Release your worries before bed by writing them down in a notepad or journal. On a separate page, write down your to-do's for the next day. When you create a list, you are less likely to worry before bed and feel more prepared for the next day.
- Try a float tank or float pod. One of the most powerful anti-stressors is floating in the dark for just twenty minutes in salted water set at body temperature. We highly recommend this practice during postpartum. A local spa or wellness center might provide this service.
- Putting gentle pressure on certain acupressure points can help you restore balance and make you feel good right away. Test out the following circuit or just a few of the suggestions. See which ones help reduce that overwhelming feeling. Press on these points as often as needed, even multiple times a day. Each time, massage the point for thirty to

sixty seconds, especially before bed.

1. Begin with the right-hand web space (between thumb and first finger)

2. Right wrist crease, palm side, below the pinky

3. Right elbow crease, on the outside of the elbow and the end of the crease, not on the bone

4. Left elbow crease as described above

5. Left wrist crease

6. Left-hand web space

7. Left ankle bone—four fingers above the ankle bone, on the inside of the leg and in the soft tissue depression below the bone

8. Left toe web between the big and second toes

9. Right toe web

10. Right ankle bone point (see #7)

◆ You can rejuvenate your energy by trying one of the following restorative postures. The Alexander Technique, which retrains habitual movement patterns and postures, suggests that you simply lie on your back with feet on the floor with knees bent and hands on your belly. Staying in this position while focused on your diaphragm breathing promotes rest and relaxation. The following restorative yoga poses can be equally effective. Doing any of these activities with the music you love amplifies the anti-inflammatory mechanism and promotes calmness.

Exercise: Restorative Child's Pose

EQUIPMENT: 3 to 4 pillows and 2 to 3 towels.

START POSITION: Get onto hands and knees on a towel/mat on the floor or on your bed.

SEQUENCE:

STEP 1. Go into a kneeling position and place one or two pillows under both buttocks so that the pillows are between your buttocks and your calves. Place a towel roll across your hips so that the towel is in the crease of your hips. Sit back so your buttocks reach down to your heels with knees apart. You can place your hands out in front of you supported by the bed or on another pillow, or place your hands at your sides, shoulders supported by a towel roll or the mattress. Place your forehead on the floor or bed with neck in neutral alignment.

STEP 2. Breathe into the back and sides of your lower ribs, relax your body and hips, as you hold this position for as little as 3 minutes or for as long as you feel comfortable.

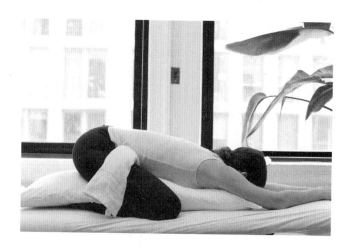

Exercise: Reclined Butterfly Leg Posture

EQUIPMENT: Multiple pillows.

Lay pillows in a shingled fashion, one overlapping the other, so that you can lie on them from your back all the way up to your head in a semi-reclined position. Place 2 to 3 pillows under your knees. Put your feet together so that the soles are touching and knees are apart, supported on the pillows. Place a couple more pillows under your arms so that they are at your sides with palms up. Allow for the chest and the hips to stay open in this supported pose as you breathe in and out, focusing on the sides and back of the lower ribs. Hold this position for as little as 3 minutes or for as long as you feel comfortable. If you drift off to sleep, that's perfectly okay.

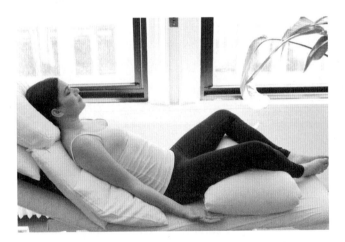

MOVEMENT

Throughout your pregnancy, the exercise program was specifically created to support your internal structure so that pregnancy and delivery would be easy. But now we are ready to do something entirely different. In order to get your body back, you have to rebuild and activate your foundational muscles, which you may be more able to connect with now that you're no longer pregnant. These are the same muscles that were supporting your growing belly and can now be recruited to promote good posture, good form, and good alignment and also close a diastasis. You may have done these exercises for the first time as a pregnant woman, and now we will be doing them with modifications and progressions to help you get back to a flat belly or get one for the first time.

Because you're doing the program in a specific, progressive pattern, you are building yourself back according to the order that your muscles involuntarily fire. This helps you prevent musculoskeletal complaints such as lower back pain, pelvic floor pain, and cervical strain/pain because when you go to push a door open, lift up your child, or even push a stroller, there's a specific order of the deep muscle system that should actually turn on. You're training your muscles in a layered fashion so that when you go out and do other activities or sports that you love, you have rebuilt your structure to do those other things safely and effectively.

For instance, Lisa came to see Patricia ten weeks postpartum, complaining of lower back pain and leaking urine when sneezing and during high impact exercise, like jumping. She thought she would just have to live with the urinary incontinence because she delivered two big babies vaginally, back to back. She feared that she wasn't going to lose the thirty pounds she gained during this pregnancy, and she began working out, focusing on sit-ups and running as soon as her doctor cleared her just a few weeks after the birth. The weight was sluggish to come off, although she had shed some of it.

Patricia also noticed that Lisa was "bearing down" with her external oblique abdominal muscle when doing abdominal exercises. This action alone increased interabdominal pressure, created back tension, and didn't allow her pelvic floor to contract appropriately for bladder control. Patricia taught her a different way to contract her abdominals and paired it with diaphragmatic breathing strategies. By doing so, she was able to support her lower back to eliminate pain and contract her pelvic floor properly to eliminate incontinence/urine leakage. Patricia showed Lisa how her navel was dropping from the poor compressive strategy. Then they modified Lisa's exercise routine, swapping the sit-ups for movement that stabilized the core and elongated her body to reduce compression until she was stronger and more resilient. Over the next few months, Lisa gradually regained a flat tummy and achieved her pre-pregnancy weight.

The Get Your Body Back Exercise Routine

You will be ready to progress from the forty day routine to the new post-partum routine following a checkup with your physician six weeks after delivery, except if you are recovering from a C-section; then you should wait for the ten-week mark. Once you are cleared, the following exercises can be part of your daily routine for the next twelve weeks. Then, once you are able to get back to more aerobic activity, or slowly transitioning back to the sport you love, you can continue to follow this routine at least three times a week. By doing so, you will continue to address the connection to your deep muscle system, which will keep you feeling good and doing all of the things that you love to do.

You can work with this exercise program for as long as you want and as long as you see benefit. Remember, your ligaments and soft tissues will continue to be lax ten months after you stop breastfeeding. If you return to your regular exercise regimen too early, you may start to feel neck or back pain because your deeper system is still not active enough, and those exercises don't necessarily isolate those muscles enough. So connect with your body and enjoy the experience of a different type of exercise program that will build a strong foundation to grant you the freedom to do what you like going forward.

Thirty-Plus Minutes of Aerobic Activity

You can resume walking thirty-plus minutes a day and work toward increasing your pace. Start slowly: if you feel that you can't tolerate more than fifteen minutes at the beginning, that's okay. Every three days, add five minutes until you get to thirty minutes of continuous walking. Be wise, take your time, and transition slowly because if you do too much too soon, you might create a strain or prevent steady progress. Jumping back into activity too early may also create bad breathing habits that can prevent you from actually achieving your goal. Aim for feeling a little bit winded during your walk, where it's hard for you to talk.

A pedometer, or the step counter on your phone or watch, might provide the right motivation to get you back to a full thirty-minute walk. In one study of women who had C-sections, the women who utilized a step counter took significantly more steps compared to the control group. Better still, these women reported a significantly easier physical and mental postpartum recovery.[3]

Modify Exercises to Improve a Diastasis

If you suspect that you have a diastasis or see a cone form as you engage your abdominals, use your hands to approximate the abdominal muscles in the start position of each exercise. By bringing the tissues together either with one hand or two hands, you are able to facilitate the connectivity of the fibers.

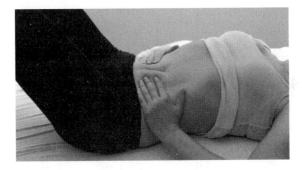

See which cues work best to generate tension in the softest areas of your abdomen. As you are doing the exercises, monitor your abdominal tension by palpating on the softer areas with your fingertips.

Notice if the areas become firmer, the depth decreases, or the gap narrows. If you feel the gap widen, or the depth increase, then you are not using an appropriate strategy and may need to see a physical therapist trained in diastasis rehabilitation.

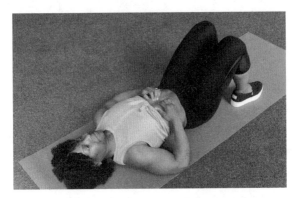

Twenty-Plus Minutes of Eccentric Strengthening

Continue with the following exercises for as long as they feel good and you feel supported.

- Pelvic Floor and Diaphragm Breathing Coordination (page 356)
- Pelvic Self-Correction (page 197)
- Scapular Protraction and External Rotation on Wall (page 287)
- Deep Neck Flexors (page 66)
- Pelvic Rotation on Hands and Knees (page 129)
- Step Forward Arm Lift (page 173)
- Sidebending with Twists (page 271)
- Sun Salutation into Downward Dog Marching (page 206)
- Foot Doming (page 70)

Afterward, add the new ones described below. Many of the new exercises have hand-hold modifications to aide with diastasis support and progressions to make them slightly more challenging as your musculature returns. When you are up for it, and diastasis is not an issue, you can add back the third trimester upper body strengthening exercises (pages 269, 275, 280, 281, 283, 287).

Equipment Needed

- Hand mirror
- Inflatable beach ball
- Pillows
- Resistance band
- Sturdy chair
- Towels
- Yoga block or similarly sized book
- Yoga mat

Exercise: Thread the Needle

EQUIPMENT: Yoga mat (optional) or bed.

PURPOSE: This exercise will help you feel looser in your midback as you move around. The midback area often gets very restricted when breastfeeding because it stiffens to accommodate larger breasts and continuous sitting [Thoracic Core].

START POSITION: Get into the all fours position with spine neutral, either on a mat on the floor or on top of your bed. If you have wrist discomfort, use your fists instead of flat hands.

SEQUENCE:

STEP 1. Bend your right elbow while balancing on both knees and the left hand; make sure to keep the left shoulder blade lifted.

STEP 2. Reach the right arm across the body, behind the left supporting arm, and let your gaze follow your right arm as long as it is comfortable.

STEP 3. Hold that reach for 2 to 3 breaths as you inhale through your nose and into the back and sides of your left lower ribs, expanding more with each inhale.

STEP 4. Repeat on the other side. Perform 5 reps for each side, alternating sides.

PROGRESSIONS:

a. Raise your right arm up to the sky at the start, instead of a bent elbow, to increase the range of motion at the beginning of the exercise.

b. Extend your range of motion at the endpoint of the exercise to where you're reaching arm's shoulder drops down to the bed/mat.

c. Hold the position for more breaths as long as your form can tolerate it.

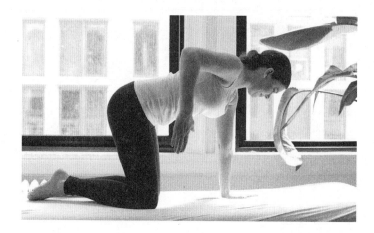

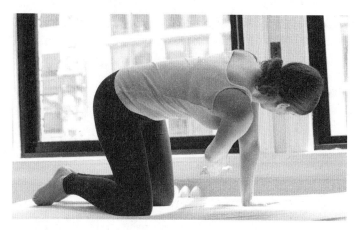

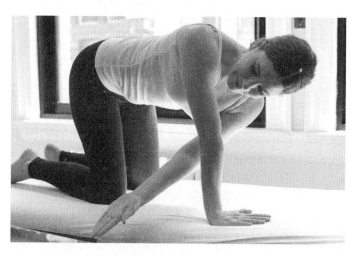

Exercise: Ball Squeeze Pelvic Floor/Transversus Coordination

EQUIPMENT: An inflatable beach ball or pillow; yoga block or similarly sized book; chair.

PURPOSE: To coordinate your pelvic floor, diaphragm, and transversus abdominis together to rebuild your core for deep support for everyday activities. This exercise specifically addresses both a prolapse and diastasis [Lumbar and Thoracic Cores].

START POSITION: Sit tall in a sturdy chair and place a yoga block or book between your calves. Hold the ball or pillow at your chest with both hands.

SEQUENCE:

STEP 1. Inhale through your nose into the back and sides of your lower ribs. On your exhale, draw all 4 points of your pelvic floor up like an elevator going up about 2 floors, as you squeeze the ball with both hands. You will feel your transversus (lower belly) engage naturally.

STEP 2. Hold this position for a full exhale and then *fully* relax, returning the ball/pillow to your lap. When beginning these stabilizer exercises, it is hard for the body to completely relax, and the muscles can stay gripped. Be mindful to completely relax your pelvic floor and abdominals between repetitions.

STEP 3. Repeat 10 times.

PROGRESSIONS:

a. Switch from a seated position in the chair to kneeling on both knees.

b. Do 2 sets of 10 repetitions.

c. Engage your transversus on the exhale and continue to squeeze the ball or pillow while you inhale and exhale. Rest on the inhale and reset. Continue for 10 reps, 1 to 2 sets.

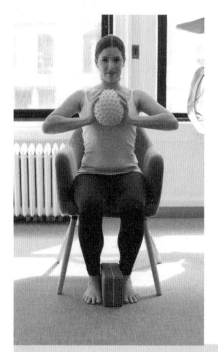 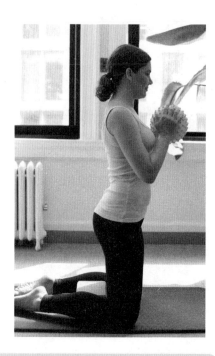

Exercise: Transversus Abdominis Activation Series

PURPOSE: This series will rebuild a solid foundational core so that you can perform safe body mechanics and future activities. This exercise specifically addresses both a prolapse and diastasis [Lumbar and Thoracic Cores].

The transversus abdominis (TrA), the deepest core muscle, is the only muscle that will help to flatten the belly and, if necessary, will be instrumental in closing a diastasis. The transversus acts like a corset, sucking the belly in. It runs from the deepest part of the front of the abdomen all the way around to the deep muscles of the lower back. When it engages, it slides across like a belt, tightening the tummy without creating bulges. It works together with the pelvic floor and diaphragm (the top and bottom of the abdominal cylinder) to provide complete support and control.

Start this series by performing exercise #1. Progress to exercise #2 after two weeks, as long as you are feeling that you have mastered the first exercise.

Then move through the series in similar two week increments. If it is difficult to connect with your transversus or pelvic floor, try elevating the hips with pillows, like you did in the inverted diaphragm breathing posture.

1. Transversus Abdominis Activation

EQUIPMENT: Yoga mat, hand mirror.

START POSITION: Lie down on your back on a mat on the floor. Keep both knees bent, feet on the floor, and breathe diaphragmatically. Keep chin down, back of neck lengthened, and head relaxed on the mat. You may use a towel roll or pillow under your head if you need that support.

SEQUENCE:

STEP 1. Exhale, gently activate the transversus by using one of the transversus cues that resonated for you in the past:

- Draw the area above your pubic bone toward your spine.
- Draw your hip bones together or apart.
- Lift the pelvic floor (imagine that you are stopping the flow of urine, lifting the vagina, or draw your tailbone/coccyx to your pubic bone).
- Count out loud (slurring numbers continuously) as you exhale. This activates the TrA involuntarily.
- Pull back your skin from your pubic bone to your navel as if you were protecting it from an imaginary zipper that is zipping up really tight jeans.
- Breathe in and hold the rib cage up and exhale half the air out while drawing the lower belly in and up.

Or, as you exhale, draw all four points of the pelvic floor up followed by drawing the area above your pubic bone in and up toward your spine. Use a hand mirror to monitor your navel—it should stay still and never move downward. Hold the transversus contraction as you exhale. If you suspect a diastasis, utilize the hand positions to cinch the tissues.

STEP 2. Continue to breathe and keep the transversus contraction engaged for roughly 10 seconds.

STEP 3. Rest and mindfully relax the whole abdomen and pelvic floor. Repeat 10 times.

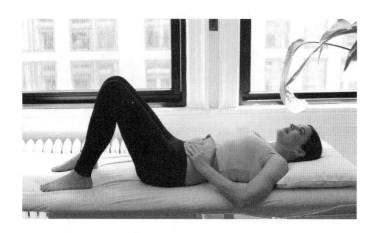

2. Transversus Abdominis Activation with Bent Knee Fall Out

SEQUENCE:

STEP 1. Perform all the steps of the previous Transversus Activation exercise.

STEP 2. On the next inhale, allow the right bent knee to open out to the side, away from your left leg. Open the leg as far as you can control, with abdominals staying engaged and your pelvis staying flat on the ground.

STEP 3. Exhale and deepen your abdominal contraction and engage your right inner thigh as you gently return the leg back to neutral. Monitor your abdominals to prevent bulging, coning, or navel dropping. Use the hand position that seems to give you the support you need to keep good tension if you have a diastasis. Limit yourself to 20 percent of your maximal effort when engaging and moving. As the exercise becomes easier, allow the leg to move a little farther away from your core.

STEP 4. Perform 10 slow reps with the right leg, and then repeat with the left.

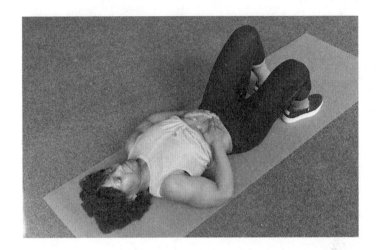

3. Transversus Abdominis Activation with Heel Raise

EQUIPMENT: Yoga mat, towel, or yoga block.

START POSITION: Perform all the steps of the Transversus Activation exercise #1.

SEQUENCE:

STEP 1. Slowly lift the right heel up while maintaining a level pelvis, not allowing your body to move except for the heel that is lifting. Hold the position for 5 seconds and then lower. You will be holding the transversus muscle activation the whole time while breathing diaphragmatically. Use the hand position that seems to give you the support you need to keep good tension if you have a diastasis.

STEP 2. Lift the left heel for 5 seconds and lower. Repeat this sequence one more time on each side while continuing to breathe. Some women like placing a hand on the lower rib cage to remind them to keep their diaphragm breathing going.

STEP 3. Rest and release the abdomen. Repeat the alternating heel lifts so that you do 2 heel lifts on each side, followed by a rest, and then reset. Perform 10 sets.

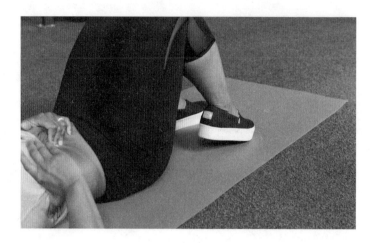

4. Transversus Abdominis Activation with Resistance

EQUIPMENT: Yoga mat, towel, or yoga block.

START POSITION: Lie down on your mat on the floor with both knees bent, feet on the floor. Place a rolled towel or yoga block between your knees.

SEQUENCE:

STEP 1. Perform all the steps of Transversus Activation exercise #1. If you see a bulge, dropping of your navel, or coning when doing this exercise, skip to exercise #5.

STEP 2. Once the transversus abdominis is activated on your exhale, press both hands at your thighs like you are pushing the knees away. This gentle pushing action will create an isometric contraction of your other abdominal muscles, while the transversus stays activated.

STEP 3. Hold this isometric resistance for 5 to 10 seconds while you continuously inhale and exhale from the diaphragm. You want to begin with mild resistance and work up to more resistance as tolerated, as long as no bulging, coning, or dropping of the navel occurs.

STEP 4. Completely relax in between reps, and perform 10 reps.

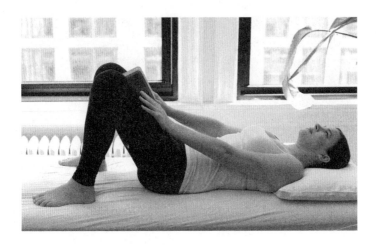

5. Transversus Abdominis Activation with Marching

EQUIPMENT: Towel or yoga mat.

START POSITION: Place a towel or yoga mat on the floor and lie down on your back with knees bent, with or without a pillow under your head.

SEQUENCE:

STEP 1. Engage your most effective transversus abdominis cue on your exhale.

STEP 2. Maintain that contraction and slowly lift and lower one knee toward your chest, followed by the other. Keep diaphragmatically breathing with the cue engaged throughout the exercise. Make sure your pelvis stays level and doesn't tip as the leg lifts and that your lower back doesn't lift up as you lower the leg. Your lower back and pelvis should remain neutral.

STEP 3. After completing one knee toward your chest on each side, rest and completely relax the abdomen. Reset your cue with breathing and repeat for a total of 10 sets.

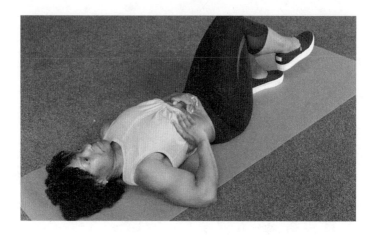

6. Transversus Abdominis Activation with Diagonal Resistance

EQUIPMENT: Yoga mat, towel, or pillow.

START POSITION: Lie down on your mat on the floor with both knees bent, feet on the floor. Head is resting on the floor or pillow with chin down and back of neck lengthened. Perform all the steps of the Transversus Activation exercise [#]1.

SEQUENCE:

STEP 1. Exhale as you bring the right knee to the chest, followed by the left knee to go into a 90–90 tabletop position. If it feels better, place an additional towel roll between your knees.

STEP 2. Keep breathing as you reach your right hand across to your left thigh and resist the knee coming in for an isometric contraction.

STEP 3. Hold that position for 5 seconds as you exhale and then rest. Switch hands and resist with right hand on left thigh on your next exhale. Repeat 10 times on each side. Rest by lowering one leg at a time to the floor. If the 90–90 tabletop position creates a bulge or you are straining to keep your legs in that position, go back to knees bent, feet on floor, and simply resist the knee coming up toward your chest with the opposite hand for 5 seconds; do 10 reps on each side.

- Hold the resistance for 10 seconds as you continually breathe and repeat 10 alternating reps, for 1 to 2 sets.

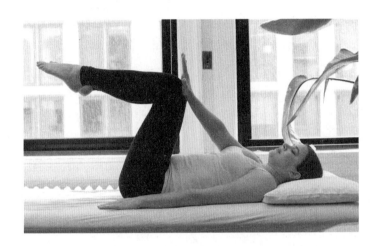

7. Transversus Abdominis Activation with Diagonal Resistance and Lengthening

This is the most challenging of the series. If it is difficult to keep your spine still, or your abs get shaky/fatigued, go back to #6 for a few more weeks. Be wise and err on the conservative side when challenging your core at this time.

EQUIPMENT: Mat on the floor.

START POSITION: Lie down on your mat on the floor with both knees bent, feet on the floor. Head is resting on the floor with the chin down and the back of the neck lengthened. Perform all the steps of the first Transversus Activation exercise to activate your transversus properly.

SEQUENCE:

STEP 1. Exhale as you bring the right knee to the chest and resist the knee coming in with your left hand on the right thigh.

STEP 2. Lengthen the left leg up toward the ceiling and open the right hand up above the head forming a long diagonal line. Keep breathing. Adjust the angle of the straight leg based on how much you can control, keeping your lower back neutral (not lifting off the floor) and your pelvis level. Hold the resistance in this position for 3 to 5 seconds.

STEP 3. Bend the left knee, and switch arms to press the right hand on the left thigh and extend right leg out and left arm up and back.

STEP 4. Alternate each side, resting the abdomen when you get to the 90–90 tabletop position with your legs (both knees bent in toward chest). Always hold the resistance for 3 to 5 seconds and alternate so that you do 10 reps on each side.

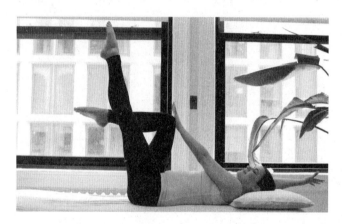

PROGRESSIONS:

a. Hold the resistance longer, up to 10 seconds, to challenge yourself further, breathing throughout.

b. Increase the number of repetitions to 2 sets of 10 reps on each side.

c. Lower the leg at whatever angle from 90 degrees (pointing up to ceiling) until parallel to the floor. It is not recommended to go below 45 degrees in the first 6 to 9 months after giving birth. The higher the leg toward the ceiling, the easier it will be; the lower it goes (45 degrees or close to being parallel to the floor), the more challenging it will be to maintain proper activation and good form.

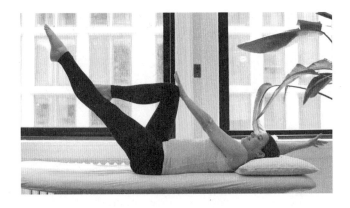

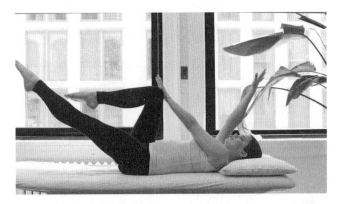

Exercise: Mini Glute Bridge with Towel Squeeze

EQUIPMENT: A towel or yoga block, yoga mat.

PURPOSE: Strengthen the gluteal muscles, integrating inner thighs and core to improve pelvic support and centering [Lumbar Core].

START POSITION: Lie on your back on a mat on the floor with knees bent, feet on the floor. Place a rolled-up towel or yoga block between your knees.

SEQUENCE:

STEP 1. Exhale, squeeze the towel with both knees equally, pressing through your heels to activate the lower glute, and raise pelvis mildly off the mat (approximately 3 inches). Keep toes down on the mat and make sure pelvis stays level: your right and left prominent pelvic bones are in a straight line. Hold that position for an inhale and exhale and lower on the exhale and relax. **STEP 2.** Repeat 10 times.

PROGRESSIONS:

a. Repeat for 2 sets of 10 repetitions.
b. Hold the bridge for 10 to 15 seconds before lowering. Perform 10 to 20 reps.
c. Go up a little higher in the bridge, hold 10 seconds, and perform 10 to 20 reps.
d. Add an alternating heel lift: when you are able to sustain the bridge, for 10 to 15 seconds, you can progress to squeezing the towel, lifting to a bridge and performing 4 alternating heel lifts (right, left, right, left). Lower and repeat for 10 to 15 sets.

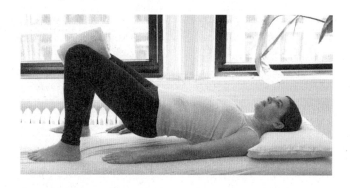

Exercise: Neutral Spine Squat with Band and Block

EQUIPMENT: Resistance band and yoga block or small pillow; chair (optional).

PURPOSE: Strengthen legs and hips while integrating core and neutral spine mechanics [All Cores].

START POSITION: Standing tall, tie a medium resistance band around your thighs. Place a block or book between your feet. If you feel unsteady, you may place your hands on a chair back or wall for support.

SEQUENCE:

STEP 1. Inhale through your nose into the back and sides of your lower ribs and gently go into a flat back squat, allowing hips to move backward, keeping back flat and chin in, like you have an apple at your chest. Gaze out on the floor in front of you so your neck stays in-line with rest of your spine; there should not be any wrinkles in the back of the neck. Feel the legs and hips working against the band and block/book as you keep your knees tracking over your second toes.

STEP 2. On your exhale, press into your heels (keeping toes on the floor) and feel the lower glutes and hip muscles activate as you rise.

STEP 3. Repeat for 10 slow reps, 1 to 2 sets.

PROGRESSIONS:

a. Perform the squat and hold it for 10 seconds; repeat 10 times, for 1 to 2 sets.

b. Go into a slightly deeper squat, holding for 10 seconds, 10 times, for 1 to 2 sets.

c. You may progress to longer hold times or 5 more repetitions every 3 to 5 days as tolerated until you reach a 20-second hold for 20 to 30 reps.

d. Add double arm pullbacks to the squat. At the bottom of the squat, row both arms back, squeezing shoulder blades together and opening the chest. You may do this with no resistance or tie a medium resistance band to something sturdy at chest level or on a doorknob for a more intense pullback.

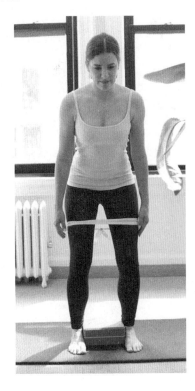

The Wise Woman's Postpartum Stretching Program

Reintroduce the following stretches as long as they feel good and you limit the range of motion. Stop at the first resistance; do not stretch into joint extremes. Remember, your ligaments will continue to be loose for ten months if you are not breastfeeding and for ten months after you stop breastfeeding.

- Quads
- Calves
- Hamstrings
- Hip Rotators
- Pecs

- Cat/Cow
- Book Opening
- Child's Pose (original version)

If you sense stiffness in your body, add the ball release techniques (see pages 198, 251-253, 321) and self-release techniques from the bed rest activities section (see pages 251-255).

Transitioning Back to Your Favorite Exercise Activities

Clear returning to any of these activities with your doctor. We do not recommend starting any activity, besides the exercise program in this chapter until at least twelve weeks postpartum, and if you are being conservative, six months.

- **Running.** Your readiness to transition back to running will depend on your level of activity before pregnancy and what type of birth you had. If you had no complications with birth and if you're not feeling any pressure or prolapse in your pelvic floor, start with a fast pace walk for the first two to three weeks before you start back to your run. Begin slowly and gradually increase distance and/or speed. Be mindful of your breathing.
- **Strength training/free weights.** When you're lifting the baby often, you are creating a forward drag or curve in the body, as you are primarily working the muscles in the front part of your neck, spine, and joints.

To counteract this, exercise good posture and use resistance bands for a couple of weeks to get your tone back. Resistance bands allow you to focus on working the muscles without weighing the joints down with a free weight that could potentially pull on your still, hyper-mobile, lax body. If you do weights too soon, your structure is still lax, and you can pull on some of the connective tissue, nerves, and ligaments, and force a compressed, hunched posture.

+ **Sit-ups.** We do not promote sit-ups for the first year postpartum because your internal organ systems are still moving around, and you may have a diastasis that takes time to resolve. Sit-ups can promote significant pressure in the exact tissues that have already been stretched during pregnancy. What's more, you don't need to do sit-ups to have a flat belly, especially if you stick with this exercise program.

+ **Yoga/Pilates/group classes.** Do not return to classes if you sense that you have a diastasis. If you don't have pain, incontinence, or signs of a diastasis, your rate of return will be based on how much you were doing before pregnancy. When you do return to classes, remember that your body is a little different than it was before. You may not want to do the most challenging exercises, at least for a few weeks, since they can actually work your core in the wrong way. If you're breastfeeding, you also may want to take it down a notch because you're still lax. As long as you're engaging the muscles with the exercises in this chapter, then you are laying the groundwork to return to your previous classes. Plan on transitioning slowly and maybe not doing the full class, or sit out during the most challenging parts. Make sure your instructor knows that you just had a baby, and position yourself near a mirror to make sure that you are hyper diligent about paying attention to your form.

+ **Recorded classes.** Hold off participating in your old routines if there is no instructor who is watching your movements. While you are still a little bit lax, your body awareness isn't necessarily there, and you may be putting yourself in a harmful position. Once you get your bearings again in a live class, and an instructor was able to correct you if that's what you needed, you should feel free to go back to a recording, with a mirror nearby!

◆ **Indoor cycling.** Biking is a great activity postpartum since your pelvis is supported by the seat. Look for bike shorts that are padded or purchase a padded seat cover, because you might still be tender at your pelvic floor. Transition slowly with a stepwise progression. Watch your spine, neck, and head position when you're on the bike because you can drift your head forward even more than it did before baby. When you start to feel that you're failing to keep your head in place or your posture is slouching, then it's time to take a break or take it back a notch and reset.

Building Great Postpartum Body Mechanics

The stress and strain of tending to baby can lead to pain if you aren't careful. Follow these guidelines, in addition to those in the previous chapter, and practice proper postures when standing and sitting (using a flat back squat for getting in and out of a chair). If you feel your legs, glutes, and arms working as you handle baby, it is a fantastic sign that you are performing more neutral spine mechanics to prevent injuries.

Exercise: Getting Baby from Floor

Reverse these steps for the best way to put your baby down on the floor:

STEP 1. Kneel to the floor with a deep, flat back. Cradle your hands under baby's head and buttocks and use your arm strength to pull her close to you.

STEP 2. Come up to high kneeling position with your spine in neutral/flat-back posture and head in line with spine.

STEP 3. Come all the way up to your knees and swing one leg in front of the other.

STEP 4. Lunge forward maintaining your neutral spine mechanics and with baby hugged in toward your chest/center. Rise up using your leg and hip strength. You can coordinate your breath by exhaling as you do this.

STEP 5. Stand tall with baby in front of you, supported in the center of your body.

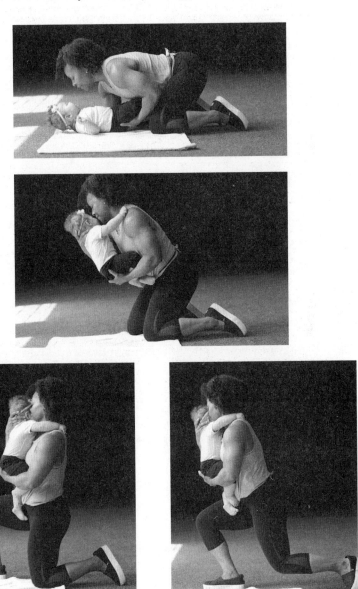

Exercise: Taking Baby Out of Tub

For the first few months, you can bathe baby at hip level on a countertop or in a deep sink. There, you can be relatively upright with a straight spine. Make sure you are wearing sturdy footwear, or slippers or socks with treading, to avoid slips from soapy water spills. Once your baby is bigger and more mobile, place the baby tub inside a larger bathtub. Use the same mechanics of getting baby down to the floor to get him into the tub.

To get your baby out of a low tub:

STEP 1. Put a padded mat on the floor right up against the tub. Place a towel over the padded mat. Drape baby's towel across your chest, over both shoulders.

STEP 2. Get into a double kneeling position with flat back and deepen the hip crease as much as is needed to be able to pick up baby with a slight bend in your arms. Keep head in-line with spine. Support baby to a sitting position so it is easier to lift out of the tub under their arms and buttocks.

STEP 3. As you slowly come up to a high kneeling position on both knees, bring baby close to your body. Wrap the baby in their towel.

STEP 4. Swing one leg in front of the other and rise up. Maintain a flat back, neutral spine position, head in-line with spine, chin relaxed down, and baby hugged up against your chest/center.

If you are having difficulty doing this movement with a neutral spine or you don't feel strong enough to do it in this way, you may need to work up your strength. The best way to do this is to practice this exercise with a similarly weighted object as your baby. Put the object in front of you on a mat and from the deep-hip-crease kneeling position with flat back, lift the object, come up to high kneeling, feeling your glutes and abs. Always keep head in-line with spine and the chin down. Perform 10–15 repetitions every other day to build up your strength.

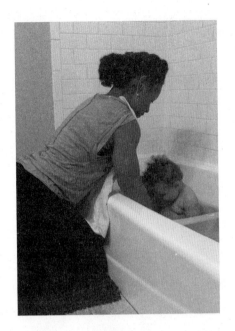
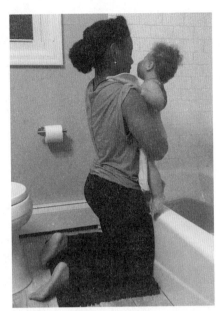
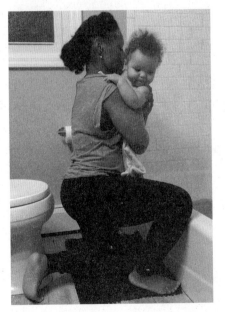
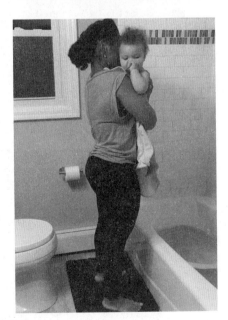

Exercise: Getting Yourself Up from the Floor

There are multiple ways to get up off the floor safely and efficiently; we like this technique because it best prevents injury by promoting neutral mechanics and uses the legs and hips.

STEP 1. Sit tall on the floor in whatever position you like.

STEP 2. Swing legs around so that one leg is bent behind you, and one bent in front of you, with knees resting on the floor.

STEP 3. Exhale and rise up to both knees keeping spine straight and using glutes and legs. You may slide the two legs close to each other if you feel unsteady in the wider kneeling position.

STEP 4. Swing one leg in front of you. Place the front foot on the floor in front of you and keep the back knee on the floor (staggered kneeling position).

STEP 5: Transfer your weight onto your front leg, keeping back flat and creasing the front hip. If you feel unsteady, place both hands on your front thigh/knee.

STEP 6: Rise up tall with ribs aligned over your belly and feet hip width apart.

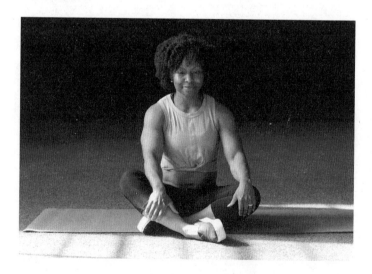

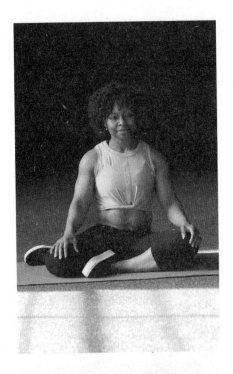

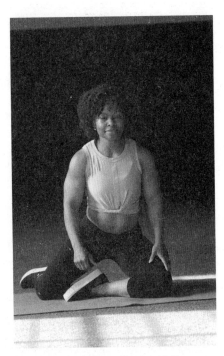

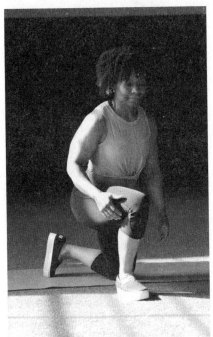

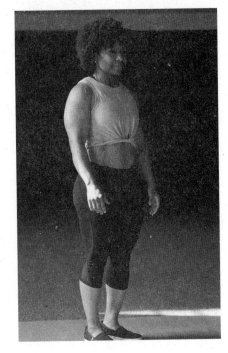

Focus on Proper Posture When You
Go Back to Work

If you are returning to work or working on a computer from home, continue to practice good posture. Most desk chairs are too deep for women to sit in properly. When you are sitting in front of a computer, use a vertical pillow(s) to support your lower back up to your shoulder blades. Sit in the chair keeping your knees approximately one hands-width distance from the seat. The pillow can fill the space between your back and the back of the chair. Make sure that both feet are on the floor or a stool. This positioning will keep your weight more grounded through the legs and will reduce spinal tension.

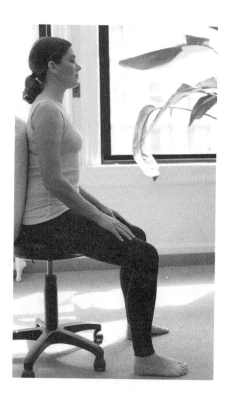
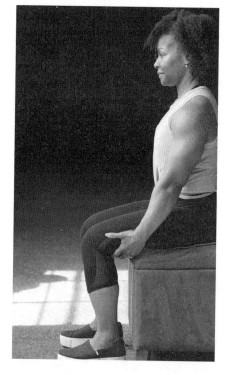

Make sure to keep your chest open, arms supported with your elbows bent at roughly 90 degrees, and the screen at a comfortable level to keep your neck in-line with your spine, chin down, with upper portion of screen at eye level. If you have a laptop, it will be a bit more challenging to get your arms at an angle that is comfortable and your head in-line with the computer. You may need to use an external keyboard and put your screen on book(s).

Additionally, watch out for developing a pressure belly when standing and follow the instructions outlined earlier in the chapter to prevent this from happening. For example, make sure to keep your ribs over your hips to prevent your hips from sliding forward, causing compression to your spine and your lower tummy to pooch out. And, when you are standing for a while, like when you are working at a standing desk, instead of sinking into one hip or the other, feel your weight evenly on both feet or put one foot up on a book or step stool in front of you. A Naboso mat (pictured here) is textured and can help to keep you in a parasympathetic state by improving the energy flow in your feet.

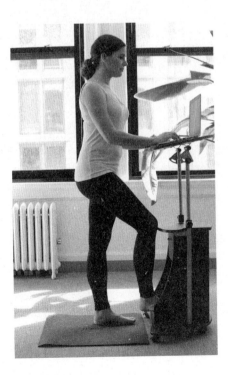

WISDOM

Who is your ultimate mother role model? What attributes does she have? Begin to adapt some of your actions to be in line with those attributes as you spread your wings to become that beautiful, balanced butterfly floating through life no matter what it may bring. For instance, if the ultimate mother for you is a wise woman who is calm and patient and can coast through challenging times, work on how you react to the little missteps of daily life so that when relationships or work or your children get more challenging, you won't react as strongly or feel tested.

As the wise woman you have become, you know to check in with yourself. Do you feel grounded, whole, and supported? Have you become disconnected from your wisdom? When we feel disconnected, we may need to reach out for support. Call a friend, family member, or even a therapist whenever you need to regain the connection with your inner wisdom again: like a stalled car needing a boost, see who will be your emotional jumper cables. What type of support do you need? What is lacking, keeping you feeling less balanced? Where are you doing okay? Are you thriving? It is your time to lean on supportive, positive people in your life as you exit the cocoon and stay in expansive butterfly mode, and then in turn, you can be the one to support them again one day.

Every Mother Can Be a Wellness Ambassador

You are now not only a wise woman, you are becoming a wise mother. After you've healed and begin getting back into both new and old routines, use all that you have learned in this book to create a positive shift toward wellness. The lessons that you learned, combined with your intuition, can make you the wellness ambassador of your home. Share your wellness lifestyle and habits with the rest of your family, your friends, and even your community. Pay it forward and involve everyone in the responsibilities of making healthier choices that nourish the mind, body, and spirit—and it can start in the kitchen and out in nature.

If you've adopted a more organic diet, continue to cook this way for your family, including your new baby. If you've learned the value of daily quiet time, let others in your home enjoy it as well. By adopting and sharing positive habits, you'll make a positive impact on society. Ultimately, you will spend more time doing the things you love and less time dealing with sickness and anxiety. The truth is, the lessons in this book are not just for pregnancy; they'll really last a lifetime and can impact many generations to come.

Remember, you hold all of the answers you seek. This journey, from pregnancy, through birthing, and finally motherhood, is a period of time for peace, joy, and abundance. Bathe in your own wisdom, support others along the way and ultimately celebrate all the gifts you have received. You are a wise woman, you are safe, and you are loved.

RESOURCES

Books

Blackburn, Elizabeth, Epel, Elissa, *The Telomere Effect: A Revolutionary Approach to Living Younger, Healthier, Longer*, Grand Central Publishing, 2017

Lee, Diane, *Diastasis Rectus Abdominis: A Clinical Guide for Those Who Are Split Down the Middle*, 2017 (self-published: Learn with Diane Lee)

Morrison, Jeffrey, *Cleanse Your Body, Clear Your Mind*, Hudson Street Press, 2011

Norman, Laura, *Feet First: A Guide to Foot Reflexology*, Simon & Schuster, 1988

Northrup, Christiane, *Women's Bodies, Women's Wisdom: Creating Physical and Emotional Health and Healing*, Bantam, 1996

Ou, Heng, *The First 40 Days: The Essential Art of Nourishing the New Mother*, Harry N. Abrams, 2016

Panda, Satchin, *The Circadian Code: Lose Weight, Supercharge Your Energy, and Transform Your Health from Morning to Midnight*, Rodale Books, 2018

SantoPietro, Nancy, *Feng Shui and Health: The Anatomy of a Home*, Harmony, 2002

Spatafora, Denise, *Better Birth: The Ultimate Guide to Childbirth from Home Births to Hospitals*, Wiley, 2009

Stassinopoulos, Agapi, *Wake Up to the Joy of You: 52 Meditations and Practices for a Calmer, Happier Life*, Harmony, 2016

Websites

In order to give you the most up-to-date information, visit www.patricialadis.com. This website offers typical dosages for the medications/supplements we recommend, as well as other pertinent information moms- and dads-to-be need.

Use promo codes when listed for discounted products and services

- Air filtration: www.intellipure.com (code wisewoman)
- Baby safety: www.babysafeproject.org
- Balls for labor and to relieve muscle tension: www.yamunausa.com
- Belly support: www.babybellypelvicsupport.com ; www.baobeimaternity.com
- Belly wrap: www.belliesinc.com
- BMI index: https://www.nhlbi.nih.gov/health/educational/lose_wt/BMI/bmicalc.htm.
- Breastfeeding bracelets: www.budhagirl.com (Wise Woman Bangle Set)
- Breathing services: www.breathingsciencenetwork.com/breathewell
- Cell tower information: www.antennasearch.com
- Dance photography: Lois Greenfield: www.loisgreenfield.com

- Doula: Chantal Traub CD, LCCE, CCCE, www.chantaltraub.com; Rosemary Foundation for Maternal Care: https://www.rosemaryfoundation.com/
- Environmental Working Group: www.EWG.org
- Fashion compression socks: www.rejuvahealth.com
- Feng Shui: https://www.andiesantopietro.com/
- Fitness equipment (resistance bands, physioballs, etc.): OPTP.com, gravityfit.com
- Insole support: Spenco: www.spencofootwear.com, Superfeet: www.superfeet.com,
- Institute for Functional Medicine: www.ifm.org/functional-medicine
- Lactation consultants: https://uslca.org/resources/find-an-ibclc , La Leche League: https://www.llli.org/
- Mayan Abdominal Massage: mbodimentmassage.com
- Meditation: www.choosemuse.com
- Men's organic skincare: om4men.com (code wise)
- Mental health support: Seleni.org
- Mold detection: www.jillcarnahan.com
- Nature Benefits: www.zachbushmd.com & walkwithwalsh.com; @thejenniferwalsh
- Nursing pillow: www.mybrestfriend.com
- Organic gardening: zachbushmd.com, Farmersfootprint.us
- Parasympathetic support mat: Naboso: naboso.com (code wisewoman)
- Parenting: @momommies and @unionsquareplay
- Pelvic core ball apparatus: www.pelvicsolutions.com/
- Perinatal/postpartum fitness classes: www.fitforbirth.com; www.pronatalfitness.com/
- Prenatal/postpartum chiropractic information: www.drrandijaffe.com
- Personalized microbiome mapping: Viome.com (code wisewomanguides)
- Physical therapist: aptaapps.apta.org//APTAPTDirectory/FindAPTDirectory.aspx
- Postpartum health coach/food: wewelltogether.com
- Postpartum Support International: postpartum.net
- Prenatal yoga: www.prenatalyogacenter.com
- Skincare: immunocologie.com (code wisewoman), Aimee Raupp Beauty: https://aimeeraupp.com/aimee-raupp-beauty-natural-hormone-balancing-skincare/
- Stability/wobble cushion: www.appleround.net
- Stress-reduction education: 1440.org
- Supportive neck pillow: www.kateklein.com/ (code wisewoman)
- Wellness educational platforms: www.first1000daysofwellness.com, www.globalwellnessinstitute.org/initiatives/first-1000-days/
- Women's health physical therapy: Diane Lee: www.dianeleephysio.com, Liz Simon: www.terrawellnesspt.com
- Women's Health Physical Therapy National Directory: www.pelvicrehab.com/?utm_source=hermanwallace.com&utm_medium=referrral&utm_content=findapractitioner

NOTES

Introduction

1. Glenn Verner, Elissa Epel, Marius Lahti-Pulkkinen, Eero Kajantie, Claudia Buss, Jue Lin, Elizabeth Blackburn, Katri Räikkönen, Pathik D Wadhwa, Sonja Entringer, Maternal Psychological Resilience During Pregnancy and Newborn Telomere Length: A Prospective Study, Am J Psychiatry. 2020 Sep 11;appiajp202019101003. doi: 10.1176/appi.ajp.2020.19101003. Online ahead of print.

2. https://www.nytimes.com/2018/09/06/well/family/diet-and-exercise-may-stem-weight-gain-of-pregnancy-but-should-begin-early.html?searchResultPosition=1

Part I

1. Moore, T., McDonald, M. & McHugh-Dillon, H. (2015). Early childhood development and the social determinants of health inequities: A review of the evidence. Published by: Parkville, Victoria: Centre for Community Child Health at the Murdoch Childrens Research Institute and the Royal Children's Hospital.

2. Rosalind J. Wright, MD, MPH, Psychological Stress: A Social Pollutant That May Enhance Environmental Risk, Am J Respir Crit Care Med. 2011 Oct 1; 184(7): 752–754. doi: 10.1164/rccm.201106-1139ED PMCID: PMC3208651, PMID: 21965012

3. Nestler, Eric J. Transgenerational Epigenetic Contributions to Stress Responses: Fact or Fiction? PLoS Biol. 2016 Mar; 14(3): e1002426. Published online 2016 Mar 25. doi: 10.1371/journal.pbio.1002426, PMCID: PMC4807775, PMID: 27015088

4. J. Denham, Exercise and epigenetic inheritance of disease risk, 2017 Scandinavian Physiological Society. Published by John Wiley & Sons Ltd

5. Tom P Fleming, Adam J Watkins, Miguel A Velazquez, John C Mathers, Andrew M Prentice, Judith Stephenson, et. al., Origins of lifetime health around the time of conception: causes and consequences, The Lancet, Vol. 391, No. 10132, p1842–1852 Published: April 16, 2018

6. Phipps WR, Martini MC, Lampe JW, Slavin JL, Kurzer MS. Effect of flax seed ingestion on the menstrual cycle. J Clin Endocrinol Metab. 1993 Nov;77(5):1215–9.

7. Tafuri S, Cocchia N, Vassetti A, Carotenuto D, Esposito L, Maruccio L, Avallone L, Ciani F, Lepidium meyenii (Maca) in male reproduction. Nat Prod Res. 2019 Dec 5:1–10. doi: 10.1080/14786419.2019.1698572. [Epub ahead of print]

8. Antoine E, Chirila S, Teodorescu C. A Patented Blend Consisting of a Combination of Vitex agnus-castus Extract, Lepidium meyenii (Maca) Extract and Active Folate, a Nutritional Supplement for Improving Fertility in Women. Maedica (Buchar). 2019 Sep;14(3):274–279. doi: 10.26574/maedica.2019.14.3.274.

9. Czeizel AE, Dudas I, Fritz G, Tecsoi A, Hanck A, Kunovits G. The effect of periconceptional multivitamin-mineral supplementation on vertigo, nausea and vomiting in the first trimester of pregnancy. Arch Gynecol Obstet 1992;251:181–5.

Part II

1. Yafeng Zhang, MS, Rita M. Cantor, PhD, Kimber Macgibbon, RN, Roberto Romero, MD, Thomas M. Goodwin, MD, Patrick Mullin, MD, MPH, and Marlena S. Fejzo, PhD, Familial Aggregation of Hyperemesis Gravidarum, Am J Obstet Gynecol. 2011 Mar; 204(3): 230.e1-230.e7. Published online 2010 Oct 25. doi: 10.1016/j.ajog.2010.09.018

2. Hinkle SN, Mumford SL, Grantz KL, Silver RM, Mitchell EM, Sjaarda LA, et al. Association of nausea and vomiting during pregnancy with pregnancy loss: a secondary analysis of a randomized clinical trial. JAMA Intern Med 2016;176:1621–7.

3. Flaxman SM, Sherman PW. Morning sickness: adaptive cause or nonadaptive consequence of embryo viability? Am Nat. 2008 Jul;172(1):54–62. doi: 10.1086/588081.

4. https://www.ncbi.nlm.nih.gov/pubmed/11041443

5. Bronson, S., Bale, T. The Placenta as a Mediator of Stress Effects on Neurodevelopmental Reprogramming. Neuropsychopharmacol 41, 207–218 (2016). https://doi.org/10.1038/npp.2015.231

6. Oerther S, Lorenz R., State of the Science: Using Telomeres as Biomarkers During the First 1,000 Days of Life. West J Nurs Res. 2018 Mar 1:193945918762806. doi: 10.1177/0193945918762806. [Epub ahead of print]

7. Chekroud SR, Gueorguieva R, Zheutlin AB, Paulus M, Krumholz HM, Krystal JH, Chekroud AM. Association between physical exercise and mental health in 1·2 million individuals in the USA between 2011 and 2015:

a cross-sectional study. Lancet Psychiatry. 2018, Sep;5 (9):739–746. doi: 10.1016/S2215-0366(18)30227-X. Epub 2018 Aug 8. PMID: 30099000

8. https://www.figo.org/news/pollution-exposure-pregnancy-affects-babys-asthma-risk-0015187

9. Bornehag CG, Lindh C, Reichenberg A, Wikström S, Unenge Hallerback M, Evans SF, Sathyanarayana S, Barrett ES, Nguyen RHN, Bush NR, Swan SH., Association of Prenatal Phthalate Exposure With Language Development in Early Childhood. JAMA Pediatr. 2018 Dec 1;172(12):1169–1176. doi: 10.1001/jamapediatrics.2018.3115.

10. Hu XC, Dassuncao C, Zhang X, Grandjean P, Weihe P, Webster GM, Nielsen F, Sunderland EM. Can profiles of poly- and Perfluoroalkyl substances (PFASs) in human serum provide information on major exposure sources? Environ Health. 2018 Feb 1;17(1):11. doi: 10.1186/s12940-018-0355-4. PMID: 29391068; PMCID: PMC5796515.

11. Herbert P. Susmann, Laurel A. Schaider, Kathryn M. Rodgers, Ruthann A. Rudel, 2019 Dietary Habits Related to Food Packaging and Population Exposure to PFASs, Environmental Health Perspectives 127:10 CID: 107003 https://doi.org/10.1289/EHP4092

12. https://www.ncbi.nlm.nih.gov/pubmed/18467962

13. Clapp JF 3rd, Kim H, Burciu B, Schmidt S, Petry K, Lopez B. Continuing regular exercise during pregnancy: effect of exercise volume on fetoplacental growth.Am J Obstet Gynecol. 2002 Jan;186(1):142–7. PMID: 11810100

14. http://clinical.diabetesjournals.org/content/23/4/165.full

15. Abu-Saad, K. (2010). Maternal Nutrition and Birth Outcomes. Epidemiologic Reviews, 32.

16. Satokari R, Grönroos T, Laitinen K, Salminen S, Isolauri E. Bifidobacterium and Lactobacillus DNA in the human placenta. Lett Appl Microbiol. 2009 Jan;48(1):8–12. doi: 10.1111/j.1472-765X.2008.02475.x. Epub 2008 Oct 17.

17. Power ML, Holzman GB, Schulkin J. A survey on the management of nausea and vomiting in pregnancy by obstetrician/gynecologists. Prim Care Update Ob Gyns 2001;8:69–72. (Level III)

18. Jednak MA, Shadigian EM, Kim MS, Woods ML, Hooper FG, Owyang C, et al. Protein meals reduce nausea and gastric slow wave dysrhythmic activity in first trimester pregnancy. Am J Physiol, 1999 Oct;277(4):G855–61. doi: 10.1152/ajpgi.1999.277.4.G855.

19. McParlin C, O'Donnell A, Robson SC, Beyer F, Moloney E, Bryant A, et al. Treatments for hyperemesis gravidarum and nausea and vomiting in pregnancy: a systematic review. JAMA 2016;316:1392–401. (Systematic Review)

20. Kayleigh E. Easey, Maddy L. Dyer, Nicholas J. Timpson, Marcus R. Munafò, Prenatal alcohol exposure and offspring mental health: A systematic review, Drug and Alcohol Dependence, Vol 197, 2019, 344–353, ISSN 0376-8716, https://doi.org/10.1016/j.drugalcdep.2019.01.007.

21. Koelsch, Fuermetz, Sack, et al. Effects of music listening on cortisol levels and propofol consumption during spinal analgesia. Frontiers in Psychology. 2011; 2: 58

22. Decreases depression: Maratos AS. Gold C. Wang X, Crawford MJ. Music Therapy for depression. Cochrane Database Syst. Rev. 2008 Jan 23"1): CD004517. Review.

23. Kuhn D. The effects of active and passive participation in musical activity on the immune system as measured by salivary immunoglobulin, A. J Music Ther. 2002 Spring: 39 (1):30–9.

24. Harmat L. Taka'cs J. Bo'dizs R. Music improves sleep quality in students. J Adv Nurs. 2008 May:62(3): 327–35.

25. Khalfa S, Bella SD, Roy M, Peretz I, Lupien SJ., Effects of relaxing music on salivary cortisol level after psychological stress., Ann N Y Acad Sci. 2003 Nov;999:374–6.

Part III

1. Hamdiye Arda Sürücü, Dilek Büyükkaya Besen, Mesude Duman, Elif Yeter Erbil, Coping with Stress among Pregnant Women with Gestational Diabetes Mellitus, J Caring Sci. 2018 Mar; 7(1): 9–15. Published online 2018 Mar 1. doi: 10.15171/jcs.2018.002, PMCID: PMC5889800, PMID: 29637051

2. Soomro MH, Baiz N, Huel G, Yazbeck C, Botton J, Heude B, Bornehag CG, Annesi-Maesano I; EDEN mother-child cohort study group. Exposure to heavy metals during pregnancy related to gestational diabetes mellitus in diabetes-free mothers. Sci Total Environ. 2019 Mar 15;656:870-876. doi: 10.1016/j .scitotenv.2018.11.422. Epub 2018 Nov 29

3. www.ncbi.nlm.nih.gov/pmc/articles/PMC5645148/

4. www.ncbi.nlm.nih.gov/pmc/articles/PMC4515446/

5. Henry, JD, Rendell, PG, A review of the impact of pregnancy on memory function, Journal of Clinical and Experimental Neuropsychology, 29:8, 793–803, DOI: 10.1080/13803390701612209

6. Field, T. Pregnant Women Benefit From Massage Therapy. Journal of Psychosomatic Obstetrics and Gynecology, 1999. Mar;20(1):31–8.

7. Field, T.. Massage Therapy Effects on Depressed Pregnant Women. Journal of Psychosomatic Obstetrics and Gynecology, 2004, Jun;25(2):115–22.

8. Tarr B, Launay J, Dunbar RIM. Music and social bonding: "self-other" merging and neurohormonal mechanisms. Frontiers in Psychology. 2014;5:1096. doi:10.3389/fpsyg.2014.01096.

9. "Global Wellness Institute, Move to be Well: The Global Economy of Physical Activity, October 2019."

10. Tang YY, Hölzel BK, Posner MI. The neuroscience of mindfulness meditation. Nat Rev Neurosci. 2015 Apr;16(4):213–25. doi: 10.1038/nrn3916. Epub 2015 Mar 18. Review. PMID: 25783612

11. Travis F, Parim N. Default mode network activation and Transcendental Meditation practice: Focused Attention or Automatic Self-transcending? Brain Cogn. 2017 Feb;111:86–94. doi: 10.1016/j.bandc.2016.08.009. Epub 2016 Nov 2. PMID: 27816783

12. Hansen CJ, Stevens LC, Coast JR. Exercise duration and mood state: how much is enough to feel better? Health Psychol. 2001 Jul;20(4):267–75.

13. Bruce KD, Cagampang FR, Argenton M, Zhang J, Ethirajan PL, Burdge GC, Bateman AC, Clough GF, Poston L, Hanson MA, McConnell JM, Byrne CD. Maternal high-fat feeding primes steatohepatitis in adult mice offspring, involving mitochondrial dysfunction and altered lipogenesis gene expression. Hepatology. 2009 Dec;50(6):1796–808. doi: 10.1002/hep.23205.

14. Gorzynik-Debicka M, Przychodzen P, Cappello F, Kuban-Jankowska A, Marino Gammazza A, Knap N, Wozniak M, Gorska-Ponikowska M. Potential Health Benefits of Olive Oil and Plant Polyphenols. Int J Mol Sci. 2018 Feb 28;19(3). pii: E686. doi: 10.3390/ijms19030686.

15. Stapleton, L. R. T., Schetter, C. D., Westling, E., Rini, C., Glynn, L. M., Hobel, C. J., & Sandman, C. A. (2012). Perceived partner support in pregnancy predicts lower maternal and infant distress. Journal of Family Psychology, 26(3), 453–463. https://doi.org/10.1037/a0028332

Part IV

1. https://www.webmd.com/baby/guide/bed-rest-during-pregnancy#1

2. Soultanakis HN, Artal R, Wiswell RA. Prolonged exercise in pregnancy: glucose homeostasis, ventilatory and cardio-vascular responses. Semin Perinatol 1996;20:315–27.

3. Georgieff M.K., Rao R. & Fuglestad A.J. (1999). The role of nutrition in cognitive development. In: Handbook of Developmental Cognitive Neuroscience (editors Nelson, C.A, Luciana, M.). Cambridge, MA: MIT Press; p. 491–04.

4. Mennella, J. A. (2014). Ontogeny of taste preferences: basic biology and implications for Health. American Journal of Clinical Nutrition, 99(suppl):704S–11S.

5. https://www.acog.org/clinical/clinical-guidance/committee-opinion/articles/2018/05/optimizing -postpartum-care

6. García González J, Ventura Miranda MI, Manchon García F, Pallarés Ruiz TI, Marin Gascón ML, Requena Mullor M, Alarcón Rodriguez R, Parron Carreño T, Effects of prenatal music stimulation on fetal cardiac state, newborn anthropometric measurements and vital signs of pregnant women: A randomized controlled trial. Complement Ther Clin Pract 2017 May:61–67. MeSH PubMed ID: 28438283

Part V

1. Sharma, D. Golden hour of neonatal life: Need of the hour. matern health, neonatol and perinatol 3, 16 (2017). https://doi.org/10.1186/s40748-017-0057-x

2. World Health Organization. Implementation Guidance: Protecting, Promoting and Supporting Breastfeeding in Facilities Providing Maternity and Newborn Services—The Revised Baby-Friendly Hospital Initiative. Geneva: World Health Organization, 2018. Report No.: CC BY-NC-SA 3.0 IGO.

3. Zwelling E. Overcoming the challenges: maternal movement and positioning to facilitate labor progress. MCN Am J Matern Child Nurs. 2010;35(2):72–80. doi:10.1097/NMC.0b013e3181caeab3

4. Christina Marie Tussey, Emily Botsios, Richard D. Gerkin, Lesly A. Kelly, Juana Gamez, Jennifer Mensik, Reducing Length of Labor and Cesarean Surgery Rate Using a Peanut Ball for Women Laboring With an

Epidural, J Perinat Educ. 2015; 24(1): 16–24. doi: 10.1891/1058-1243.24.1.16, PMCID: PMC4748987 PMID: 26937158

5. https://www.ncbi.nlm.nih.gov/pmc/articles/PMC2742151/

Part VI

1. Hu S, Belcaro G, Hosoi M, Feragalli B, Luzzi R, Dugall M. Postpartum stretchmarks: repairing activity of an oral Centella asiatica supplementation (Centellicum®). Minerva Ginecol. 2018;70(5):629–634. doi:10.23736/S0026-4784.18.04254-5

2. Deoni, S.C.L., et al. (2013). Breastfeeding and Early White Matter Development: A cross-sectional study. NeuroImage, 82: 72-86.

3. Vitora, C. G., et al. (2015). Association between breastfeeding and intelligence, educational attainment, and income at 30 years of age: a prospective birth cohort study from Brazil. The Lancet, 3(4): e199-e205.

4. Vitora, C. G., Barros, A. J. D., Franca, G. V. A., Horton, S., Krasevec, J., Murch, S., Sankar, M. J., Walker, N., & Rollins, N.C. (2016). Breastfeeding in the 21st century: Epidemiology, mechanisms, and lifelong effect. The Lancet, 387, 475-489.

5. Bezirtzoglou E, Tsiotsias A, Welling GW. Microbiota profile in feces of breast- and formula-fed newborns by using fluorescence in situ hybridization (FISH). Anaerobe. 2011; 17:478–82.

6. Pannaraj PS, Li F, Cerini C, et al. Association Between Breast Milk Bacterial Communities and Establishment and Development of the Infant Gut Microbiome. JAMA Pediatr. 2017;171(7):647–654. doi:10.1001/jamapediatrics.2017.0378

7. Schwarz, E. Duration of Lactation and Risk Factors for Maternal Cardiovascular Disease. (2009). Obstetrics & Gynecology, 113(5).

8. Black, M. M., & Aboud, F. E. (2011). Responsive feeding is embedded in a theoretical framework of responsive parenting. The Journal of Nutrition, 141(3), 490-494.

9. Mitra AK, Mahalanabis D, Ashraf H, Unicomb L, Eeckels R, Tzipori S. Hyperimmune cow colostrum reduces diarrhoea due to rotavirus: a double-blind, controlled clinical trial. Acta Paediatr. 1995;84(9):996-1001.

10. Davidson GP, Whyte PB, Daniels E, Franklin K, Nunan H, McCloud PI, Moore AG, Moore DJ. Passive immunisation of children with bovine colostrum containing antibodies to human rotavirus. Lancet. 1989;2 (8665):709-12.

11. https://nervedoctor.info/daily-toxin-intake-how-many-toxins-are-you-accumulating/

12. Landrigan PJ, Sonawane B, Mattison D, McCally M, Garg A. Chemical contaminants in breast milk and their impacts on children's health: an overview. Environ Health Perspect. 2002;110(6):A313-A315. doi:10.1289/ehp.021100313

13. Fromme H, Mosch C, Morovitz M, Alba-Alejandre I, Boehmer S, Kiranoglu M, Faber F, Hannibal I, Genzel-Boroviczény O, Koletzko B, Völkel W. Pre- and postnatal exposure to perfluorinated compounds (PFCs). Environ Sci Technol. 2010 Sep 15;44(18):7123-9. doi: 10.1021/es101184f. PMID: 20722423.

14. https://www.asbestos.net/legal/laws/legislation/asbestos-bans/

15. Gandhi OP, Morgan LL, de Salles AA, Han YY, Herberman RB, Davis DL. Exposure limits: the underestimation of absorbed cell phone radiation, especially in children. Electromagn Biol Med. 2012;31(1):34-51. doi:10.3109/15368378.2011.622827

16. https://www.postpartum.net/

17. Park, E.M., Meltzer-Brody, S. & Stickgold, R. Poor sleep maintenance and subjective sleep quality are associated with postpartum maternal depression symptom severity. Arch Womens Ment Health 16, 539–547 (2013). https://doi.org/10.1007/s00737-013-0356-9

18. Cheng CY, Pickler RH. Effects of stress and social support on postpartum health of Chinese mothers in the United States. Res Nurs Health. 2009;32(6):582-591. doi:10.1002/nur.20356

Part VII

1. Cai T, Gacci M, Mattivi F, et al. Apple consumption is related to better sexual quality of life in young women. Arch Gynecol Obstet. 2014;290(1):93-98. doi:10.1007/s00404-014-3168-x

2. O'Malley et al. BMC Pregnancy and Childbirth (2018) 18:196, https://doi.org/10.1186/s12884-018-1838-6

3. Ganer Herman, Hadas MD; Kleiner, Ilia MD; Tairy, Daniel MD; Gonen, Noa MD; Ben Zvi, Masha MD; Kovo, Michal MD, PhD; Bar, Jacob MD, MSc; Weiner, Eran MD Effect of Digital Step Counter Feedback on Mobility After Cesarean Delivery, Obstetrics & Gynecology: June 2020 - Volume 135 - Issue 6 - p 1345-1352 doi: 10.1097/AOG.0000000000003879

INDEX

F

ABOUT THE AUTHORS

Patricia Ladis, PT, CBBA, is a licensed physical therapist and behavioral breathing analyst to professional athletes, dancers, and pregnant women. She is founder of WiseBody PT, and the co-founder of The First 1000 Days of Wellness, a global educational platform for practitioners, spas, and consumers to promote perinatal wellness and prevent non-communicable diseases in future generations. Patricia was the co-founder of KIMA Center for Physiotherapy & Wellness, one of New York City's most highly regarded PT and wellness centers. Patricia was also a professional dancer and as a physical therapist has been helping pregnant dancers and athletes get back on stage or sport after pregnancy since 1999. She has worked with the Rockettes, various Broadway shows including *Fosse, Lion King,* and *Movin' Out,* the American Ballet Theatre, and Paul Taylor Dance Company, and currently consults with the United States Tennis Association (USTA) and Women's Tennis Association (WTA). Patricia is building a new protocol for women returning to sport after pregnancy (WTA, IOC) and has designed the exercise program for the first-ever postpartum exercise study coming out in 2021 with the Hospital for Special Surgery and the Weill-Cornell Medical Center. She has appeared in articles in *Forbes, Vogue, Men's Health, Thrive Global* and *Ladies' Home Journal.* TV appearances include NBC and CBS, and she regularly appears on Sirius XM's Doctor Radio. As an active delegate of the Global Wellness Summit and chair of the First 1000 Days Initiative for the Global Wellness Institute, Ladis has support from wellness centers around the world, including Six Senses, Canyon Ranch, Rancho La Puerta, and Borgo Egnazia. Visit her website at patricialadis.com.

Anita Sadaty, MD, is a holistic practitioner and founder of Redefining Health Medical, a women-focused medical practice that combines conventional medical training with an integrative functional medicine approach. A graduate of Cornell Medical and a board-certified ob-gyn, Dr. Sadaty is also recognized as a Certified Medical Practitioner by the Institution for Functional Medicine. She was a founding member of the Kresser Institute ADAPT Functional Medicine Training program in 2016. In addition to maintaining a full-time private practice, Dr. Sadaty is involved in residency training education at Northwell Hospital and is a clinical assistant professor at Hofstra Medical School. She serves as an expert reviewer for women's reproductive health articles featured in Verywellhealth.com and was recently named as one of the best obstetrics and gynecology physicians on Long Island, New York, in Best of Long Island. She has appeared in numerous newspaper articles, magazines, and professional publications to discuss various topics in women's health. Visit her website at www.drsadaty.com.